Whole Person Promotion, Women, and the Post-Pandemic Era:

Impact and Future Outlooks

Michelle O. Crosby
Corvinus University, Hungary

Julianna Faludi
Corvinus University, Hungary

A volume in the Advances in Religious and Cultural Studies (ARCS) Book Series

IGI Global
PUBLISHER of TIMELY KNOWLEDGE

Published in the United States of America by
IGI Global
Information Science Reference (an imprint of IGI Global)
701 E. Chocolate Avenue
Hershey PA, USA 17033
Tel: 717-533-8845
Fax: 717-533-8661
E-mail: cust@igi-global.com
Web site: http://www.igi-global.com

Library of Congress Cataloging-in-Publication Data

Names: Crosby-Nagy, Michelle O., editor. | Faludi, Julianna, 1977- editor.
Title: Whole person promotion, women, and the post-pandemic era : impact and future outlooks / Michelle Crosby, and Julianna Faludi, editors.
Description: Hershey PA : Information Science Reference, [2022] | Includes bibliographical references and index. | Summary: "This book will aim to provide the latest empirical research findings in COVID era effects, with the household as the central unit of analysis, and helps activists who want to improve their understanding of how old institutions persist and are even reinforced during times of crisis as well as generate a discussion about to what extent there is variation in experiences, how satisfied we are (or not) with these dynamics,"-- Provided by publisher.

Identifiers: LCCN 2022001280 (print) | LCCN 2022001281 (ebook) | ISBN 9781668423646 (hardcover) | ISBN 9781668423653 (paperback) | ISBN 9781668423660 (ebook)
Subjects: LCSH: COVID-19 Pandemic, 2020---Social aspects. | COVID-19 Pandemic, 2020---Economic aspects. | Women--Social conditions--21st century. | Women--Economic conditions--21st century.
Classification: LCC RA644.C67 W56 2022 (print) | LCC RA644.C67 (ebook) | DDC 362.1962/414--dc23/eng/20220303
LC record available at https://lccn.loc.gov/2022001280
LC ebook record available at https://lccn.loc.gov/2022001281

This book is published in the IGI Global book series Advances in Religious and Cultural Studies (ARCS) (ISSN: 2475-675X; eISSN: 2475-6768)

British Cataloguing in Publication Data
A Cataloguing in Publication record for this book is available from the British Library.

All work contributed to this book is new, previously-unpublished material.
The views expressed in this book are those of the authors, but not necessarily of the publisher.

For electronic access to this publication, please contact: eresources@igi-global.com.

Advances in Religious and Cultural Studies (ARCS) Book Series

ISSN:2475-675X
EISSN:2475-6768

Editor-in-Chief: Nancy Erbe, California State University-Dominguez Hills, USA

MISSION

In the era of globalization, the diversity of the world and various cultures becomes apparent as cross-cultural interactions turn into a daily occurrence for individuals in all professions. Understanding these differences is necessary in order to promote effective partnerships and interactions between those from different religious and cultural backgrounds.

The **Advances in Religious and Cultural Studies (ARCS)** book series brings together a collection of scholarly publications on topics pertaining to religious beliefs, culture, population studies, and sociology. Books published within this series are ideal for professionals, theorists, researchers, and students seeking the latest research on collective human behavior in terms of religion, social structure, and cultural identity and practice.

COVERAGE

- Human Rights and Ethics
- Impact of Religion on Society
- Politics and Religion
- Group Behavior
- Gender
- Sociology
- Cross-Cultural Interaction
- Globalization and Culture
- Social Stratification and Classes
- Cults and Religious Movements

IGI Global is currently accepting manuscripts for publication within this series. To submit a proposal for a volume in this series, please contact our Acquisition Editors at Acquisitions@igi-global.com or visit: http://www.igi-global.com/publish/.

The Advances in Religious and Cultural Studies (ARCS) Book Series (ISSN 2475-675X) is published by IGI Global, 701 E. Chocolate Avenue, Hershey, PA 17033-1240, USA, www.igi-global.com. This series is composed of titles available for purchase individually; each title is edited to be contextually exclusive from any other title within the series. For pricing and ordering information please visit http://www.igi-global.com/book-series/advances-religious-cultural-studies/84269. Postmaster: Send all address changes to above address.

Titles in this Series

For a list of additional titles in this series, please visit:
http://www.igi-global.com/book-series/advances-religious-cultural-studies/84269

Global and Transformative Approaches Toward Linguistic Diversity
Sarah E. DeCapua (University of Connecticut, Storrs, USA) and Eda Başak Hancı-Azizoglu (Mediterranean (Akdeniz) University, Turkey)
Information Science Reference • © 2022 • 383pp • H/C (ISBN: 9781799889854) • US $215.00

Promoting Diversity, Equity, and Inclusion for Women After the COVID-19 Pandemic
Siham El-Kafafi (Arrows Research Consultancy Limited, New Zealand)
Information Science Reference • © 2022 • 335pp • H/C (ISBN: 9781668437995) • US $215.00

Global Perspectives on the LGBT Community and Non-Discrimination
Augustine Edobor Arimoro (University of Roehampton, UK)
Information Science Reference • © 2022 • 290pp • H/C (ISBN: 9781668424285) • US $215.00

Examining the Relationship Between the Russian Orthodox Church and Secular Authorities in the 19th and 20th Centuries
Bogdan Ershov (Voronezh State Technical University, Russia) and Igor Ashmarov (Voronezh State Institute of Arts, Russia)
Information Science Reference • © 2022 • 283pp • H/C (ISBN: 9781668449158) • US $205.00

Reciprocity and Its Practice in Social Research
Jahid Siraz Chowdhury (University of Malaysia, Malaysia) Haris Abd Wahab (University of Malaya, Malaysia) Rashid Mohd Saad (University of Malaya, Malaysia) Hasan Reza (Indiana University, USA) and Mokbul Morshed Ahmad (Asian Institute of Technology, Thailand)
Information Science Reference • © 2022 • 300pp • H/C (ISBN: 9781799896029) • US $205.00

For an entire list of titles in this series, please visit:
http://www.igi-global.com/book-series/advances-religious-cultural-studies/84269

IGI Global
PUBLISHER of TIMELY KNOWLEDGE

701 East Chocolate Avenue, Hershey, PA 17033, USA
Tel: 717-533-8845 x100 • Fax: 717-533-8661
E-Mail: cust@igi-global.com • www.igi-global.com

Table of Contents

Detailed Table of Contents

The authors seek to critically reflect on the meaning of work in a globally emancipated society. They start by arguing that work is a central issue for human societies, whether to produce socially useful goods, to provide basic needs or as the making, objectification, and safeguarding of ontological humanization of Mankind itself – even if in the field of socialist politics this centrality has been overshadowed by programs mainly focused on the defense of assistentialism, philanthropy, or even charity. To conceive work today, in the current stage of the capitalist society, we have to mobilize several concepts, methods, and areas of knowledge, among which the authors highlight critical sociology, global labor history, and psychodynamics of work. Finally, they argue about what would be the fundamental aspects of work in an emancipated society.

Section 2
The Double Movement and Whole Personhood

Teresa Panico, University of Naples Federico II, Italy
Stefano Pascucci, Business School, University of Exeter, UK
Elise Lobbedez, Emlyon Business School, France
Teresa Del Giudice, University of Naples Federico II, Italy

Since the mid-1990s, three million people living in the metropolitan area of Naples (Italy) have been facing one of the most dramatic socio-ecological crises witnessed in Western Europe. This is a crisis orchestrated by Mafia-like organizations (e.g., the Neapolitan Mafia also known as Camorra) and their interest in the illegal management of waste disposal and incineration in the shadow of a weak state, a phenomenon often referred to as the "Land of Fires." In this chapter, the authors attempt to inductively theorise from this prolonged socio-ecological crisis as an exemplar process of embeddedness of market economies in diffused illegal and violent social and economic relations. They use the Land of Fires to extend the notion of "embedded economy," building on the work of Karl Polanyi. The authors argue that this process of social embeddedness through illegal and violent practices are particularly intense in contexts of socio-ecological crises, where the expropriation of land and destruction of nature is coupled with the disarticulation of the role of the state by criminal organizations.

Measures to curb the COVID-19 pandemic forced many young professionals to work from (often small and sometimes shared) homes. On the basis of in-depth interviews in the Netherlands, this chapter aims to unpack how working from home in times of COVID-19 affects the whole personhood of young knowledge workers. Three important insights are provided. First, when it comes to around boundary sculpting practices, many respondents' boundary negotiations between personal and professional spheres entail personal, collective, temporal, and spatial borders. Second, interpersonal connections prove to be of vital importance because a lack of face-to-face interactions not only causes a lack of interpersonal contact and emotional connection to colleagues, but also a lack of tacit knowledge. Third, additional spheres like the public sphere are crucial for providing motivation and inspiration. This research shows that working from home can be detrimental to the whole personhood of young professionals.

Against the background of the global COVID-19 pandemic, this chapter presents an in-depth vision of the relationship between music-making and the domestic life of Portuguese artists. The chapter presents and discusses data from an international project related to the Portuguese reality. Then, on the basis of some 40 semi-structured interviews with Portuguese musicians, the author reflects on the impacts of the pandemic on their musical careers and potential impacts on music-making processes more generally, as well as on family and domestic life. Finally, the chapter highlights the scarcity of this kind of research in the Portuguese reality, making it imperative that other dimensions of music-making and artists' lives are explored and made perceptible, not just the economic losses suffered.

This chapter analyzes gender-based violence in Mexico before and during the COVID-19 pandemic. Various indicators related to the 2030 Sustainable Development Goals, particularly Goal 5, "Achieve gender equality and empower all women and girls," are analyzed. The fuzzy ordering method of Subjective Preferences is used to perform two multidimensional analyses, a global analysis that identifies the position of Mexico with regards to other countries in the American continent and an analysis that identifies the position of each of the states of the Mexican Republic. The results allow the authors to identify the countries with the lowest and highest prevalence of gender-based violence as well as the states of the Mexican Republic with the lowest and highest prevalence of gender-based violence.

Since the times that Karl Polanyi named "the great transformation" and up to the pre-COVID-19 era, the market has played the central role in organization of the society. Such a system has affected women more profoundly: to be officially paid, they had to compromise professional and family life. The COVID-19 pandemic lockdowns added even more burden to them, returning education and childcare to the household realm. This chapter draws on the rich empirical data featuring post-Yugoslav and post-Soviet female immigrants' experiences of the COVID-19 pandemic in Austria and Hungary. The analysis reveals the ways in which experiences with previous global crises that represented radical changes influenced their resilience throughout the COVID-19 pandemic.

Preface

The challenges of the lockdown inspired the article by the editors: 'Digital Economy of the Sourdough' (Faludi & Crosby, 2021), and subsequently, this edited volume reflects the role of crises and shocks such as the COVID-19 global pandemic in accelerating and illuminating various social tensions as the result of our system of global capitalism. In times of crisis, researchers are implored as a condition of their moral duty to provide consultation, encourage, and warn. Such activities assume a common language and standard instruments for analyzing our society. The current tools at our disposal involve one type of exchange (monetary) and one means of business exchange (the market). Still, they are unfortunately quite limited tools in assisting people with conceptually "inventing" their lives.

This book was evoked to reflect and analyze the structures behind the social tensions illuminated by crises – such as the COVID-19 pandemic, war, and financial situation – and the 'great' transformations of our times – digitization, the perceived threat of automation, and mismanagement of resources and waste. Although COVID-19 seems to be in the recent past now, the consequences of the lockdowns are being borne by societies. The lessons learned from the latter reveal the vulnerabilities of our current socioeconomic systems; thus, this book proposes a forward-looking framework to build upon for the future. The perspective of this book is that of the individual – the whole person – ideally nested in an equal and fair system of existence – the household, the organization, and the regional and the global economy. The chapters of this book grasp the different dimensions of how this completeness of the whole personhood is corrupted by violence, precarity, forced migration, and uneven global structures. What binds these factors together is the goal of developing a forward-looking frame of resilience, governance, and fairness. To this end, the devastating impact of these crises is viewed through their effect on regional economies and the interconnectedness of the global economy that frames the positions individuals might take. Such situations are defined on the one hand by the drastically changing new division of labor and the unprecedented collapse of spheres. Therefore, the unit of analysis varies from the individual to the organization, institution, or system. To provide a concise understanding of the phenomena, we rely on the conceptual framework proposed by Karl Polanyi that encompasses the remarkable transformation of today and the prevalent social tensions ingrained in our societies for centuries.

ORGANIZATION OF THE BOOK

The book is organized into two sections and nine chapters. Section 1 explores the relevance of Polanyi's The Great Transformation in the context of digital capitalism; defines the whole personhood; develops a frame for organizing resilient societies from an institutional and a community perspective and illustrates how local crises reflect the effects of the global double movement. Section 2 gives empirical examples of how the COVID-19 pandemic has affected women in different spheres and what lessons women can learn to overcome the challenges. Finally, a historical analysis of emancipated societies gives a scenario about how to build the future based on real social sustainability and decent work, closing the book.

Michelle O. Crosby
Corvinus University, Hungary

Julianna Faludi
Corvinus University, Hungary

REFERENCES

Faludi, J., & Crosby-Nagy, M. (2021). The Digital Economy of the Sourdough: Housewifisation in the Time of COVID-19. *TripleC*, 113–124. doi:10.31269/triplec.v19i1.1222

Acknowledgment

The Editors would like to thank the Contributors, the Reviewers and the Publishers of this book. We also thank the many reviewers and advisors helping to shape the Chapters with their valuable comments and suggestions.

Introduction

WHOLE PERSONHOOD AND THE DOUBLE MOVEMENT – TOWARD A UNIFIED FRAMEWORK

The Concept of Whole Personhood

Investigating how individuals navigate personal, public, economic, political, social and personal spheres is one of the means of understanding the dynamics that exist between the agency of individuals and those of the forces of structure. Furthermore, the economic field and the role of money and labor in it define the latter and the extent to which alienation extends and how individuals are restricted in their wholeness (in actions and choices). The concept of Whole Personhood departs from the approach of the role of labor by defining the individual's place in the socioeconomic system. For understanding how labor shapes the different formations of whole personhood, the authors of this book rely on the concept of commodification by Polanyi. The concept of whole personhood is not a universal mold that defines an ideal type of human existence, and it does not offer a radical restructuring of the system – rather, it is a frame based on choice, individual action, and a decommodified space for human existence.

To this end, we may need to reconsider the role of labor in the life of an individual and how the economic arrangements of capitalism define this across time (Chapter 4 by Varela & della Santa), as well as investigating digitization (Chapter 1 by Faludi, and Chapter 6 by Mols & Wijngaarden) and intersectionalities (Chapter 2 by Dén-Nagy, Chapter 8 by Pinto-López, Montaudon-Tomas and Yáñez-Moneda). Commodification, an expanding process, is capturing ever more physical space that is essential for human existence, including land (nature), thereby shrinking the array of choices (explored in Chapter 5 by Panico and Pascucci). Individuals navigating the pressure of collapsing spheres develop resilience (Chapter 9 by Tepavcevic) and expand their creativity (Chapter 7 by Guerra) as a result of their struggle for decommodified private spaces. The following sections will locate the concept of whole personhood within the frame of the double movement.

How the Great Transformation Transforms Whole Personhood

The Double Movement

Recognition of Polanyi's seminal work, *The Great Transformation* (TGT), peaked by the beginning of the twenty-first century (Dale, 2010). We can identify the vast interest in conceptualizing the current transformations, marked by crises, by the third decade of this century based on Polanyi's core concepts, as laid out in his book. TGT encompasses the story of market capitalism from its birth during the industrial revolutions in England to its growth and deepening global interconnectedness that ended in collapse in the 1930s. The main related conflict was derived from a dialectic process that Polanyi coined 'the double movement' – a process that pushed markets to expand, but also to encounter emergent forces that would limit their influence – hence the countermovement. These forces have produced an array of societal arrangements shaped by various political economies. Polanyi concluded in TGT that liberal capitalism collapsed in the 1930s, while scholars since the post-WWII period have been examining the dimensions of liberal capitalism.

Disembeddedness was the concept used in TGT to describe the process which resulted in social relations becoming embedded in the economy, while before the deep transformative forces of commodification emerged, the economy was more integrated, thus embedded into society (Beckert, 2009). This suggests that, ideologically, the price-mechanism of the market regulates each and every sphere of human life, and humans must adjust – an extreme that may not be reached. The effects of disembeddedness, according to the meaning attached to it in TGT, were elaborated by Polanyi in a later work (1957) that suggested that as a consequence the distinct spheres of politics and the economy have subverted society.

The double movement as a synchronic and dialectic process (Goodwin, 2018: 1275) created unresolvable tensions within liberal economies, while the Great Depression acted as a catalyst for change, followed by governmental policies aimed at ameliorating the severe consequences thereof. Now globalization has evolved into its most profound and interconnected form, with the market integrating labor on a global scale. Despite the forces that are promoting the reorganization of regional systems of labor, new forms of precarity – particularly in the areas of digital work –indisputably challenge the global division of labor, as well as that of the household and the private sphere, and individuals are being called on to navigate this.

The 'Soft' and the 'Hard' Polanyi

To derive the two fundamental strands of scholarship that interpret the concept of embeddedness, we first need to locate the discourse about the double movement within the broader Polanyian framework. The 'hard' reading of Polanyi suggests a critical but reformist approach towards the radical interpretation of capitalism, resulting in its overthrow as an economic and political system. The 'soft' view of the double movement tends to accept the former as part of the natural dialectics of the capitalist system, associated with cycles of the disembeddness and re-embeddness of the economy into society, whereby market liberalization is followed or accompanied by decommodification in cycles that regulate access to processes of commodification (Goodwin, 2018), albeit not interconnected (Peck, 2013).

The 'hard' take on the double movement suggests that market capitalism is based on the fundamental contradiction of individuals' 'supportive' social relations in society and the unlimited expansion of capitalist markets (Lacher, 1999; Levitt, 2006). It is also clear that the interpretation of the double movement depends on the particular path and position within the world system that the given economy takes. For example, Goodwin (2018) highlights that scholars may question the degree of decommodification that takes place before neoliberal reform in some economies – and that countermovements in Latin America have been social forces that emerged as a result of a developmentalist state, and are aimed at protecting vulnerable groups (thus being initiatives that defend against the dismantling of regimes or traditional customs, but could become offensive or destructive in nature in terms of creating new forms of organizing). From a methodological perspective the 'hard' view of the double movement is context dependent in its approach and toolkit, while the 'soft' view allows for the anchoring of milestones in series of events that help with analyzing unfolding processes.

Embeddedness: From Commodification to Networks

The fundamental difference in how the double movement is interpreted provides an understanding of how the two fundamental strands that elaborate the concept of embeddedness developed. The 'hard' reading focuses on the problem of commodification that results in disembedding the economy from societal relations. The 'soft' interpretation is based on Polanyi's later work, the *Economy as Instituted Process* (Polanyi, 1957a), which suggests that the processes of economic and political organizing are embedded in the economy, thus are socially determined. Not until Granovetter (1985) was an efficient attempt to operationalize the concept of embeddedness made by elaborating the theory of social bridging across the spheres, with trust developing in networks. Economic exchange is a set of micro-interactions – the economy is built on the architecture of such trusted networks. Taking the concept further, Hess (2004) stressed that actors are defined by their cultural, social, etc. heritage, thus act in a socially embedded way. One great contribution of the scholarship on network embeddedness is how it has highlighted the positive and negative implications of social capital. Being based on trust and community formation, network embeddedness can be beneficial and efficient, but it may also lead to negative effects and distortions in the economy and harm to society, creating bottlenecks, criminal alliances, and environmental degradation (see Chapter 5 by Panico & Pascucci).

Overarching the concerns related to network embeddedness and its 'soft' contribution to understanding the micro- and meso-contextual elements of economic organizing, interest in the commodification-driven perspective about embeddedness is considered particularly relevant for understanding labor commodification processes in the context of great transformations (Wood et al., 2019).

The Connection of Embeddedness and Whole Personhood

Labor and Commodification

Polanyi claimed when analyzing British economic history that the double movement started in the 1830s with the reform of British labor legislation (Dale, 2010). Until then, the process of the expansion of market relations and the commodification of human power resulted in labor; of nature in land; and in money becoming a unit of trade and source of capital accumulation – these processes unrestricted and indeed enabled by governmental forces. The expansion of the commodification of labor and land caused the dimension of 'nature' (including livelihoods, personal boundaries and lives, communities and households, personal and social time) to shrink – and also engendered economic threats such as unemployment, while the structural-existential threat of shocks points to the continuing relevance of revisiting questions connected to the regulation of labor and the meaning of work. The integration of labor into the market was an extremely powerful force in the wake of the twentieth century, but it is also in the twenty-first century in the context of the globalized division of labor and digital capitalism.

Whole personhood has a myriad of dimensions that must be considered when envisioning how to organize economic activity in order to balance the process of the (de)commodification of labor and creating conditions in which individuals can make choices and thrive. Theorizing these dimensions leads to the macro, meso, and micro-level investigations discussed in the present book.

To connect the dimensions of personal needs and organizational governance, Tortia and Sacchetti (Chapter 3) – in departing from the 'soft' reading of embeddedness and moving toward the Granovetterian frame that describes the role of social ties in forming the economy – propose a model of embedded governance. They argue that the precondition for self-realization in a context of production lies in institutional design which allows for the production of organizational routines that satisfy needs and involves interaction with the external societal environment. Old wine in a new bottle – new institutionalism meets the concept of embeddedness with a twist.

The precarity of digital work arrangements and the implications of working from home during the COVID-19 pandemic are explored in Chapter 6 (Mols & Wijngaarden) on a particularly vulnerable group of young professionals, while in Chapter 7 (Guerra) describes how musicians are facing the challenge of the intersection of employment structures in cultural production with the market for cultural goods.

Working from home, particularly due to the enforced nature of this during the COVID-19 pandemic, has expanded previous discussions about the blurring boundaries between life and work. Simultaneous existence and activity in professional and private realities is what is described as the convergence and divergence of spheres by Mols and Wijngaarden (Chapter 6). Precarious positions are being enforced due to the need to work from home, in addition to other vulnerabilities.

Forms of Integration, Embeddedness, and Dysfunction in Society

Polanyi (1957) later suggested that economies organize themselves around three phenomena: redistribution, reciprocity, and market exchange. The main indicator of which of the latter is dominant depends on how societies access land, water, clothing, shelter, or income for daily sustenance.

Important here is understanding how markets are being organized. The main "transactional modes" or allocation systems that organize economies involve redistribution and reciprocity – these economic systems are indeed deeply social and cultural and tend to be embedded. With redistribution in the context of capitalism the market is the main institution, and the most disembedded form of this is laissez-faire market exchange.

The connection between the concepts of the double movement and forms of integration is the countermovements that aim at expanding forms of organization based on redistribution and reciprocity. A plurality of movements is characteristic of the double movement, rather than a singular process for or against the market – concludes Goodwin (2018, p. 1285).

The power of the theory with regard to economic integration and the countermovement may be illustrated by the case study of waste in Naples. Although Chapter 5, *Land of Fires...* (Panico & Pascucci) puts under scrutiny (through the lens of network embeddedness) the roots of the dysfunctionality of waste management, an interpretation that stems from 'hard' Polanyian scholarship confirms previous findings about the relevance of radical countermovements that aim at the decommodification of land and nature, the defense of heritage and vulnerable groups, and the creation of new forms of organizing – as summarized by Goodwin (2018).

Waste may be viewed from the logic of ‘production of use’ in the household system (analogous with the ancient Greek household) rather than ‘production for gain’ (the latter produced for market exchange and monetary purposes). Waste management should be part of the redistribution system organized by the state and local governance, with waste ideally being collected and managed without (or at least minimizing) environmental harm and health risks, similarly to with the non-market allocation systems. In the chapter Land of Fires, dysfunctionality stems from the corruption of the marketization of waste. The government assumes the role of price-making (following North, and classical institutionalists). There are no exactly defined property rights for waste, which is exchanged according to a specific market mechanism. These property rights in part should belong to the ‘producers of waste’ in terms of determining how waste is dealt with in a legal and non-harmful way – which is what the countermovement of locals and NGOs is trying to enforce. The ‘profits’ of the market exchange between the local government and the mafia and other illegal actors presently go into their pockets, so it is in their interest to maintain the market, using violence if necessary. Waste – if commodified – should be driven by fair exchange. Instead, the market for commodified waste harms local society and the environment. Therefore, this market is a classic example of disembeddedness – market interests involving violence to the detriment of people and environment.

The commodification of waste may also be a metaphor for nature when linked to land, according to Polanyi’s concept of fictitious commodities. The latter is not being produced and invested into, unlike a ‘normal’ commodity. The ‘legal’ market for waste is codified by legislation and approved by Rome. Waste is a fictitious commodity similar to land as it has an impact on the nature and the lands of communities – and in order to marketize waste, farmers’ land is involved.

Some societies may pretend such tension does not exist as a driver of migration (Chapter 9 by Tepavcevic); some societies prioritize one type of production over another, causing physical violence (Chapter 7, Pinto-López, Montaudon-Tom and Yáñez-Moneda); and some may believe that promoting both is achievable, and seek balance. We argue that “Contemporary societies that are shaped by digital capitalism in the social media age do not focus on biological human reproduction but on capital accumulation mediated by digital technologies” (Faludi & Crosby-Nagy, 2021). Further, during the pandemic the household returned to its original conceptualization as a firm, temporarily erasing and then re-creating a source of need fulfillment (Chapter 6 by Guerra), including by the corporation (Chapter 3 by Sacchetti & Tortia). Finally, we argue that if it is the case that a resolution of the tension between social reproduction and capital accumulation is what can contribute to or explain Polanyi’s forms of integration, then what is central in society is work, not the market (Chapter 4 by Varela and della Santa).

It is not the intention of the authors of this book to take a stand regarding the 'soft' versus 'hard' reading of Polanyi's ideas, thus coming to conclusions about the need for reforming or overthrowing capitalism. It is our intention to unveil persistent patterns of economic and political organization that reproduce socioeconomic tensions. The following chapters shed light on how crisis-triggered shocks are enhancing contradictory forces of commodification and evoking countermovements that create new paths of existence.

Julianna Faludi
Corvinus University, Hungary

REFERENCES

Beckert, J. (2009). The social order of markets. *Theory and Society*, *38*(3), 245–269. doi:10.100711186-008-9082-0

Dale, G. (2010). *Karl Polanyi: The Limits of the Market* (1st ed.). Polity Press.

Engels, F. (1891). The Origin of the Family, Private Property and the State. In *Marx & Engels Collected Works* (Vol. 26, pp. 129–276). Lawrence and Wishart.

Faludi, J., & Crosby-Nagy, M. (2021). The Digital Economy of the Sourdough: Housewifisation in the Time of COVID-19. *TripleC*, 113–124.

Goodwin, G. (2018). Rethinking the Double Movement: Expanding the Frontiers of Polanyian Analysis in the Global South. *Development and Change*, *49*(5), 1268–1290. doi:10.1111/dech.12419

Granovetter, M. (1985). 1985: Economic action and social structure: The problem of embeddedness. *American Journal of Sociology*, *91*(3), 481–510. doi:10.1086/228311

Hess, M. (2004). 'Spatial' relationships? Towards a reconceptualization of embeddedness. *Progress in Human Geography*, *28*(2), 165–186. doi:10.1191/0309132504ph479oa

Lacher, H. (1999). Embedded Liberalism, disembedded markets: Reconceptualising the pax Americana. *New Political Economy*, *4*(3), 343–360. doi:10.1080/13563469908406408

Levitt, K. P. (2006). Keynes and Polanyi: The 1920s and the 1990s. *Review of International Political Economy*, *13*(1), 152–177. doi:10.1080/09692290500396768

Peck, J. (2013). For Polanyian Economic Geographies. *Environment and Planning A. Economy and Space*, *45*(7), 1545–1568. doi:10.1068/a45236

Polanyi, K. (1957a). The Economy as Instituted Process. In *Trade and Market in the early empires: Economies in history and theory*. The Falcon's Wing Press.

Polanyi, K. (1957b). *Trade and Market in the Early Empires: Economies in History and Theory*. The Free Press.

Wood, A. J., Graham, M., Lehdonvirta, V., & Hjorth, I. (2019). Networked but Commodified: The (Dis)Embeddedness of Digital Labour in the Gig Economy. *Sociology*, *53*(5), 931–950. doi:10.1177/0038038519828906

Introduction

In 2020, the COVID-19 crisis uncovered hidden social tensions. Special attention was paid to the distribution of unpaid household labor, which has remained grossly unequal across European societies (Vargha et al., 2017). This all too frequently invisible inequality was especially visible during the 2020 global lockdown. Women whose jobs were "digital" were expected to work from home, while simultaneously assuming their unpaid labor tasks. A remarkable feature of the lockdown was the widely accepted solution to these expectations of multi-tasking. Women had to either stop working and leave their jobs so that they could focus on taking care of children and assisting them with home-schooling, or attempt to do it all.

This general trend developed into an expectation that women be available across multiple spheres of the economy, all now concentrated in the household. These spheres included the economic (performing at work), social (caretaking), educational (homeschooling), and institutional (house chores). Moreover, the immediate economic effects of the COVID-19 lockdowns were felt most strongly by industries with predominantly female workers, such as the service sector, retail, tourism, caretaking, and other informal work. Unemployment rates rose across economic sectors, and the gendered data reveals that this trend has hit women especially hard, confining them to the household, depriving them of income, and deepening current structures of dependence. Jobs that sent employees "digital" shifted the "location of production" to the household. As a result, this central social unit has become a critical issue for those interested in gender equality.

In her study on the discovery of unpaid work, British economist Susan Himmelweit finds women's unpaid work to be "a costless resource to exploit", highlighting the gendered effect of shrinking state social interventions (Himmelweit, 1995). Perez (2019, p. 244) points out that, in the UK, social spending cuts contributed, above all, to a rise in female unemployment, which increased by 20% due to the 2009 recession. More than ten years later, the pandemic had crushed societies even more (Perez-Mayo, 2019). The modern-day "catch-allness" of mothers can be seen in contract types, wages, social ties, and a long list of other realities which provide insights into the "status" of women (Baxter & Kane, 1995), which is still low and far from equal.

Karl Polányi, Countermovements and Instituted Processes

In his major works, especially *The Great Transformation*, Karl Polányi initiates the conversion of social interventions by first elaborating on the idea of instituted processes. Polányi writes:

Ultimately that is why the control of the economic system by the market is of overwhelming consequence to the whole organization of society: it means no less than the running of society as an adjunct to the market. Instead of the economy being embedded in social relations, social relations are embedded in the economic system (Polányi, 1957, p. 60).

Many studies in political science, along with an entire branch of science and technology studies (Bijker Wiebe & Pinch Trevor, 2012) have supported an interpretation of Polányi's description of instituted processes as *embeddedness*. One of these has been to characterize the economy during the 19th-century industrialization, and again during the era of Thatcherism in the United Kingdom, as capitalist periods witnessing an attempt to *dis*-embed the economy from social relations, including weakening labor organizations such as trade unions. This approach can be seen in the typologies elaborated by the *Varieties of Capitalism* research and its extensions (Bohle & Greskovits, 2012). In these works, state interventions are interpreted as protection from market forces, also known as *counter-movements*.

Polányi elaborates on the forms of economic integration a society can have. These forms are *reciprocity*, *redistribution*, and *exchange*. Each of these, Polányi writes, occurs at a different level. Economies might be classified according to the dominance of one of these forms over another, for example, an economy might be characterized as featuring more exchange than redistribution and some might serve as countermoving mechanisms (Szelényi & Mihályi, 2021).

For this edited volume, various support mechanisms are referenced that serve to protect the people from market forces or restrain the market, with the acknowledgement that these features are not limited to institutions, but could be mechanized in other forms. Specifically, we would like to extend the idea to the concept of countermovements and the role of women in the *bourgeois family*, given that the family unit serves as the ultimate or penultimate counter-movement. The pandemic proved this point where women were both expected to supply social protection and showcase pride in their unpaid work, as symbolized by the image of baked sour-dough bread (Faludi & Crosby, 2021).

Women as Economic and Social Engine

We are exposed more directly to the importance of the household and the bourgeois family in the work *Capitalism, Socialism and Democracy* and specifically Joseph Schumpeter's chapter on Decomposition. In the context of the drive towards his general thesis, which is that society will evolve out of capitalism as a passing stage from feudalism towards something else, he articulates one of the significant aspects of self-destruction: the decline in social reproduction.

With the decline of the driving power supplied by the family motive, the businessman's time horizon shrinks, roughly, to his life expectancy. And he might now be less willing than he was to fulfill that function of earning, saving, and investing even if he saw no reason to fear that the results would but swell his tax bills. He drifts into an anti-saving frame of mind and accepts with an increasing readiness anti-saving theories that are indicative of a short-run philosophy (Schumpeter, 1943, p. 161).

Capitalism will destroy itself because once people start to calculate the costs and benefits of having children, then couples will have fewer children. This dynamic is seen in today's European societies and is even treated as a crisis in Hungary (Fodor, 2022).

In order to realize what all this means for the efficiency of the capitalist engine of production, we need only recall that the family and the family home used to be the mainspring of the typically bourgeois kind of profit motive (Schumpeter, 1943, p. 160).

Schumpeter goes on to help the audience understand that unless the outsourcing of the hosting of guests, and child-rearing using social infrastructures or alternatives can be made undesirable, the role of the family shall disappear.

He writes:

As regards the style of life, capitalist evolution decreases the desirability of and provides alternatives to, the bourgeois family home. I have previously adverted to the Evaporation of Industrial Property; I have now to advert to the Evaporation of Consumers' Property (Schumpeter, 1953, p.158).

The average family of bourgeois standing tends to reduce the difficulties of running the big house and the big country place by substituting for it small and mechanized establishments plus a maximum of outside service and outside life—hospitality, in particular, being increasingly shifted to the restaurant or club (Schumpeter, 1943, p. 159).

COVID-19 was both a test as well as an expression of the forging of the return to the household and bourgeois family as central, and this was experienced globally, resulting in significant relational tensions ranging from domestic violence to the dissolving of pairs. The absence of so-called "alternatives" proved to be quite dividing among society, especially surrounding school closures with one faction demanding social infrastructure and the other accepting online schooling and sacrificing their own work-life. And of course, we shouldn't forget the middle, consisting of the sour-dough superwoman, baking bread and working at the same time. This bridge from Schumpeter to modern life manifested in household labor division during the pandemic.

CONCLUSION

Women's role in the absorbing of shocks to the economy and society is a modern-day expectation of women and a role seen very visibly during the COVID-19 crisis. This role can be interpreted as a counter-movement in itself, in the sense that protections from market forces or the need to correct or redistribute is enabled or facilitated by the smoothing effect of unpaid household labor. Incentivizing women to reproduce or providing support to women with cash emphasizes their difference as being specialized in reproduction or unpaid labor. Here we are presented with a situation of paradox. While an essential facet of any kind of society, unpaid labor is at the same time, consistently marginalized and undervalued. However, when we broaden our imagination about the mechanisms of societies beyond exchange rates and fiscal levers, to social forces, tensions, and interactions, then dialogue about social change can begin. We hope this book can contribute to the desperately needed sparks required for clashing current structures into upheaval.

Michelle O. Crosby
Corvinus University of Budapest, Hungary

REFERENCES

Baxter, J., & Emily, W. K. (1995). Dependence and Independence: A Cross-National Analysis of Gender Inequality and Gender Attitudes. *Gender & Society*, *9*(2), 193–315. doi:10.1177/089124395009002004

Bijker, W., Hughes, T., & Pinch, T. (Eds.). (2012). *The Social Construction of Technological Systems: New Directions in the Sociology and History of Technology. Anniversary edition*. The MIT Press.

Bohle, D., & Greskovits, B. (2012). *Capitalist Diversity on Europe's Periphery*. Cornell University Press.

Faludi, J., & Crosby-Nagy, M. (2021). The Digital Economy of the Sourdough: Housewifisation in the Time of COVID-19. *TripleC, 19*(1), 113–124. doi:10.31269/triplec.v19i1.1222

Fodor, E. (2022). More Babies for the State: The "Carefare" Regime of Anti-Liberal Hungary. *New Labor Forum, 31*(1), 34–41.

Himmelweit, S. (1995). The Discovery of 'Unpaid Work': The Social Consequences of the Expansion of 'Work.'. *Feminist Economics, 1*(2), 1–19. doi:10.1080/714042229

MacIver. (1957). *The Great Transformation* [The Political and Economic Origins of Our Time]. Beacon Press.

Perez-Mayo, J. (2019). Inequality of Opportunity, a Matter of Space? *Regional Science Policy & Practice, 11*(1), 71–87. doi:10.1111/rsp3.12181

Schumpeter, J. (1943). *Capitalism, Socialism and Democracy*. Harper.

Szelényi, I., & Mihályi, P. (2021). Karl Polanyi: A theorist of mixed economies. *Theory and Society, 50*(3), 443–461. doi:10.100711186-020-09403-3

Vargha, L., Gál, R. I., & Crosby-Nagy, M. O. (2017). Household Production and Consumption over the Life Cycle: National Time Transfer Accounts in 14 European Countries. *Demographic Research, 36*(32), 905–944. doi:10.4054/DemRes.2017.36.32

Section 1

The Great Transformation, Whole Personhood, and Resilient Societies

Chapter 1
Automation and Platform Capitalism:
The Great Transformation

Julianna Faludi
Corvinus University, Hungary

ABSTRACT

The morphology of the current transformation of the 21st century can be examined with the tools of Polanyi's analysis of the great transformation (TGT). The previous profound socio-economic transformation was connected to the Industrial Revolution that created industrial-urban societies. The first Industrial Revolution was localized as the most eloquent example in England 1750-1850, overarching only a century and followed by further waves of industrial revolutions stretching the new socio-economic system toward a globalized order. There is no doubt that the changes of the 21st century are unprecedented and far-reaching. The considerations about which changes exactly are transforming our global realities are manifold but can be grouped at least into two main strands: those concerned about the transformation of socio-economic systems to preserve and to redefine ecological systems and those that focus on the impact of the digital or platform economy reformulating fundamental institutions, such as markets, governance, and ownership.

INTRODUCTION

Earlier profound socioeconomic transformation was connected to the Industrial Revolution which created industrial-urban societies (Polanyi 1944) and culminated in the 'conservatism' of the 1920s that ended in the Great Depression. The first

DOI: 10.4018/978-1-6684-2364-6.ch001

Industrial Revolution was localized in its clearest example in England from 1750-1850, spanning only a century, but being followed by further waves of industrial revolution that expanded the new socioeconomic system into a globalized order. There is no doubt that the changes of the twenty-first century are also unprecedented and far-reaching. Debates about which changes exactly are transforming our global realities are manifold, but they can be classified into two main strands – those related to the transformation of socioeconomic systems and the preservation and redefinition of ecological systems, and those which focus on the how the impact of automation and the digital economy is reformulating fundamentally important institutions such as markets, governance, and ownership in a context of platform capitalism and hyper-globalization.

The so-called digital revolution has turned out to be a trigger for evolutionary processes in the context of global capitalism. The digital revolution, an abrupt technological paradigm shift, was connected first to the spread of the internet, which implied a shift in social interaction, news, and information consumption patterns – the first visible and much-discussed change. The technology-assisted metamorphosis of the political, economic, and social spheres has resulted in the emergence of platform capitalism. These profound transformations involve new institutional arrangements of markets and political agency, and the (re)distribution of power, democracy and autonomy, as information technologies are tightly linked to political systems. Just as the industrial revolution was the long-term context for short-term political conflict (Novy 2020), the process of the digital revolution is creating the underlying structure for a series of politically and economically framed events.

Following the method of connecting short-term events to underlying structures, in methodological terms the COVID-19 pandemic is taken as a political-economic rupture – with specific reference to the harsh governmental responses in the form of lockdowns, especially during the first waves of the pandemic, which came as a shock. This rupture on the one hand caused immediate damage to social and economic systems, and on the other accelerated digitalization and platformization processes. It involved a game of temporality – obtaining time on the inter-governmental level to freeze the devastation to the social system, while accelerating the profound digital transformation in the economy and further commodification of labor. Automation and the disruptive innovations in the field of Artificial Intelligence (AI) are impacting all spheres of work, from factories to online services and beyond, questioning the fundamental frames of work such as knowledge, skills, working conditions, and forms and approaches to organizing work. The enhanced commodification of labor is tightly connected to the redrawing of boundaries of public and private spheres (Faludi and Crosby 2021) and abrupt changes in the labor market.

HYPERGLOBALIZATION AND THE POWER OF TECH GIANTS – BACKGROUND

The process of long-term change, called The Great Transformation (TGT), is a socioeconomic evolution explained in the seminal work by Polanyi (1945). It is an undercurrent-type movement that is not visible to the eye at a first glance. What is visible is the moment of radical rupture in elements of the political-economic fabric. This short-term change can accelerate the ongoing profound transformation (Novy 2020). Current forms of capitalism are being theorized from diverse angles such as global, digital (Schiller 2000) and platform capitalism (Srnicek 2016), as well as transnational information capitalism (Fuchs, 2008) to describe the nexus of state-capital-society relations on a transnational scale. This chapter applies the notion of platform capitalism to highlight the importance of the growth of tech giants that bridge national economies, and the prospective consequences of the expansion of the AI-driven economy. Platform capitalism has emerged, with companies providing platforms for new businesses to innovate and grow ecosystems. These processes first redefined patterns of economic interaction, creating space for new business models and ways of organizing economic activity. Second, with the expansion of social media platforms, social interactions and ways of living and organizing have fundamentally changed on the level of micro-interactions, further expanding into direct business-to-consumer models on a global scale, creating a new culture. Platforms have grown into tech giants that monopolize the market, profiting from precarious work conditions (Srnicek 2016; Gray and Suri 2019). The process of hyper-globalization infers the existence of an economy that relies on outsourced and hard-to-trace supply-chains, industrialized agriculture, and corporations with nation-size wealth and cross-national power. Hyper-globalization is driven by cross-border economic integration, global social media communications and technology-driven transformations based on Artificial Intelligence (Rodrik 2011; Kessler and Subramanian 2013). The global economic system that has emerged and evolved since the Industrial Revolution is known to be the driver of the 'great acceleration' – the process of impacting the Earth System – that has accelerated to an unprecedented extent since the 1960s (Steffen et al., 2006) – highlighting the scale of growth potential and related impact, including the devastation presently being caused. An important strand of social theory is examining how planetary co-existence and profound socioecological change can be sustained (Novy, 2020; Barnthaler et al. 2020), involving re-embedding the economy as a counterweight to the great acceleration. The possibilities for de-commodification and the counter movement to create structures of co-existence within the contemporary reality of platform capitalism are yet to be analyzed. The current transformative forces of the twenty-first century are connected to the gradual shift in production toward automation and artificial general intelligence. The new forms of division of labor and class structure are defined by emergent technologies such as advanced industrial robotics, machine learning, and artificial intelligence. These processes, coined the Fourth Industrial Revolution (Schwab 2016), are transforming the way socioeconomic life is organized through the integration of human lives and technologies. Most importantly, the progress of Artificial Intelligence affects numerous domains of human existence beyond its economic functionality and may render a competitive advantage to national states in the form of economic power. Those who succeed in training better AI solutions, rendering them more knowledgeable and adaptive, will be the driver of the global economy in the future.

The growth of tech giants is attributed to the power of information society (Webster 2002) of the network economy. These companies have applied management strategies based on the acquisition and diversification of their portfolios; buying up competitors, and creating monopolistic conditions for business ecosystems through ownership. The servitization of the economy – the shift from selling to renting goods – has been a trend since the late 1970s and was accelerated by digital platformization. Traditional companies like Rolls-Royce and Zipcar have shifted toward deploying the potential of digital platforms (Srnicek 2017). The new digital business models have connected different economic agents and capitalized on the marketplace. By defining the standards of the market, platforms control the entry points for businesses. As a consequence, the emergent centralized platform capitalism accumulates political and public power while eliminating competition. The concentration of capital of the tech giants had been causing problems related to tax-avoidance and the lack of inter-governmental regulation long before the shock caused by the pandemic. Moreover, the labor rights and conditions of work at these companies have been scrutinized since the 'sharing economy' became subject to criticism (Murillo et al. 2017).

The severe lockdown measures of the first waves of the pandemic in 2020 shifted work, social life, and entertainment entirely to digital platforms. As a result, global tech giants benefited from their role in organizing the economy on a supra-national scale and their stock value has come to rival the wealth of nations. In February 2021, Amazon was the third biggest employer in the world with 1.2 million workers worldwide, and the value of Google-owned Alphabet outstripped that of Hungary's economy in 2019 (Jolly, 2021). The pandemic-related crisis has contributed to unprecedented growth of newcomers such as Zoom and preexisting corporations as Microsoft, e-commerce platforms such as Etsy, Amazon, cloud services such as Snowflake, Alphabet, and streaming services such as Netflix and Disney, which entered the streaming market. The revenue of the latter companies grew unprecedentedly from 2019 to 2021 due to the work-from-home shift and the opportunity of attracting people's attention through more screen time. In fact, the expansion of online services (payment, ecommerce, cloud, fintech, etc.) into uncharted and less dominant territories substantially contributed to this growth. (Gartenberg, 2022).

The reallocation of economic value to platform corporations increased their role in the redistribution of public power as they directly and indirectly structure the work and life spaces of humans. Platform corporations extract benefits from the labor force, citizens' purchasing power, and the infrastructure of national economies, while their profits accumulate outside these states. In contrast, the domestic service sector of national economies shrunk during the lockdowns, diminishing their share of local economies, leading to imbalance. The dominance of a handful of corporations over industries across nations is raising questions about the need for the re-distribution of power in the form of a 'new social contract' (Ross 2021) that can promote a new equilibrium of governance.

The mass-scale displacement of the workspace to the home during lockdowns not only contributed to the acceleration of digitization processes but also triggered the relocation of public services (schooling, care work, social services) to households. Moreover, the surveillance of home-office arrangements and state measures has reordered the boundaries of private-public-corporate time and space, questioning human agency to shape space and social relations. Protective regulations – despite the promising steps and efforts of the European Union on this matter – aimed at protecting people from the devastation caused by corporate control and the loss of the commons in the digital space are being designed, but lag behind.

The role of national and supra-national governance in regulating a market mechanism that now spans international boundaries is an evolving question. Unfolding events show the power of big tech to control information flow and the efforts of national governments to regulate and restrict access to social platforms.

It was not just the seismic effect of the pandemic that triggered the growth of big tech, but the underlying trends of automation and the sophistication of big-data-based artificial intelligence (AI) strategies. AI has seamlessly proliferated into all areas of the digital reality of humans in much more sophisticated ways than mere product recommendations. The market for AI associated social media annual adjustment is predicted to grow in the near future to 2,197.1 Million USD by 2023 (Markets and Markets, n.d.[1]), and the tech giants that own big data have a comparative advantage in this area. AI and machine learning are important drivers of the acceleration of automation and robotization that is taking over human work in all sectors of the economy.

Susskind (2020) suggests that the concentration of economic power is the issue that the twentieth century had to deal with, yet more concern is being raised about the political power associated with the growth of big tech in the twenty-first century due to its impact on justice and democracy. To understand the depth of the transformation being created by platform capitalism, we need to dissect its traces in the twentieth century. To this end, in what follows current transformations are analyzed from the perspective of the universal power of the forces of market creation and the dual movement examined by Polanyi involving the case of the Industrial Revolution and the Great Transformation that led to the collapse of some of the major paradigms of the nineteenth century (Polanyi, 1944).

AUTOMATION AND UNEMPLOYMENT FROM A HISTORICAL PERSPECTIVE

Despite critical arguments suggesting that social inequalities and the logic of class divisions are persistent in the context of capitalism and constructs such as network society and information society (Castells 2000) may not cover class division dynamics, we still suggest that economic systems need their societies as a context, similarly to how Polányi (1944) suggested that industrial society provided the context for economic and political forces to create markets for fictitious commodities and new modes of industrial production. This chapter relies on the term information society to describe the context for the hyper-globalization processes of digital- and later platform capitalism.

The problem of the future of work is often boiled down to the simple question whether automation and robotics will create unemployment. The uncertainty and anxiety that exists in relation to employment is reinforced by economic crises and by pessimism about the role of technologies in production. This view of technology as a substitute for labor and a threat is rooted in the Industrial Revolution. But even the Luddites of the nineteenth century who destroyed machinery did not do so to simply obstruct industrial transformation – the production of textiles shifting from workshops to factories – but due to the absence of a system of social security; the economic and social precarity of working conditions in times of crisis. The act of the destruction of machinery was one of collective bargaining (Hobsbawm 1952). During this most active period of the Industrial Revolution (1795-1834), the free labor market was organized – the last of the markets to be established under the new system (Polanyi 1944: 81). It was beneficial to mobilize labor for emerging industries – such as through the enclosure movement – although this led to devastating social destruction.

In the wake of the nineteenth century, the crisis of 1810-12 was triggered by war and export bubbles related to the unpredictability of the market that caused disruption and massive unemployment in the textile industry, especially the cotton industry (Heckscher 2018). It was unemployment that triggered technophobic acts rather than the technological advancement itself that caused unemployment.

Following Polanyi, the problem that underlay these events (crisis, war, export-related problems) was a transformational one: a regular labor market had to be created that attributed market value to labor. In fact, modes of production were transforming and introducing new technologies for at least two reasons: to enhance productivity, and to leverage the risk of employability which stemmed from the lack of wage-labor market regulation. The Industrial Revolution as a whole did not take destroy jobs – the disruption was caused by how and when the labor market was created. Polanyi points out that this process involved the creation of a market for land and money in the first phase, and it was only later that the conditions for people to sell their labor for market value were institutionalized. As a result of the first Industrial Revolution several new economic classes emerged (Polanyi 1944: 84), but the most important of these were the classes of employers and of workers. The division of labor and of breaking down production processes into smaller tasks had two important consequences (among others). First, the phenomenon of deskilling and low-skilled jobs; second, the fact that well-defined routinized tasks could be undertaken using machinery (Leijonhufvud 2007). These processes encouraged mass production and new ways of organizing the economy that involved innovation in management. In sum, despite the substitution effect of machinery, new jobs were created.

At the turn of the twentieth century, the rise of organizations that ate up the supply chain occurred, providing vast employment for the bureaucracy and the managerial class. The system of Fayolism involved developing layers of administrators and floor managers to surveil and coordinate production. At the same time, the scientific management of Taylor (2008(1911)) based on time and motion studies (Gilbreth 2008(1911)) involved the further deskilling and dehumanization of the worker, later partially substituted by automation. The dreaded Fordian system was one of the first to use automated machines. Eventually, although the conveyor belt remained, jobs involving soft skills and specialized knowledge increased in importance, along with human-centered management. Assembly lines were abolished in Sweden by Volvo in the late 1980s-1990s, and automation replaced by teams of workers assembling entire cars (Benanav, 2020).

Throughout the waves of the second industrial revolution, innovation in the transportation of goods, management and accounting systems, as well as legal forms of organizing for production spurred the growth in the number of entrepreneurs (Chandler 1977). The rise of large corporations and the growth of bureaucracy created managerial capitalism (Chandler 1984) with the emergence of the "organization man" (Whyte 1956) and the white-collar "salesman world," consisting of "cheerful robots" replacing the autonomous individual and implying that the way factory and office work is organized may involve dehumanization (Mills, 1951). Mediocracy, risk avoidance, and the moral mazes produced by organizational culture proliferated into everyday life (Jackall, 1984). It was no surprise that the automation of white-collar job processes occurred at an early stage (Ford 2015). Computing technology was experimented with to substitute routinized skilled work based on human-trait behavior during the first waves of the application of artificial intelligence (Susskind 2020).

In sum, technological advancement since the industrial revolutions has challenged the employment structure, jobs have been taken over by machines, and new jobs have been created by the growing bureaucratic sector, as well as by the expanding service sector – which may be dreadful and monotonous in both areas. The substitution of monotonous jobs or tasks by automation increases productivity and creates jobs in other domains through a process of complementarity (Susskind 2020).

That industries emerge, grow, and die out is a natural economic phenomenon (Schumpeter 2014 [1942]) and jobs emerge and disappear as a consequence. But the main problem of shifting from one industry or system of production to another is connected to locality and skills. People who lose their jobs may live some distance from where new industries emerge, and the skills required in an older field of industry might not be sufficient for a new one – the root cause of structural unemployment.

Breaking down tasks into routines is a way toward deskilling, but it is also an opportunity for technology to step in (Lejionhufvud 2007). Machinery started to take over routine tasks from workers back in the nineteenth and twentieth centuries (Susskind 2020), and deskilling along with industry shifts may leave some unemployed, while in times of crisis a combination of factors lead to mass unemployment. The most eloquent collapse, the Great Depression, put workers on the streets as a consequence of several market inefficiencies, but mostly due to a laissez-faire market economy (Polányi 1945) that deprived workers of labor security. Although it was tempting to attribute the extent of this to "technological unemployment," as propagated by Keynes (1931), among others, Polanyi viewed the Great Depression as one event among a series of events that included World War I, the interwar period, fascism, and World War II – the culmination of the 'planned' 'laissez faire' policies of governments that led to market forces overwhelming society (Kuttner 2020). The response to the crisis, the New Deal, was an attempt to counteract market forces and heal the wounds of a society permeated by severe inequality. The war economy during World War II was able to hide the structural problems that led to the crisis. The new jobs required new skills, and structural unemployment left low-skilled workers on the brink. What we are witnessing today is that automation has a class dimension, and the lives of the less educated and the vulnerable are at stake.

ARE ROBOTS TAKING JOBS TODAY?

Industrial production is the first and foremost site of the growth in automation and robotics today. Automation technologies include industrial and social robots, self-service kiosks, artificial intelligence, chatbots, face recognition technology, voice-controlled technologies, wearable and implanted technologies, additive manufacturing (3D printing), and the internet of things, among others. The substituting force of automation displaces workers locally and may cause frictional technological unemployment (Susskind 2020). Acemoglu and Restrepo (2020) examined a dataset covering a decade and found that industries that adopted robots employed fewer workers, raising the level of unemployment in the localities of the respective industrial plants. Further, the increase in the productivity of the factories lowered the average wage of a worker. The effect of technology on devaluing human labor expressed in wages and in physically crowding out people from their workplaces has a devastating impact on local society. Some industries, however, grow on a national scale due to the complementary effect of automation, demanding labor force in a location that may attract people. Despite this, displaced workers may not be able to meet the new demand for labor for several reasons, including the mismatch of place or skills (Susskind 2020). The substituting force of technology may be predicted for groups of jobs and skills. From a test of such predictions based on a survey of adult skills between 2012-2014, Georgieff and Milanez (2021) found that jobs associated with a high risk of automation in manufacturing, sales, clerical, and agricultural occupations contributed to a decline in employment. Employment growth was lower in high-risk occupations (6%) compared to low-risk occupations (18%). The study confirmed that workers with a low level of education were particularly at risk of displacement by automation as they were increasingly employed in jobs associated with high risk.

The profound transformation that occurred in previous centuries points to a desire to raise productivity and enhance workers' performance using technology – a general and overarching driver of technological innovation. But apart from this push to increase productivity, any disturbance in the labor market can trigger technological substitution. Such disturbances may be connected to labor market regulation or a critical event such as Brexit (which may trigger the modernization of UK manufacturing, and an increase from 75 to 101 robot density units within five years by 2020; see below); or the COVID-19 lockdowns that led to a temporary loss of foreign labor. A further cause may be the demographics of the available labor force. The latter was found to be one of the reasons for the variation in the rate and impact of automation across countries, as demonstrated by Acemoglu and Restrepo (2018). The authors reveal that in rapidly aging countries such as Germany, France, Italy, Japan, and South Korea, the relative shortage of middle-aged production workers triggered the adoption and development of robotics. These countries have invested into technology and became exporters of robotics to other countries, such as the United States, which is experiencing less rapid demographic change. Predominantly Japan is the world's first robot manufacturing country. According to Acemoglu and Restrepo (2018) the demographic factors associated with the labor market explain why European countries are often ahead of the US in robotics.

The labor market and disturbance in production caused by the COVID-19 has tended to accelerate automation as companies reduce their reliance on human labor and contact between workers (Georgieff and Milanez 2021). This shift is not only occurring in manufacturing. Early evidence from during the pandemic showed that just over 80% of employers were accelerating the digitization of their work processes and expanding their use of remote work; and 50% were set to accelerate and augment the automation of jobs at their companies (World Economic Forum, WEF 2020, p.14). In addition, more than one-quarter of employers were expected to temporarily or permanently reduce their workforce.

Coming back to the question whether automation will lead to the loss of jobs, we may examine how the top ten countries associated with the highest level of automation deal with employment. Data are taken from the International Federation of Robotics[2] that measures the number of robots per 10,000 workers in an industry. The ranking shows that manufacturing is mostly robotics-based in Singapore (almost three times as intensively as in the third-ranking country, Japan) and South-Korea. Unemployment in these two countries is slightly higher than in Japan. This suggests a well-functioning labor market and a sound growth rate based on productivity. In general, the unemployment rates of the most automated countries are moderate (Table 1) – only in Sweden has there been a relatively high rate of structural unemployment since the mid-1990s, especially among youth and the migrant population. This suggests that long-term unemployment is not connected directly to the substituting force of technology. Similarly, Hong Kong, and the US also experienced a slowdown due to the severe outbreaks of COVID-19, resulting in a high spike in the unemployment rate. (Heer, 2021)

According to the IFR, worldwide robot density almost doubled between 2015 and 2020, which might be attributed to the natural growth of technology adaptation in the manufacturing industry, along with the turn toward automation to eliminate reliance on human labor in manufacturing (see above). Manufacturing is shifting at a faster pace and automated production has saved some industries from complete shutdown, increasing the need for further automation.

Table 1. Top 10 automated countries and unemployment rate in 2019-2021

Top 10 Automated Countries by Robot Density in 2019	Unemployment Rate in %		
	2021	**2020**	**2019**
Singapore (918)	3.5	3.0[5]	2.3
South Korea (868)	3.7	3.9	3.84
Japan (364)	2.8	2.8 (WB)	2.4 (WB)
Germany (346)	3.2	5.9 and 4.6[8]	5
Sweden (272)	8.2	6.67	6.48
Denmark (243)	5.1	4.85	4.91
Hong Kong (242)		5.8 (WB)	2.9
Chinese Taipei (234)	3.64	3.9	3.8
USA (228)	5.3	8.3	3.68
Belgium (214)	5.7	5.69	5.59
Luxembourg (214)	5	5.24	5.36

(data source: IFR, 2019); (source: Statista, and other OECD as indicated in the table, Singapore: (Ministry of Manpower, 2022)[3], South-Korea: (The World Bank, 2022), Japan: (Statistics Bureau of Japan, n.d.)

The underlying causes of unemployment are deeper economic crises and longer recoveries. Benanav (2020) demonstrated that weak demand for human labor is related to the economic slowdown rather than to technological development. To see the connection with technological advancement, Graetz and Michaels (2017) studied recoveries from 71 recessions across industries and countries between 1970-2011. They found that industries more exposed to robotization did not experience slower employment recovery than others. Recent recessions were associated with slower GDP recovery, but not with slower employment recovery across the 17 countries. However, with respect to the US economy, recovery was associated with weak employment growth. This is in line with the 'long recovery' argument that, since the 1980s, a longer period of jobless recovery has been observed after times of recession (examined using US data by Benanav 2020). This claim is supported by the findings of Jaimovich and Siu (2020) who demonstrated that, in the US, despite the recovery in output, employment was slow to rebound, which tells us about the 'bigger pie' effect of an increase in productivity associated with fewer jobs over the examined 35 years. In sum, longer jobless recoveries are rather connected to structural unemployment and profound problems with education and skills as well as wage gaps and growing inequalities than technological investment.

The new division of labor implies division between humans, robots, and algorithms, with new skills needed for the transition to automation. Economic estimations based on platform and employment data published by the World Economic Forum

(2020) identified the skills and occupations that are liable to be needed in the forthcoming years (2020-2025). These suggest the need for vast re-skilling programs and the recruitment of a better educated, younger labor force. From agriculture to transportation – across selected sectors of the economy – the forecast foretells the adoption of encryption and cybersecurity- (28%), cloud computing- (17%), humanoid robot- (11%), non-humanoid robot- (10%), IoT (9%), AI- (8%), and distributed ledger technology (11%) by the surveyed companies (WWEF 2020: p. 27). Machines are expected to take over more tasks related to information and data processing, administering, and even reasoning, decision-making, managing, and advising. The latter will be developed due to the opportunities provided by machine learning. There will be an increase in demand for data scientists, machine learning specialists, and developers, but also mechanics and machine repairers as well as strategic advisors. The emerging job clusters will be centered around engineering, marketing, content production, and sales, among others, absorbing a variety of jobs that are clustered today under accounting, real estate, legal-, purchasing-, support- or community and social services. The new bigger clusters will unify skills applicable to a diversity of domains. Most importantly, the report highlights the skill gaps in local labor markets as barriers to the adoption of new technologies consistently across the 20 countries in which, among the emerging professions, skill shortages are most acute. Job transition challenged by skills mismatch may cause disruptions in the adaptation of new technologies, while comparative advantage will be obtained through by the capability to attract new talent. Among other obstacles are the shortage of investment capital, the regulatory framework, and a insufficient understanding of opportunities of the leadership of organizations (WEF, 2020, p. 29-33).

The wage-productivity gap shows how this gap has substantially grown in the US since the 1970s due to anti-worker deregulatory pushes (such as the deregulation of industry financial policies). The gap (thus the fruit of the surplus of productivity growth) has benefited two areas – highly paid corporate employees and top management, and shareholders' assets, concentrating wage income at the top, according to the Economic Policy Institute. (2021) The consequences are twofold: a growing gap in wages (inequality) and a shift of income from labor to capital owners. A similar phenomenon has been found for 24 OECD countries (OECD 2018), suggesting that technology and trade had a negative impact on real median wages, albeit strong variation across countries is explained by domestic policies. Technological acceleration is not the root of labor insecurity, but a response to problems related to the labor-wage gap, frictional and structural unemployment, and the demand for productivity-driven growth.

CONCLUSION. RE-EMBEDDING THE ECONOMY: AN OUTLOOK

Automation in the World Production System

The society of automation will be associated with a new employment structure and will operate using regulations and work contracts that favor hybrid and remote working arrangements, with redefined human-machine-human interactions and ways of living. Technological determinists envision the greater productivity of home-workers and satisfaction with their work-at-home-arrangements, as well as the 'equalizing' effect of digital technologies that reduce gender, age, and race disparities. The automation of industrial plants has local effects. Therefore, government intervention needs to address the problem of reduced wages and unemployment locally. Polanyi defines this as "a decline of production and earning" in the domestic sphere, representing disequilibrium, typified as the "tension of classes" (p. 218) that indicates a struggle of social forces in domestic politics. The policies of preserving current economic structures and supporting the repatriation of production might support national economies (such as the Reshoring Initiative, ongoing since 2010 in the US). Automation as a means of repatriation of production may have a local stimulatory effect. Although the shift from offshore to domestic production has been an explicit policy initiative in several countries, Noreau (2021) found that enterprises are more prone to nearshore to geographically closer suppliers. The supply shortages during the pandemic pushed larger national economies to reinforce domestic production. Repatriation can cause temporary labor shortages, as producing previously outsourced components may require skills that are locally unavailable. The substituting force of automation can bridge these types of labor shortages. However, it must be considered that the cost of investing in robotics is associated with sound returns on investment only in industries that have a reliable and long-term market for their products.

In an era of hyper-globalization and economic and social connectedness, it is even more true that technological change in any part of the world production system will impact social structures and global inequality. Shifting production from manual-labor-intense industries and countries without creating new opportunities and relieving social costs locally will mean shifting the risk and cost of industrial and social change to supplier economies. The automation shift may disproportionately affect vulnerable classes on a global scale. Any inclusive innovation policy aimed at 'localizing' economies should involve a long-term strategy based on policies that promote skills and education adjustment to fit shifting occupational schemes.

Universalism and Platform Capitalism

Robots, algorithms, and machine learning are designed to complement human labor, to take over routinized tasks, and to place humans into domains where they can creatively thrive with or without jobs – suggests the positivist view of technology. But others warn of the opposite effects. The twenty-first century's transformation of the division of labor is creating a new logic of distribution and hierarchies in terms of new forms of the division of labor and power among humans, robots, and algorithms. Workers at Amazon warehouses are complementing the work of robots at conveyor belts with manual and routinized work, measured using per-hourly metrics. Algorithms are taking over the jobs of managers in surveilling and reporting on workers – in white-collar jobs too. At the same time, Amazon is an example of how a company may be built on low-paid digital ghost work, and was among the first in 2005 to crowdsource workers on-demand for the content development of their platform (through Amazon Mechanical Turk). Crowdsourcing is a way of breaking down tasks: instead of hiring a temporary supplier to manage an entire project, microtasks are complemented by distributed workers (following Mturk). Despite the innovative nature of the business models, large profits and company growth are based on the deployment of global labor-market pooling that uses a low-paid and alienated labor force. The case of Uber (Rosenblat 2018) illustrates how a platform giant used the advantages of algorithms to create a nexus of contracts associated with precarious working conditions and 'faceless bosses' who are the future of organizational hierarchies. Platforms extract value from workers yet do not offer social protection due to the contractual structure they employ, corresponding to the frames of hyper-exploitation (Srnicek 2017, Murillo 2017). Gray and Suri (2019) studied the shadow workforce behind companies like Amazon, Uber, Google, LeadGenius, Instagram, Facebook and others (2019), and found that crowd workers were undertaking underpaid remote work without social security, resulting in an ability to engage in collective bargaining. Ghost work jobs are typically anonymous complementary tasks that cannot be completed by algorithms such as proofreading, editing, or content-driven tasks such as filtering out inappropriate content. Ghost-workers are often people who are shut out of more desirable jobs for structural reasons such as their being minorities, young mothers, early retired professionals, etc. Moreover, some machine learning uses the labour of ghost-workers as a behavioral template for development.

Technological platforms like Apple, Microsoft, Airbnb, Facebook and Google, Ebay, etc. have connected entrepreneurs with consumers and created monopolies by capitalizing on data extraction and the cross-subsidizing of their activities. Post-pandemic reality has seen the rise of omnichannel commerce, remote work, and digital content consumption. These processes give way to a further rise in digital entrepreneurship. Mushrooming platform-based small and medium enterprises are targeting a global consumer base and audience. Services operating in real time, more than ever before, are becoming accessible and affordable globally. Just as a new entrepreneurial class emerged out of the "remnants of old classes" which served the interests of the community as a whole (Polanyi, p. 162), so the new digital entrepreneurs are accounting for their share of the economy. Digital entrepreneurship is expanding with a variety of missions and business models, across borders, and often with a socially engaged focus. This represents a unique opportunity for emerging platforms to create an infrastructure for social digital entrepreneurship, as inclusive technologies are crucial for re-embedding the economy.

Platform capitalism points towards the development of what Polanyi called 'universalism' (Polanyi 1945) – an overarching structure driven to dominate the world economic order. Although this is more explicit in the case of states that Polanyi used as various examples of universalism, the logic of tech platforms of creating a universal market with regulatory frameworks defined by monopolies, based on a global labor market, is somewhat definitive. The gold standard is the great symbol of universalism that would represent a means of balancing the 'foreign economy' through 'undirected trade' (Polanyi, 1945:8), suggesting the dominance of the free market on the international scene. However, in contrast to the universalism of the free market, Polanyi praised regional economic instruments for abolishing unemployment, adjusting currencies, and 'to coordinate domestic employment and living standards' through trade policies within a purposefully managed national system (1945:7). Regionalism, a variety of socioeconomic systems nested in their context, is what Polanyi argued for to control the external economy.

The role of the state and co-operation based on regionalism are crucial for establishing frameworks associated with regulatory forces that can foster indie platforms that unite social initiatives and entrepreneurs; platform cooperatives owned by workers, beneficiaries, or small enterprises that may combat the phenomenon of precarious work conditions. Non-standard employment or atypical work should be associated with social security and labor regulations, just like those that 'standard' workers have. One of the efforts in this domain is the European Commission's decision to develop and implement regulation for digital platforms (Digital Services Act and Digital Markets Act) that would prohibit unfair practices associated with users and workers. The EC adopted Platform-2-Business Regulation, which protects the rights of small businesses with respect to big tech platforms (in effect since 2020) (EUR-LEX, 2019). Digital cooperatives are being designed to unite the digitally self-employed and to create new and fair forms of economic organizing. However, the social and economic goals of the new entrepreneurialism need better orchestration backed up by financial instruments. Community-driven and responsible digital platforms could coordinate and facilitate these processes to grow knowledge, visibility, and engagement for re-embedding the economy within a hyper-globalized socioeconomic fabric.

Isolation, Regionalism and the Great Transformation Today

Whether regionalism or the hyperglobalization of economic organizing will predominate is a question that is coming to the fore. The political power of platforms belonging to tech giants is being disrupted by nation-states seeking to protect the political and economic interests of their markets. Examples range from China's 'Great Firewall' policy to the Trump administration's attempts to block social media like TikTok and WeChat due to concerns about the treatment of the data of US citizens (the Biden administration continued to investigate potential regulations of data protection and third-party auditing), to Iran's ban on social media platforms such as Signal, which emerged as a rival app to the (formerly named Facebook) Meta-purchased WhatsApp, considered to be leaking user data. Just like with other forms of media and the press, censorship has been used to shut down social media (in Iran since 2009). The hybrid wars of the late twentieth and early twenty-first century have grown into particularly ferocious military and information wars, as occurred in the case of Russia and Ukraine. Information war is taking place across the globe, while economic sanctions operate on a global scale. Due to attempts to restrict and bring under surveillance communication channels and sources of information, social media bans are harming various branches of industry and individual small and medium enterprises. As a counter-movement, users are rushing to subscribe to VPN services to evade the regulatory forces that are affecting the market and harming the right to freedom of speech and access to information. Banking systems, cards, and regular monetary exchange mechanisms are being blocked across states, while cryptocurrency systems are being established partly to replace them. Regionalism borders on isolationism and, as Polanyi warned, may end up in chauvinism if economic co-operation does not rely on administration and finance but on 'confidence' (Polanyi, 1945: 5). Can these events be interpreted as 'adjustments of single countries to the great transformation,' and as the old world order collapsing in the advent of a new era (Polanyi, 1944: 236), such as happened with the New Deal, or the withdrawal from the gold standard along with the cutting of social services by the British Government of the time, or the fixing of currencies among countries shaken by the Depression? The 1930s saw the collapse of a global liberal market agenda and scattered state intervention policies, along with isolation. In Novy's interpretation, this 'great transformation' "was the consequence of liberal resistance to policy reforms that offered social protection" - the "anti-globalist turn of the 1930s" (Novy 2020: 61) that culminated in the "complete paralysis" of economic and political systems, and when the "time was ripe for the fascist solution" (Polanyi,

1944: 244). Currently unfolding events that have culminated in the recent war and severe isolationism on a global scale suggest a profound analysis of Polanyi's claims.

The Great Transformation of the hyper-globalized economy in an era of platform capitalism is driven by the profound disruptions and trends of market forces associated with a long period of recovery after the global financial crisis of 2008. Platform capitalism is a form of social and economic organizing, but not the cause of the current great transformation. Neither the automation of manufacturing, nor AI and the machine-learning-based automation of services may be blamed for labor market disruption such as unemployment or global inequalities. The interdependencies of a hyper-globalized economy are created by free market forces, as well as by how "capitalist's built industry into a fortress from which to lord the country" (Polanyi, 1944: 244) – and the emergence of corporations with concentrated economic power that can "lord" the world. The risk associated with tech giants is the outreach of this power that is so clearly visible in the context of hybrid wars, and the crashing economies. Digital platforms are spaces for organizing the local economy (local services, the promotion of immaterial and material goods, virtual marketplaces, etc.). Social media platforms can create narratives, induce or filter hate speech, influence masses, and engage in war with the representatives of states and economic regions. In contrast, the state-driven surveillance efforts of citizens can be supported or blocked by social media. Platforms can curtail or enhance freedom of speech. YouTube, part of Google, has served as a medium for supporting independent thinkers, intellectuals, and journalists in the context of state propaganda in Russia. After the outbreak of the war, monetizing content on YouTube was blocked for Russian users, threatening the existence of entire crews of journalists who were working on providing reliable and independent information, in contrast to the official narrative that denies the fact of the war itself. The volume of these platforms in terms of the opportunities and the number of users is undeniably connecting the dots in the world. Isolation may lead to state measures aimed at surveilling and controlling such platforms.

Following Polanyi, regional economics suggests that peace may be based on the coordination of domestic employment, price mechanisms, and long-term industrial collaboration with other governments. Large common markets may be based on democratic and safe cooperation and the freedom of individuals. Solidarity is based on the democratic consensus of free individuals expressed through the regulation of labor, wages, land, as well as transactions that occur outside of the free market. In conclusion, the future agenda of policy-informing research may focus on the impact of automation on global inequalities in relation to global stakeholders and local labor markets; regionalism in the context of platform capitalism; and the causes and effects of the transformations that are increasing the current trend towards isolationism.

REFERENCES

Acemoglu, D., & Restrepo, P. (2018). The Race between Man and Machine: Implications of Technology for Growth, Factor Shares, and Employment. *The American Economic Review, 108*(6), 1488–1542. doi:10.1257/aer.20160696

Acemoglu, D., & Restrepo, P. (2020). Robots and Jobs: Evidence from US Labor Markets. *Journal of Political Economy, 128*(6), 2188–2244. doi:10.1086/705716

Bärnthaler, R., Novy, A., & Stadelmann, B. (2020). A Polanyi-inspired perspective on social-ecological transformations of cities. *Journal of Urban Affairs*, 1–25. doi:10.1080/07352166.2020.1834404

Benanav, A. (2020). *Automation and the Future of Work*. Verso.

Castells, M. (2009). *The Rise of the Network Society* (2nd ed.). Wiley-Blackwell. https://www.wiley.com/en-us/The+Rise+of+the+Network+Society%2C+2nd+Edition%2C+with+a+New+Preface-p-9781405196864

Chandler, A. D. (1977). *The Visible Hand: The Managerial Revolution in American Business*. The Belknap Press of Harvard University Press.

Chandler, A. D. (1984). The Emergence of Managerial Capitalism. *The Business History Review, 58*(4), 473–503. doi:10.2307/3114162

Ford, M. (2015). *Rise of the Robots Technology and the Threat of a Jobless Future*. Basic Books. https://www.uc.pt/feuc/citcoimbra/Martin_Ford-Rise_of_the_Robots

Fuchs, C. (2008). *Internet and Society: Social Theory in the Information Age*. Routledge. http://fuchs.uti.at/wp-content/uploads/Internet+Society.pdf

Gartenberg, C. (2022, February 11). *Big Tech's 2021 earnings were off the chart*. The Verge. Retrieved from https://www.theverge.com/2022/2/11/22925859/big-tech-companies-2021- earnings-record-revenue-apple-amazon-alphabet-meta

Georgieff, A., & Milanez, A. (2021). *What happened to jobs at high risk of automation?* doi:10.1787/1815199X

Gilbreth, F. B., & Kent, R. T. (1911). *Motion Study: A Method For Increasing The Efficiency Of The Workman*. Kessinger Publishing, LLC.

Graetz, G., & Michaels, G. (2017). Is Modern Technology Responsible for Jobless Recoveries? *The American Economic Review, 107*(5), 168–173. doi:10.1257/aer.p20171100

Gray, M. L., & Suri, S. (2019). *Ghost Work: How to Stop Silicon Valley from Building a New Global Underclass*. Houghton Mifflin Harcourt. https://books.google.hu/books?id=u10-uQEACAAJ

Heer, C. (2021, January 27). *Robot race: The world's top 10 automated countries*. IFR International Federation of Robotics. Retrieved from https://ifr.org/ifr-press-releases/news/robot-race-the-worlds-top-10-automated-countries

Hobsbawm, E. J. (1952). The Machine Breakers. *Past & Present*, *1*(1), 57–70. doi:10.1093/past/1.1.57

Jackall, R. (1988). Moral Mazes: The World of Corporate Managers. *International Journal of Politics, Culture, and Society*, *1*(4), 598–614. https://www.jstor.org/stable/20006876

Jaimovich, N., & Siu, H. (2020). Job Polarization and Jobless Recoveries. *The Review of Economics and Statistics*, *102*(1), 129–147. doi:10.1162/rest_a_00875

Jolly, J. (2021, February 6). Is Big Tech now just too big to stomach? *The Guardian*. Retrieved from https://www.theguardian.com/business/2021/feb/06/is-big-tech-now-just-too-big-to-stomach

Keynes, J. M. (n.d.). *Economic Possibilities for our Grandchildren*. Harcourt Brace.

Kuttner, R. (2020). Karl Polanyi and the Legacy of Red Vienna. In B. Aulenbacher, A. Novy, A. Thurner, M. Marterbauer, & K. Polanyi (Eds.), *Karl Polanyi. The Life and Works of an Epochal Thinker* (Vol. 1, pp. 98–101). Falter Verlag.

Labour Force Survey. (n.d.). *Statistics Bureau of Japan*. Retrieved from https://www.stat.go.jp/english/data/roudou/index.htm

Leijonhufvud, A. (2007). The Individual, the Market and the Division of Labor in Society. *Capitalism and Society*, *2*.

Mills, C. W. (1951). White collar; the American middle classes. Oxford University Press.

Murillo, D., Buckland, H., & Val, E. (2017). When the sharing economy becomes neoliberalism on steroids: Unravelling the controversies. *Technological Forecasting and Social Change*, *125*, 66–76. doi:10.1016/j.techfore.2017.05.024

Novy, A. (2022). The political trilemma of contemporary social-ecological transformation – lessons from Karl Polanyi's The Great Transformation. *Globalizations*, *19*(1), 59–80. doi:10.1080/14747731.2020.1850073

OECD. (2018). OECD. *Economic Outlook, 2018*(1). Advance online publication. doi:10.1787/eco_outlook-v2018-1-en

Regulation (EU) 2019/1150 of the European Parliament and of the Council of 20 June 2019 on promoting fairness and transparency for business users of online intermediation services (Text with EEA relevance). EUR-Lex. (2019). Retrieved from https://eur-lex.europa.eu/legal-content/EN/TXT/?uri=CELEX%3A32019R1150

Rodrik, D. (2011). *The Globalization Paradox: Democracy and the Future of the World Economy*. W.W. Norton. http://books.wwnorton.com/books/The-Globalization-Paradox/

Rosenblat, A. (2018). *Uberland: How Algorithms Are Rewriting the Rules of Work*. University of California Press. doi:10.1525/9780520970632

Schumpeter, J. A. (1942). *Capitalism, socialism, and democracy*. Academic Press.

Srnicek, N. (2017). Platform capitalism. *Polity*.

Steffen, W., Sanderson, R. A., Tyson, P. D., Jäger, J., Matson, P. A., Moore, B. III, & Wasson, R. J. (2006). *Global change and the earth system: a planet under pressure*. Springer Science & Business Media.

Summary table: Unemployment. (2022, June 17). *Ministry of Manpower*. Retrieved from https://stats.mom.gov.sg/Pages/Unemployment-Summary-Table.aspx

Susskind, D. (2020). *A world without work: Technology, automation, and how we should respond*. Metropolitan Books.

Taylor, F. W. (1911). *The principles of scientific management*. Harper and Brothers.

The Productivity–Pay Gap. Economic Policy Institute. (2021, August). Retrieved July 8, 2022, from https://www.epi.org/productivity-pay-gap/

Unemployment, total (% of total labor force) (national estimate) - Korea, rep. (2022, June). *The World Bank*. Retrieved from https://data.worldbank.org/indicator/SL.UEM.TOTL.NE.ZS?locations=KR

Webster, F. (2014). *Theories of the Information Society* (4th ed.). Routledge.

Whyte, W. H. (1956). *The organization man*. Doubleday.

ADDITIONAL READING

Adler, P., & Heckscher, C. (2018). Collaboration as an Organization Design for Shared Purpose. In Research in the Sociology of Organizations. doi:10.1108/S0733-558X20180000057004

Bensman, J. A., & Vidich, A. J. (1971). *The New American Society: The Revolution of the Middle Class*. Quadrangle. https://www.amazon.com/New-American-Society-Revolution-Middle/dp/B0016CFBT6

Braverman, H. (1998). *Labor and Monopoly Capital: The Degradation of Work in the Twentieth Century*. https://www.amazon.com/Labor-Monopoly-Capital-Degradation-Twentieth/dp/0853459401

Radziwill, N. M. (2018). The Fourth Industrial Revolution. *The Quality Management Journal*, *25*(2), 108–109. doi:10.1080/10686967.2018.1436355

Chapter 2
Social Theories and Whole Personhood During the COVID-19 Pandemic:
A Polanyian Perspective

Ildikó Dén-Nagy
Trigon Research Ltd., Hungary

ABSTRACT

Owing to the introduction of social distancing measures during the COVID-19 pandemic, the separate entities of work and family condensed entirely into one physical space for many people. Diverse challenges started to arise within the household and people had to develop coping strategies without any previous experience of such an extreme situation. This chapter explores these problems from a theoretical point of view. First, it discusses the economic value of housework, which increased and became more complex and unequally distributed during the pandemic. It then provides insights into the conception of disembeddedness and work-life balance. Finally, the chapter comments on the moral and cultural aspects of the COVID-19-related public measures, which were launched to mitigate the social impact of the pandemic. The chapter pays particular attention to Karl Polanyi's economic sociology and to the research perspectives offered by his theories in this context.

INTRODUCTION

In early 2020, the COVID-19 pandemic emerged, affecting countries across the globe and resulting in more than 500 million cases and 6.2 million deaths as of

DOI: 10.4018/978-1-6684-2364-6.ch002

May 2022 (World Health Organization [WHO], 2022). The pandemic has affected all European Union (EU) Member States and has been present on all continents. Although COVID-19 is a mild to moderate disease in most infected people, it is highly contagious and severe precautionary measures are thus required to contain any outbreaks. Protecting public health and safeguarding the health and wellbeing of its citizens has been one of the EU's top priorities throughout the pandemic. By the end of 2020, governments worldwide had launched vaccination programs, which played a crucial role in saving lives, protecting health systems, and promoting economic recovery.

However, during the first few months of the outbreak, and before the program of mass vaccination has been rolled out, governments introduced unprecedented measures to curb the rising numbers of cases. For instance, with virtually no warning, schools (from primary through to universities) worldwide started an "off-class digital working order," later referred to as 'homeschooling', which followed the concept of the "home office." In many countries, this distance learning model was indeed akin to going to school at home, with institutions providing minimal remote support. Closing the doors of schools was only the beginning: a series of lockdown events followed suit, with the announcement of a general movement control order, unprecedented isolation, contact reduction, and a severe economic shutdown. The measures imposed threatened human wellbeing (Venkatapuram, 2020) and forced a complete change in lifestyle for many (Khan, 2020; Koós et al., 2020). Work and private life condensed entirely into one physical space for many people, not only blurring the boundaries between these two areas of a person's life but also redefining the concept of work–life balance (hereafter WLB). Depending on the parameters of job and family status, diverse challenges began to arise, and people had to develop coping strategies without any previous experience of global pandemics.

Given the strength of the pandemic, the abrupt switch to enforced isolation came as a shock to some people; however, given the development of information and communication technologies (ICT), the practice of "working from home" was not entirely new. The strict barriers and mental borderlines between work and home had started already to diminish over the past few decades (Dén-Nagy, 2014). Thus, the COVID-19 lockdown arrived under circumstances in which technology made extending communication in terms of time and space possible and provided opportunities for distance working and learning. The commonplace use of ICT devices and platforms (mobile phones, computers, and the Internet) made the shift from working and teaching in a physical sphere to working in a virtual space possible, and it was accepted socially and economically in many countries.

Nevertheless, COVID-19 has had an impact on households and the family as an institution. The usual work–life distinction was overturned, and small, detached nuclear families underwent hardships as the focus was placed on protecting the most vulnerable members of society. In other words, the pandemic highlighted the weaknesses of this type of family structure (i.e., a married/cohabiting couple and their children) compared with big, interconnected, extended families. Characteristics such as resilience or flexibility become critical when considering the unexpected burdens placed on a family. Resilience is the ability of a family to withstand and rebound from crisis and adversity (Walsh, 1996). When a child becomes ill suddenly, or when a parent unexpectedly loses their job, the extended family provides protection, and a larger network steps in to help. In contrast, a disconnected nuclear family involves a set of intense relationships between few people, with no buffer if something goes wrong.

In terms of care work, a reliance on women increases their productive, reproductive, and community responsibilities (Adeniyi-Ogunyankin, 2012). This situation is exacerbated by the fact that recent data show that women still spend significantly more time on housework and childcare than men (Goodin et al., 2008). The pandemic put further pressure on already stressed, tired mothers who were struggling to balance work and child-rearing. According to a report (Organisation of Economic Co-operation and Development [OECD], 2021), the COVID-19 pandemic has had disproportionately negative effects on women in general, and mothers in particular. This is why the OECD proposes the word "momcession" rather than "shecession" to describe the recession that is shadowing the COVID-19 pandemic. This also indicates that one must focus not on the individual, but on the family or household as the arena of labor reproduction with regard to the effects of the pandemic.

While working from home became a possibility in many sectors during the pandemic, this brought about new issues for mothers, such as handling distractions (e.g., the presence of small children demanding continuous attention), getting used to a new workplace set-up (with a lack of physical separation from other family members during work hours), and consequently managing the even more blurred boundaries between work and private life (Rudnicka et al., 2020). With schools and childcare facilities closed down, coupled with the sick and elderly needing more support owing to the pandemic, the total amount of care work in households with children grew drastically. Eurofound (2020) reported that people with children were the group most challenged by the new living and working arrangements. The pandemic had the unique characteristic that lockdowns eliminated the ability for a nuclear family to seek help from outside the household (i.e., in the form of grandparents or paid help). This change affected wealthy families as well, who generally can afford to employ people to fulfill the services that an extended family used to provide.

This chapter explores the social impacts of COVID-19 from a theoretical perspective. First, the chapter discusses the most relevant approaches relating to the economic value of housework, which increased and became more complex and unequally distributed during the pandemic. It then provides insights into the conception of disembeddedness and the importance of weak ties during the COVID-19 lockdown. The third section of this chapter is dedicated to the issue of ensuring WLB in terms of whole-personhood. Finally, the chapter comments on the moral and cultural aspects of the COVID-19-related public measures that were designed to mitigate the social impacts of the pandemic.

Each section pays particular attention to Karl Polanyi's economic sociology and the research perspectives offered by his theories. From a level of abstraction, however, the discussion will also move to the domain of middle-range theories to provide implications for empirical researchers.

THE VALUE OF HOUSEHOLD LABOR

The question of valuing unpaid, invisible household labor has rarely been more topical than it is today. International studies (Matulevicius et al., 2021; Alon et al., 2020; Collins et al., 2021) show that gender inequality in paid work, in the division of childcare, and in household work and quality of life were prevalent during the lockdown (Yerkes et al., 2020; Thelwall & Thelwall, 2020). Given that women traditionally do a disproportionally larger share of care work, as well as other household duties (Goodin et al., 2008), they are also likely to be more affected by the increase in care duties during the pandemic. A Hungarian study showed that although men have increased their contributions to housework to roughly the same rate as women, in absolute terms, women's contributions grew significantly more than men's, and the gap between men and women has increased in terms of work hours (Fodor et al., 2021). It is, however, important to consider how one can measure work surplus sourcing from the absence of state-provided care during this period and how one can interpret and value this non-economic type of production without a clear market price.

The standard economic theory makes almost no mention of the family, while the "home production" of women traditionally belonged to the non-economic sphere for many decades. Neoclassical economists focus on the marginal utility theory and on how market mechanisms allocate goods instead of the process of production itself. Scholars such as Walras (Vaggi and Groenewegen, 2003), Jevons (1871), and Wicksteed (1967) generally ignored the role of household work and divided society into "private" and "public" spheres. Marxist economists emphasized direct production and also had a dualistic view of the domains of market and non-market activities, productive and unproductive labor, the public sphere of waged work, and the hidden private sphere of the household (Jefferson and King, 2001). The economics of housework was re-evaluated in the 1970s and 1980s, when Marxist-feminists such as Benston (1989) concluded that women have a definite role in the means of production and that this is different from that of men.

Polanyi (1944) recognized that labor is a special commodity; it cannot be placed, replaced, or used on-demand without affecting the person who carries it. A labor force is a physical, moral, and psychological "human" entity that can be destroyed without the canopy of society and the cultural environment. "Fictitious commodities," such as labor, could never behave like real ones, as they have not been produced for sale. Market self-regulation is fallible.

As O'Hara (1995) argues, "Household labor has the potential to promote human communication, nutrition, emotional development, preparation for work, population growth, consumption, a latent reserve army of labor, total labor time, and work transfer in supermarkets" (p. 90). However, because it is unpaid labor, expressing its value in monetary terms is problematic. The OECD argues that domestic work is a productive contribution and that nations should include it in the National Accounts statistics, despite the fact that it does not contribute to gross domestic product (Chadeau, 1992).

The Labor Theory of Value suggests that the value of a commodity can be measured by the labor hours necessary to produce it (Smith, 1937; Ricardo, 1821). Within Marxian economics, "direct labour time ... is the determinant factor in the production of wealth" (Marx, 1973, p. 704). Smith, Ricardo, and Marx, however, found issue with quantifying this value. Instead of past labor spent on a commodity, Smith applied a utility value: everything is worth the labor it "commanded" or "saved" at present. (Smith, 1937). Although price is an indicator of value in free markets, in the case of unpaid household labor, it is difficult to calculate monetary value owing to the absence of correct market prices. Shadow pricing is an alternative technique that can be used to express value if monetary terms must be applied.

Glazer-Malbin (1976) was among the first to consider the monetary value of housework for a family, and as an estimated contribution to gross national production. She introduced a new concept, known as "work transfer," arguing that more household products and services became commodified as a result of increasing numbers of women participating in the paid labor market. Glazer (1984, 1990) analyzed healthcare services and compared the turnover of formal home health services and home care agencies with the monetary value of unpaid services by the homebound person's family and friends.

Using the "measuring rod of money," however, is not the only possibility. Goodin et al. (2008) suggest that the "measuring rod of time" could function as an alternative metric. Poverty, for instance, can be expressed in time and the authors argue that "looking at poverty in a joint time-and-money framework reveals important differences in how different socio-economic regimes impact on people's welfare" (p. 9).

Using time as a metric can be especially fruitful in relation to the social consequences of the pandemic. The lockdowns caused a de-commodification of the already "outsourced" household labor. The volume and the content of this type of work changed temporarily. Time expresses the scarcity of labor precisely because it has an absolute limit. This makes efforts comparable, and time division research can help us understand how whole-personhood can be translated into action, such as daily, weekly, or monthly routines. Time spent on different activities, such as breadwinning, child-raising, household labor, free time, or discretionary time, are important elements of whole-personhood. Individuals who have only time enough to do strictly necessary activities, such as earning sufficient income, shopping, cooking, or fulfilling biological needs (such as eating or sleeping), play no part in their own life, over which they have autonomous control. During the pandemic, women whose household burdens further increased lost their discretionary time (i.e., the amount of time one has as a leftover once necessary activities have been carried out, see Goodin et al., 2008) as well as their spare time (i.e., pure free time). This created an imbalance, in which women did not have sufficient time for all those activities that are required for basic survival (such as paid work or sleeping). Losing a job as a result of increased family commitments or neglecting a children's educational commitments (especially in the case of small children) because of work-related obligations could result not only in a high level of frustration and other unfavorable emotional and mental conditions, but also in a significant decrease in family welfare.

Any consideration of the value of household labor begs the following questions: how can people create a balance between private life and work? And how they can maintain this balance during a long-lasting global crisis? Providing household labor is not only an issue in terms of value creation and the re-production of labor, but also in terms of the domestic division of labor and creating a WLB (Paksi et al., 2008; Takács, 2008). However, prior to discussing the most relevant middle-range theories that relate to the reconciliation of private life and paid work, ground theories are further considered and insights into the economic sociological interpretations of links between market and non-market activities, as well as the hierarchical relationship between market values and social values, are provided.

EMBEDDEDNESS DURING THE PANDEMIC

Economic sociology is based on two fundamental sociological theorems. First, action is always socially determined, but it is impossible to explain it by individual motives alone. This is linked to the issues of social networks being the mediators of economic activities and the problem of embeddedness. Second, social institutions are not created automatically but are instead socially shaped. Both arguments are incompatible with neoclassical economics.

In order to understand notions of embeddedness and disembeddedness, one has to take a long view. The emergence of modern capitalism between the sixteenth and eighteenth centuries was a historical turning point for society insofar as the power relations between the economy and social relations changed irrevocably. Before this point, economies were already embedded in social relations (in the non-economic domain), but with the rise of market societies, market values and processes dominated over social values and processes. This is Polanyi's (1944) core argument: it acknowledges that the idea of a completely self-adjusting market remains a "utopia," because it cannot exist without destroying the human and natural substance of society. The word "dystopia" might also have been applied, given that Polanyi was sharply critical of social establishment based on market dominance (i.e., turning land and labor into fictitious commodities).

Polanyi's formal meaning of "economic" is about rational optimization, which aims to select the most preferred combination of scarce means. However, the substantive meaning of economic action describes how people ensure material satisfaction when interacting with the social and natural environment. Polanyi's substantive view discards all essential postulates of economics, including the scarcity postulate, profit-maximizing, or stable preferences. Embeddedness is not a separate theory in Polanyi's work, but is, rather, essential to his substantivist approach.

To summarize, the theory of embeddedness assumes that a wide range of cultural, political, or religious factors influence economic motives. In non-market societies there are no pure economic institutions, so one cannot apply formal economic models. In contrast, market societies include rational economic activities, but as market dominance increases, economic action becomes "disembedded" from society and is able to follow its own distinctive logic, which is the subject of economic modeling. Despite its relationship to the process of disembeddedness, the social environment cannot be fully erased; the market behavior becomes dominant but not exclusive (Lengyel, 2016). From this perspective, Polanyi's concept of "embeddedness" rests on the constraint of economic activities by non-economic institutions, such as kinship and religious or political institutions.

Polanyi's notion of the "disembedded economy" goes some way to explaining the relationship between women's work and economic performance. Under the conditions of a capitalist economy, work is organized according to the logic of the "formal economy" that members of society usually consider "real" work. This work is institutionalized in market exchanges and appears in the labor markets. The home is a place for productive actions as well, despite its exclusion from the formal economy. A feminist debate from the 1970s and 1980s regarding the interpretation of domestic labor from the aspect of producing value and/or surplus labor and/or surplus value argues that value and surplus value are both generated in the home because the family is like a capitalist enterprise (Folbre, 1982).

Both the feminist approach and the theory of social embeddedness propounded by Karl Polanyi recognize the importance of reproduction, and that some institutions promote it while others do not. Polanyi (1944) hypothesized that the "free market" approach ignores the social origins of economic processes. Polanyi asserted that disembeddedness as a process results in the dominance of profit-driven businesses as economic organizations, and that profit-maximizing behavior thus becomes the dominant human behavior. O'Hara (1995) argues that the "disembedded economy" can result in a destruction of family relations in favor of rational economic behavior, which may undermine long-term economic performance. Household stability is fundamental to social stability, and households, or more precisely families, can guarantee the long-term reproduction of labor power and thus the exploitation of labor by capital. The household also provides stability, confidence, and the maintenance of social relations that are necessary for capital accumulation.

Polanyi's approach of emphasizing the political and cultural aspects of embeddedness enables us to compare economic systems, describe the diverging motives of actors in mixed economies (Lengyel, 2016), and analyze abrupt changes in the institutional set-up of production as a result of the COVID-19 pandemic. However, research into this topic can usefully go beyond Polanyi's interpretation, to other theoretical literature on embeddedness, as his work has fueled new generations of economic sociologists.

Polanyi's theory was first adapted by Granovetter (1985) to the system of relationships between economic agents. In Granovetter's approach, economic activity is a complex network of business and social relationships. Granovetter's critical development of the substantive concept consists of three different levels of embeddedness, which deal not only with the institutions, but also with the economic actions and their outcomes. In addition, he interprets the relational and structural aspects of embeddedness separately. The former refers to the influence of the personal relations of the actors, while the latter refers to the structural characteristics of the whole network. Granovetter argues that the degree of embeddedness is lower in pre-capitalist societies and higher in market economies than the substantive concept suggests.

New economic sociology defines not only the relational (structural), but also the cognitive, cultural, and political aspects of the social embeddedness of economic actions (Zukin & DiMaggio, 1990). Cognitive embeddedness refers to the rules of mental processes that systematically influence rational economic calculations. These constraints have been explored in the fields of cognitive psychology, behavioral economics, and descriptive decision theory, and have shown that the assumptions made about actors in economic models (e.g., perfect rationality, complete and free information, unlimited problem-solving and computational ability, single-mindedness) are not valid in real life. In special situations, such as a pandemic, the uncertainty surrounding, and the complexity of, decision situations becomes even more apparent; thus, cognitive embeddedness becomes a highly relevant concept as a means by which to interpret an individual's coping strategies.

The cultural embeddedness of economic actions refers to the influence of social values (norms) that shape economic goals and strategies. Culture constrains economic rationality: it can prohibit the sale of certain things or propose particular economic transactions. Culture has a double effect on the economy: it shapes the conditions for self-interested economic action, and it limits free market forces (Szántó, 1994).

To summarize, an important element of embeddedness dictates that the individual actor is strongly influenced by their social relationships, while the social relationships of economic agents provide them with "social capital" (Coleman, 1990). For instance, economic transactions between parties with specific social ties can help reduce uncertainty as these relationships protect against high-risk transactions. The social capital of economic agents can be as important as physical, financial, and human capital.

Removing the individual from their personal network of relationships, or transferring this network to the digital space, has an obvious impact on the social capital that can be mobilized during times of uncertainty and risk. If the structural embeddedness is damaged, the weak ties (to adopt Granovetter's term) can ensure the mobilization of social resources. During the pandemic, families and other types of strong relationships—such as friends, teammates, and classmates—were isolated from each other, forcing these strong ties into the digital sphere and having a potentially negative impact on personal interactions, performance, and wellbeing. Colleagues, children's friends' parents, or acquaintances—in other words, the weak ties—became more important than ever. Their power lay not only in providing informal bridges between social groups but also in spreading information and providing cohesion within a physically isolated society.

From the domain of highly abstract ground theories, where formal concepts take priority over understanding social reality (Mills, 1959), more concrete sociological theorizing is explored, aiming to integrate theory and empirical research (Merton, 1968). The following section discusses the WLB middle-range theories caused by the pandemic.

WHOLE PERSONHOOD AND WORK–LIFE BALANCE

There is a wide variety of middle-range theories relating to WLB, all of which use different terminology to describe the contradictory "spheres" of life and the transformations between these domains. Sociologists have focused on the relationship between these dualistic domains, that is, work (economic) and non-work (non-economic or social), since the 1950s. Using the terms "private life," "non-work," or "family" in contrast to "work" became prevalent in sociology in the 1990s. These terms express different expectations, family-related needs, and career patterns. Referring to private life instead of family enables us to cover all types of people, such as those who are childless or child-free or those who have other familial commitments (Geszler, 2012). As regards the transactions between the two spheres (work and private life), Rantanen (2008) argues that the connection can be described by means of four parameters: (1) integration (or scope of segmentation); (2) direction (which domain affects the other); (3) context (the perspective of investigation); and (4) quality (positive or negative effects, resource withdrawals, scarcity, enrichment, or facilitation). These four parameters can be used as dimensions to categorize the theoretical approaches, or hypothesis, in the literature (e.g., Staines, 1980). Zedeck and Mosier (1990) distinguished compensation theory, instrumental theory, segmentation theory, conflict theory, and spillover theory as the most basic concepts that can guide researchers in conceptualizing the issues surrounding WLB. Compensation theory assumes that one domain can compensate for the shortcomings of the other; for instance, negative emotions at home can be compensated for with work satisfaction (Staines, 1980). Instrumental theory, on the other hand, focuses on the double utilization of assets; in other words, working to produce money makes it possible to maintain a successful private life. Segmentation theory, however, suggests that work and non-work domains are utterly distinct from each other and that the two spheres do not influence each other. Conflict theory goes even further, stating that the two life domains are separate and that commitments in one sphere can necessitate sacrifices in the other, leading to constant, irreconcilable conflicts (Evans & Bartolomé, 1984). This theory can provide a useful framework when focusing on the different roles a person wants or has to fulfill within a restricted timeframe. During the pandemic lockdowns, both aspects of everyday life could be a source of tension and had the potential to restrict an individual's ability to experience whole-personhood.

As a relatively new concept, border theory focuses on the power of the individual to shape the two connected life domains. It states that individuals undertake conscious demarcation-line management and negotiate with border-keepers (especially with regard to influential and defining members of a given domain) to establish balance in their life (Clark, 2000). However, exercising this ability can be problematic during times of emergency, when the individual is freed from everyday routines and has to face new problems or a new context in their life.

Another (prevalent) theoretical approach is the spillover theory, which evokes the permeability of the two life domains, and assumes that an individual's behaviors, emotions, attitudes, and capabilities can be easily transferred from one domain to the other (Staines, 1980). An individual can experience negative and positive work-to-life and life-to-work spillovers, as they can be a worker, a partner, a relative, and a parent simultaneously (Martinengo, 2007). Once more, these effects can occur in parallel to each other. Recognizing the nature of the relationship between the two life domains could set an interesting research agenda for investigating the WLB challenges encountered during the pandemic lockdowns. However, the classic work–nonwork arrangements such as part-time work, occasional working from home, remote working, flexible work hours, child-care arrangements, and parental leave are likely to be extended in the future, along with other, pandemic-specific dimensions that resulted in unprecedented life set-ups (e.g., working from home with small children, working from home while teaching children from home, single parent versions of these situations.) In addition, job characteristics such as job stressors, organizational restructuring, or job insecurity, and family characteristics such as spousal support and parenting stressors (Geurts & Demerouti, 2003) can also be relevant variables in any research agenda. An empirical researcher can combine these with pandemic-specific variables (e.g., the ways in which schools organized distance learning).

One of the most recent, and perhaps most pandemic-relevant, theories offers a multidimensional agency-centered approach for examining WLB (Hobson et al., 2011). Agencies and capabilities theory states that an individual can choose only from the available options. Hobson et al. (2011) collected a set of capability factors, such as care benefits, job quality, organizational culture, human capital, income, and network, which affect an individual's access to resources and their freedom to choose. They called the possibilities for alternative choices 'agency freedom'.

Other theories can be relevant as well, for instance the behavioral theory of reasoned action (Ajzen & Fishbein, 1974), which can be utilized as a framework for understanding WLB-related decisions or perceptions in the context of attitudes and beliefs, social norms, self-efficacy, intention, and behavior sequence. Social norms, for instance, may make an individual reluctant to interrupt work hours to attend to family responsibilities, especially during times of uncertainty.

This section does not intend to provide an exhaustive list and an in-depth explanation of every middle-range theory that can be connected to the pandemic, but instead focuses on the applicability of each to the context of the COVID-19 pandemic and the new challenges that arose during this time. Middle-range theories allow researchers to phrase very concrete research questions, hypotheses, and statements about conceptualization.

The following section focuses on the household—the people who share a living space and combine economic resources. However, instead of the role of the individual and the individual's challenges and coping strategies, the focus is on the role of the welfare state and how to interpret its actions and outcomes from an economic sociological perspective.

PROTECTING FAMILIES AND VULNERABLE GROUPS

In 2020, a century after the Great Depression (as analyzed by Polanyi), the world has once again witnessed a global crisis that calls for an economic and policy response. During the COVID-19 pandemic, saving lives was the most important factor, and until herd immunity could be reached (mainly through vaccination or the temporary immunity afforded by previous infection), the main objective for countries globally was to keep levels of transmission low and manageable. The World Health Organization developed guidelines for preventive measures that needed to be implemented at each stage of the pandemic (e.g., closing schools, restaurants, bars, cinemas, workplaces; wearing masks in public places; and detecting, testing, isolating, and treating cases and tracking and tracing contacts). Countries changed their regulations in response to the latest science, statistics, and lessons learned from other countries, constantly balancing epidemiological advantages and socioeconomic disadvantages. However, during this time, welfare was not the focus of governments; they were seeking to save as many lives as possible while minimizing economic losses.

In practice, this meant that the everyday lives of many people around the globe changed from one day to the next, and they had to adapt to a given situation without any recourse to financial, physical, or mental support. In Hungary, for instance, on March 11, 2020—as in many other European countries during those first critical weeks—the government declared a national emergency and, with minimal preparation, schools were brought online from March 16. This was followed on March 27 by the announcement of a general movement control order. People were left alone to deal with the isolation, reduction in human contact, and serious economic shutdown. They had no choice but to continue their daily lives, working as before and ensuring their children's education without any governmental support. Could or should governments have intervened more to help their citizens? What measures might have been appropriate in such a long-lasting but seemingly temporary state of emergency? What is the acceptable level of post-COVID compensation that might help to prevent long-term negative consequences? This section seeks to answer these difficult questions through the application of theoretical frameworks.

Duzgun (2020) argues that the Polanyian logic relates to the start of the COVID-19 pandemic. This pandemic was not only an abrupt tragedy in the history of otherwise smoothly operating capitalist systems, but an inherent consequence of the way market societies work. It was a direct result of "the fundamental contradiction between the limitedness of our planet and the endlessness of capital accumulation in a manner that perhaps no other single phenomenon has ever done in the modern history" (p. 58).

Polanyi argued that free-market policies are unworkable in the long-run and must be supplemented by "protective responses," such as familial relationships, health and safety legislation, or a social security network (Stanfield, 1986). Seccombe (1980) similarly hypothesizes that "private capital is structurally indifferent to labor power's production, and tends, without external regulation, to jeopardize and destabilize its long-term reproduction" (p. 247). These stabilizing institutional arrangements become increasingly important during an event as terrible as the pandemic.

Polanyi drew attention to the double movement of fictitious goods that accompanied the emergence of the market. In *The Great Transformation*, he pointed out that there is a constant regulative desire from the state to counteract the liberalization of markets, particularly with regard to fictitious goods such as labor, wherein there is an intent to execute protectionism (Polanyi, 1944). This protectionism is also present in societies today; when decisions are made to strengthen the position of certain groups, they are usually based on moral-cultural, rather than market, grounds. Polanyi views the periodically changing trends of increased marketization and laissez-fair intentions as "disembedding" the economy, followed by the countermovement of re-embedding the economy and strengthening social protection by applying labor laws and tariffs—the so-called "double movement" (Polanyi, 1944).

Double movement is a dialectical description of an irreversible historical development. It follows an inner scheme of development (thesis-antithesis-synthesis) (Patomäki, 2014). It is a global process, a strategy to appropriately handle the non-economic elements of life. This theory identifies the power relations of self-defensive counter-reactions correctly and in a forward-looking way. Polanyi concluded that the incentives to create a global self-regulating market are insufficient to trigger double movement at the global level. This requires an additional ideological force (Lengyel, 2016).

To understand how double movement works, one can refer to the aforementioned historical example: the expansion of the market system in the nineteenth century was a process for creating international free trade, competitive and accessible labor markets, and the spread of the gold standard. These processes were intertwined and resulted in an important global condition: from 1815 to 1914, there was a century of peace. However, the agricultural crisis and the Great Depression between 1873 and 1886 shook the economy's self-healing capacity and self-sustainability, thus making protectionism necessary (Polanyi, 1944). This global shock was thus considered sufficient in the past to undermine the perfection of the self-regulating power of markets and wake up protectionism. What kind of policy implications does this theory have in the context of a global pandemic?

According to the social-democratic literature, Polanyi envisioned a political-economic compromise, whereby for-profit businesses accept regulatory constraints (e.g., taxation, restrictive laws) and the existence of welfare institutions (Block & Sommers, 2014). For Polanyi, the attempt to regulate markets is a reasonable response to the laissez-faire market economy, which had negative consequences during the interwar period and became a source of crisis (Duzgun, 2020). During this period, the compromise was between the efficiency and wage increase, between competitiveness and job security. The welfare state led to improvements in living conditions for the laboring masses. Although society took measures to protect itself, the disorganized industrial life endangered society in another way (Polanyi, 1944). This argument was later labeled a political "inconsistency" and a theoretical "tension" in Polanyi's work (Block & Sommers, 2014).

A counter movement is brewing, however, namely increasing protection rather than market deregulation. National governments have already taken a number of fiscal, liquidity, and policy measures to increase the capacity of their health systems and help the most vulnerable individuals and economic sectors. These actions supersede those at the national level. The European Union, for instance, launched the Instrument for Temporary Support to Mitigate Unemployment Risks in an Emergency (SURE), which is available to all Member States. The aim is to mobilize significant financial means to fight the negative economic and social consequences of the pandemic. Financial assistance is available in the form of loans from the EU and is distributed to affected Member States to address sudden increases in public expenditure for the preservation of employment. SURE is a crucial element of the EU's comprehensive pandemic recovery strategy (European Commission, n.d.). This is but one example of many that aim to protect citizens and mitigate the serious socio-economic consequences of the COVID-19 pandemic.

To summarize, both during and after the pandemic there has been an emerging need for regulative forces, while fictitious commodities, such as labor, also remain affected by market forces. The question of decommodification thus became timely during the pandemic, not only from a gender equality perspective or as a result of the ecological impacts of consumption-oriented capitalism, but also from the perspective of protecting families and vulnerable groups during an emergency, and subsequently, a global economic crisis. The immunization of labor from market dependence is now on the agenda because countries must protect individuals and families and provide them with a socially acceptable standard of living that is independent of market participation. The original idea of decommodification propounded by Esping-Andersen is an egalitarian concept that "... serves to capture the degree to which an individual commands the means to satisfy his or her social and family needs independently from cash nexus" (Esping-Andersen & Kolberg, 1991, p. 78). Loosening wage dependency, however, can erode any work incentives.

Polanyi (1944) comes to the same conclusion, devoting two chapters (6 and 7) of *The Great Transformation* to his analysis on the Speenhamland Act. He analyzed a historical case study of the introduction of an unconditional basic income. The Speenhamland system was introduced in the late 18th century in England and damaged the English economy. In Polanyi's interpretation, Speenhamland shattered all the norms on which society was based and made pauperism attractive to those who would otherwise have had to work to avoid poverty. Speenhamland temporarily improved the quality of life of thousands of people, but it was ultimately considered a mistake, shedding new light on how benefits and moral harms can prevail in tandem, and how consequences can change over time. Speenhamland provided lessons on the moral tension between individual wealth and economic status when compared with acceptable and respectable actions. It can serve as a starting point for understanding the applicability and implications of universal basic income, even during a temporary, socially critical time such as the COVID-19 lockdowns. Policymakers would do well to remember that withdrawing the Speenhamland Act came as no less of a shock than its economic consequences.

CONCLUSION

This chapter delved into the relevant grand theories (Mills, 1959) and discussed more concrete middle-range theories (Merton, 1968) of economics to get closer to a sociological understanding of the effects of the COVID-19 pandemic. The consequences were, in part, short-term and manifested themselves in dramatic, sudden, but temporary alterations to everyday life during the period of social distancing. Some of these consequences, however, appear to be more long-term, and raise questions around policy.

One of the most significant effects of the lockdown was the emergence of new WLAs that will likely remain in place after the pandemic, such as the acceptance of remote working and distance learning. Households evolved from being a social unit of individuals sharing a living space to becoming a social unit working and learning together. For many people, the household provided the only physical arena for social interactions, while the rest of an individual's social network moved to the virtual sphere, causing changes in the structure and other characteristics of social ties. These new WLAs resulted in new challenges with regard to whole-personhood, and, as empirical research shows, they confirmed gender-based inequalities in household labor, making the application of a gender perspective all the more relevant.

During this historic event, the usual patterns of domestic labor division were slightly or strongly adjusted, depending on individual circumstances, and the main characteristic of the new set-up was a reduction in outsourcing. As household work moved from the market to the family, the dispute over the value of the household became topical once more. The non-economic nature of temporary home-production, and the changing distinction between the private and the public spheres require more attention. The de-commodification of household labor and the tendency toward removing it from the self-regulating power of markets make its value unmeasurable in monetary terms and make the process of value creation more critical at a societal level. The problem of WLB is discussed in more detail elsewhere and offers alternatives for researchers in relation to newly devised coping strategies (e.g. Staines, 1980; Zedeck & Mosier, 1990; Evans & Bartolomé, 1984; Clark, 2000; Geurts & Demerouti, 2003).

The pandemic ripped the family (and the individual within the family) from its social network. Questions relating to the Polanyian formal economy, such as selecting the preferred combination of scarce means, were dominated by the substantive meaning of economic action—namely how people ensure material satisfaction in their interaction with the social environment. This was also strongly influenced by the pandemic measures and will undoubtedly be influenced by post-pandemic measures.

In addition, social embeddedness became an issue. Strong ties got weaker and were partly transferred to the online sphere, while weak ties became a more important cohesive force within society. Thus, the conclusion is not that there exists an increased disembeddedness of the economy in Polanyian terms (1944), but rather that there is a loosening of the embededdness of the individual in Granovetterian terms (1985).

Here the focus lies more on the structural characteristics of embeddedness (e.g., by going online and being isolated) and on the economic influence of the personal relations of the actors. The pandemic did not cause the destruction of family relations in favor of the rational economic behavior (Polanyi, 1944), but it led to a destruction of home life, and, perhaps more importantly, the destruction of the economy to protect human health. The decrease in embeddedness was a change in the system of relationships between economic agents that raised the questions of cognitive, cultural, structural, and political aspects of social embeddedness of economic actions (Zukin & DiMaggio, 1990) and the formation of social capital (Coleman, 1990).

The long-term consequences of the COVID-19 pandemic have resulted in economic and policy responses to the post-pandemic global crisis. Polanyi's *Great Transformation* may be a warning for our generation: measures taken to safeguard society from market pressures conflict with the self-regulation of markets, and this conflict can easily exacerbate a crisis. Fictitious commodities (labor, land, money) cannot remain marketized if protectionism is to be halted; however, it is unlikely that preventing the handling of human beings as commodities is a realistic scenario in a capitalist and democratic society. This paper does not seek to pursue this argument further by rooting it in historical lessons; rather, it strives to offer possible theoretical points of departure and to raise questions for future research.

REFERENCES

Adeniyi-Ogunyankin, G. (2012). "When will I get my rest?" Neo-liberalism, women, class and ageing in Ibadan, Nigeria. *Agenda: Empowering Women for Gender Equity, 26*(4), 29–36. doi:10.1080/10130950.2012.758426

Ajzen, I., & Fishbein, M. (1974). Factors influencing intentions and the intention behavior relation. *Human Relations, 27*(1), 1–15. doi:10.1177/001872677402700101

Alon, T., Doepke, M., Olmstead-Rumsey, J., & Tertilt, M. (2020). *The Impact of COVID-19 on Gender Equality*. National Bureau of Economic Research. doi:10.3386/w26947

Benston, M. (1989). The political economy of women's liberation. *Monthly Review (New York, N.Y.), 41*(7), 31–44. doi:10.14452/MR-041-07-1989-11_5

Block, F., & Somers, M. (2014). *The Power of Market Fundamentalism: Karl Polanyi's Critique*. Harvard University Press. doi:10.4159/harvard.9780674416345

Chadeau, A. (1992). *What is a Households' Non-market Production Worth*. Organisation for Economic Co-operation and Development.

Clark, S. C. (2000). Work/family border theory: A new theory of work/family balance. *Human Relations, 53*(6), 747–770.

Coleman, J. S. (1990). *Foundations of Social Theory*. Harvard University Press.

Collins, C., Landivar, L. C., Ruppanner, L., & Scarborough, W. J. (2021). COVID-19 and the Gender Gap in Work Hours. *Gender, Work and Organization, 28*(1), 549–560. doi:10.1111/gwao.12506 PMID:32837019

Dén-Nagy, I. (2014). A Double-Edged Sword? A Critical Evaluation of the Mobile Phone in Creating Work–Life Balance. *New Technology, Work and Employment, 29*(2), 193–211. doi:10.1111/ntwe.12031

Duzgun, E. (2020). Ecology, democracy, and COVID-19. In J. M. Ryan (Ed.), *COVID-19: Global Pandemic, Societal Responses, Ideological Solutions* (pp. 54–67). Routledge. doi:10.4324/9781003142089-7

Esping-Andersen, G., & Kolberg, J. E. (1991). Decommodification and work absence in the welfare state. *International Journal of Sociology, 21*(3), 77–111. doi:10.1080/15579336.1991.11770014

Eurofound. (2020). *Living, working and COVID-19*. Retrieved March 7, 2022, from https://www.eurofound.europa.eu/publications/report/2020/living-working-and-covid-19

European Commission. (n.d.). *SURE A szükséghelyzeti munkanélküliségi kockázatokat mérséklő ideiglenes támogatást nyújtó európai eszköz (SURE)*. Retrieved May 26, 2022, from https://ec.europa.eu/info/business-economy-euro/economic-and-fiscal-policy-coordination/financial-assistance-eu/funding-mechanisms-and-facilities/sure_hu

Evans, P., & Bartolomé, F. (1984). The changing pictures of the relationship between career and family. *Journal of Occupational Behaviour*, *5*(1), 9–21. doi:10.1002/job.4030050103

Fodor, É., Gregor, A., Koltai, J., & Kováts, E. (2021). The impact of COVID-19 on the gender division of childcare work in Hungary. *European Societies*, *23*(1), 95–110. doi:10.1080/14616696.2020.1817522

Folbre, N. (1982). Exploitation comes home: A critique of the Marxian theory of family labour. *Cambridge Journal of Economics*, *6*(4), 317–329.

Geszler, N. (2012). *A munka és család konfliktusának forrásai az európai férfiak életében* [Unpublished MA Thesis]. Corvinus University of Budapest, Budapest, Hungary.

Geurts, S. A., & Demerouti, E. (2003). Work/non-work interface: A review of theories and findings. In M. J. Schabraco, A. M. Winnubst, & C. L. Cooper (Eds.), *The handbook of work and health psychology* (pp. 279–312). John Wiley & Sons.

Glazer, N. Y. (1984). Servants to Capital: Unpaid Domestic Labor and Paid Work. *The Review of Radical Political Economics*, *16*(1), 60–87. doi:10.1177/048661348401600106

Glazer, N. Y. (1990). The Home as Workshop: Women as Amateur Nurses and Medical Care Providers. *Gender & Society*, *4*(4), 479–499. doi:10.1177/089124390004004004

Glazer-Malbin, N. (1976). Housework. *Signs (Chicago, Ill.)*, *1*(4), 905–922. doi:10.1086/493308

Goodin, R. E., Rice, J. M., Parpo, A., & Eriksson, L. (2008). *Discretionary Time: A New Measure of Freedom*. Cambridge University Press. doi:10.1017/CBO9780511611452

Granovetter, M. (1985). Economic action and social structure: The problem of embeddedness. *American Journal of Sociology*, *91*(3), 481–510. doi:10.1086/228311

Hobson, B., Fahlén, S., & Takács, J. (2011). Agency and Capabilities to Achieve a Work-Life Balance: A Comparison of Sweden and Hungary. *Social Politics*, *18*(2), 168–198. doi:10.1093p/jxr007 PMID:21966697

Jefferson, T., & King, J. E. (2001). "Never intended to be a theory of everything": Domestic labor in neoclassical and Marxian economics. *Feminist Economics*, *7*(3), 71–101. doi:10.1080/13545700110103504

Jevons, W. S. (1871). *The Match Tax: A Problem in Finance*. E. Stanford.

Khan, D. B. (2020). Economic Impact of Covid-19 and Change in Value System. *LC International Journal of STEM*, *1*(2), 23–31.

Koós, B., Kovács, Zs. S., Páger, B., & Uzzoli, A. (2020). Az új koronavírus-járvány társadalmi-gazdasági hatásai és ezek területi következményei. In M. Czirfusz (Ed.), Területi kihívások és területi politikák Magyarországon, 2010-2020 (pp. 123-131). Közgazdaság- és Regionális Tudományi Kutatóközpont Regionális Kutatások Intézete

Lengyel, G. (2016). Embeddedness, redistribution and double dependence: Polanyi-reception reconsidered. *Intersections. East European Journal of Society and Politics*, *2*(2), 13–37. doi:10.17356/ieejsp.v2i2.184

Martinengo, G. (2007), *Gender differences and similarities in the work-family interface: The importance of considering family life stages* [PhD dissertation, Brigham Young University]. Theses and Dissertations.

Marx, K. (1973). *Karl Marx on society and social change: With selections by Friedrich Engels*. University of Chicago Press. doi:10.7208/chicago/9780226173788.001.0001

Matulevicius, S. A., Kho, K. A., Reisch, J., & Yin, H. (2021). Academic medicine faculty perceptions of work-life balance before and since the COVID-19 pandemic. *JAMA Network Open*, *4*(6), 1–10. doi:10.1001/jamanetworkopen.2021.13539 PMID:34129021

Merton, R. K. (1968). *Social Theory and Social Structure*. Free Press.

Mills, C. W. (1959). *The sociological imagination*. Oxford University Press.

O'Hara, P. A. (1995). Household Labor, the Family, and Macroeconomic Instability in the United States: 1940s—1990s. *Review of Social Economy*, *53*(1), 89–120. doi:10.1080/00346769500000004

OECD. (2021). *Caregiving in Crisis: Gender inequality in paid and unpaid work during COVID-19*. Retrieved March 7, 2022, from https://www.oecd.org/coronavirus/policy-responses/caregiving-in-crisis-gender-inequality-in-paid-and-unpaid-work-during-covid-19-3555d164/

Paksi, V., Sebők, Cs., & Szalma, I. (2008). A párkapcsolatban élők háztartási munkamegosztásának főbb meghatározói. *Társadalmi Regiszter*, *2*, 79–106.

Patomäki, H. (2014). On the dialectics of global governance in the twenty-first century: A Polanyian double movement? *Globalizations*, *11*(5), 733–750. doi:10.1080/14747731.2014.981079

Polanyi, K. (1944). *The Great Transformation*. Beacon.

Rantanen, J. (2008). *Work-Family Interface and Psychological Well-Being: A Personality and Longitudinal Perspective*. University of Jyväskylä.

Ricardo, D. (1821). *On the principles of political economy*. J. Murray.

Rudnicka, L., Gupta, M., Kassir, M., Jafferany, M., Lotti, T., Sadoughifar, R., & Goldust, M. (2020). Priorities for global health community in COVID-19 pandemic. *Dermatologic Therapy*, *33*(4), 1–4. doi:10.1111/dth.13361 PMID:32239578

Seccombe, W. (1980). The Expanded Reproduction Cycle of Labour Power in Twentieth Century Capitalism. In B. Fox (Ed.), *Hidden in the Household: Women's Domestic Labour Under Capitalism* (pp. 217–266). The Women's Press.

Smith, A. (1937). *The wealth of nations: An inquiry into the nature and causes*. Modern Library.

Staines, G. L. (1980). Spillover versus compensation: A review of the literature on the relationship between work and non-work. *Human Relations*, *33*(2), 111–129. doi:10.1177/001872678003300203

Stanfield, J. R. (1986). *The Economic Thought of Karl Polanyi: Lives and Livelihood*. St. Martin's Press. doi:10.1007/978-1-349-18434-7

Szántó, Z. (1994). A gazdaság társadalmi beágyazottsága. *Szociologiai Szemle*, *3*, 141–145.

Takács, J. (2008). Ha a mosogatógép nem lenne, már elváltunk volna…" Férfiak és nők otthoni munkamegosztása, európai összehasonlításban. *Esély*, *6*, 51–73.

Thelwall, M., & Thelwall, S. (2020). *Covid-19 Tweeting in English: Gender Differences*. ArXiv: 2003. 11090v1

Vaggi, G., & Groenewegen, P. (2003). Léon Walras, 1834–1910: The Notion of General Equilibrium. In G. Vaggi & P. Groenewegen (Eds.), *A Concise History of Economic Thought: From Mercantilism to Monetarism* (pp. 217–226). Palgrave Macmillan. doi:10.1057/9780230505803_21

Venkatapuram, S. (2020). Human Capabilities and Pandemics. *Journal of Human Development and Capabilities*, *21*(3), 280–286. doi:10.1080/19452829.2020.1786028

Walsh, F. (1996). The Concept of Family Resilience: Crisis and Challenge. *Family Process*, *35*(3), 261–281. doi:10.1111/j.1545-5300.1996.00261.x PMID:9111709

WHO. (2022). *WHO Coronavirus (COVID-19) Dashboard.* Retrieved May 12, 2022, from https://covid19.who.int

Wicksteed, P. H. (1967). *The Common Sense of Political Economy*. Routledge.

Yerkes, M. A., André, S. C., Besamusca, J. W., Kruyen, P. M., Remery, C. L., van der Zwan, R., Beckers, D. G. J., & Geurts, S. A. (2020). 'Intelligent' lockdown, intelligent effects? Results from a survey on gender (in) equality in paid work, the division of childcare and household work, and quality of life among parents in the Netherlands during the Covid-19 lockdown. *PLoS One*, *15*(11), e0242249. doi:10.1371/journal.pone.0242249 PMID:33253238

Zedeck, S., & Mosier, K. (1990). Work in the family and employing organization. *The American Psychologist*, *45*(2), 240–251. doi:10.1037/0003-066X.45.2.240 PMID:2178504

Zukin, S., & DiMaggio, P. (Eds.). (1990). *Structures of Capital. The Social Organization of the Economy*. Cambridge University Press.

Chapter 3
Organizational Governance, Individual Wellbeing, and Needs Theory

Ermanno C. Tortia
https://orcid.org/0000-0002-2138-1119
University of Trento, Italy

Silvia Sacchetti
University of Trento, Italy

ABSTRACT

A needs theory of governance is introduced and discussed, in which the new institutionalist economics, which consider selfishness and opportunism as the main behavioral principles, are confronted with a new theory in which the organization, as a social system, is embedded in the broader social and cultural context and in a network of social relations. It develops symbiotically with the needs expressed by its internal stakeholders and must seek to increase their welfare through the adaptation of governance rules to both needs and production goals. Institutional solutions informed by the goal of sustainably meeting needs are discovered and developed. Comparison of the two theories leads to theorizing a new layered model, reminiscent in part of Maslow's hierarchy of needs, in which different institutional layers satisfy different types of needs, from the most basic ones of survival and security to the highest ones of belonging, self-esteem, and self-actualization.

DOI: 10.4018/978-1-6684-2364-6.ch003

INTRODUCTION

This article presents a theory linking the governance of production to the well-being of individuals participating in production. Individual well-being is also a measure of governance performance. The basic idea of the paper stems from the observation that a clear and structured theoretical link between governance and individual well-being is still understudied, while governance should be evaluated in terms of its ability to sustain well-being. We take the model of human psychology proposed by Abraham Maslow (1943, 1968, 1998) as an example of how well-being can be related to the structure of the organization, as this structure emerges and evolves to meet different kinds of needs of various stakeholders, thus generating well-being. Specific reference is made to the well-being of employees, but customers can also be considered.

The initial behavioral hypothesis, drawn from Oliver Williamson's (1975, 2000) neo-institutionalist approach, is that individuals behave opportunistically if there is sufficient information asymmetry and if the sanctions are less than the benefit gained through self-seeking behavior. Governance structures are characterized by exclusive decision-making (to save internal costs) and supported by command-and-control mechanisms to impose direction, order, and punish opportunism (Sacchetti, 2015). In our approach, however, needs can influence or even define the basic organizational dimensions of formal governance and organizational routines, because when needs are better met, stakeholder well-being improves. A sense of fulfillment can lead to improved organizational behavior and even customer satisfaction. For example, an organization that is able to provide greater job protection and stability for its workforce will likely be rewarded with better organizational citizenship behaviors, professional growth, and performance (Akerlof, 1982). Therefore, we expect the evolution of governance structures to take into account the satisfaction of stakeholder needs. Consistently, we develop a theory based on multiple individual motivations, which emphasizes multiple and coexisting individual needs (needs for survival, security, belonging, self-esteem, self-actualization) as in Maslow's pyramid. These needs cannot be consistently met through opportunistic behaviors at the individual level and the use of authority at the organizational level, as research in social and organizational psychology has highlighted the importance of intrinsic motivation and the dangers associated with exclusion, direction and extrinsic incentives (cfr. Frey, 1997, in economics; Deci & Ryan, 2000). Building a theory of individual need satisfaction requires modification of the mainstream behavioral assumptions implicit in the principal-agent model and the contributions of the new institutional economics. Consequently, so does the justification of the exclusive governance structures advocated by transaction cost theory (Williamson, 1975; Jensen & Mackling, 1976). The perspective introduced here emphasizes that individual needs and their satisfaction require to be nurtured at the organizational level by structures and practices that integrate productive resources not yet by authority, but by reciprocity, cooperation and inclusive decision-making processes (Tortia & Valentinov, 2018).

In our framework, opportunism, understood as "seeking self-interest with cunning" (Williamson, 1975: 255), represents only one of the possible (and deviant) behavioral traits. From an organizational perspective, it must be understood as behavioral risk and danger, which can emerge and spread under negative organizational conditions, but which can be kept at bay when appropriate rules (involvement, constraints, incentives, and sanctions) are put in place (Ostrom, 1990).

Within a similar line of research, Hodgson (2004) cautions against the exclusivity of the explanatory role of opportunism in Williamson's approach to governance. In addition to control, he cites the promotion of education, corporate culture, and trust among employees as key functions of management. Foss and Weber (2016) argue that the centrality of opportunism in the transaction cost literature makes it difficult to explain why hierarchies are not always used. According to their approach, opportunism should not "occupy the first place" in the new institutionalist theory of the firm. Bounded rationality as a separate source of transaction costs and its interaction with different hierarchical forms is a better explanatory factor for how governance structures are implemented and how they guide the behavior of relevant stakeholder groups. The needs perspective explains opportunism as a deviation from a behavioral pattern of positive reciprocity and inclusion, a potential obstacle to the realization of cooperative behavior and the resilience of individual motivations, rather than as an ontological characteristic of all human beings (Ben-Ner & Jones, 1995). Need satisfaction represents the most fundamental function of governing production relations and defines the main organizational models through which production is realized and distributed.

The explanatory strategy proceeds as follows. First, we examine the new institutional approach to governance, drawing on Williamson's layered institutional analysis (Williamson, 2000). Next, we address the issue of needs, drawing on the seminal work of Maslow (Maslow, 1943, 1968, 1998) and relating it to the theory of social embeddedness and cultural differences in the study of the well-being of members of organizations (Polanyi, 1944; Hofstede, 1980; Granovetter, 1985). The following section presents the components of a needs theory of governance, comparing it with neo-institutional theory. Finally, we present our framework of analysis, which delves into the interaction between institutional levels and individual needs.

BACKGROUND LITERATURE

New Institutionalism

Neo-institutionalism represents one of the most influential schools in understanding opportunistic behavior facing asset specificity, contrasting interests, and asymmetric information (Williamson, 1973; Jensen & Meckling, 1976). This approach has been central to the study of resource allocation through markets and hierarchical forms of governance (Williamson, 1975), with applications including unconventional resources, as in the study of common resources (Ostrom, 1990).

The behavioral assumptions of neo-institutionalism are closely related to those developed by agency theory, namely, that individuals are self-seeking utility-maximizing. This principle was explicitly placed at the heart of the principal-agent problem by Jensen and Meckling (1976). Selfish behavioral assumptions and individual preferences for deception are also reflected in the prevailing approach to "good governance," which considers solutions to the principal-agent problem by implementing rules geared toward facilitating board and regulatory control over managers' actions (Birchall, 2014). Good governance requires the existence of processes embodied in rules and an incentive system that ensures managers' accountability to the firm's principal patrons (for a critique see Davis, Schoorman, & Donaldson, 1997; Gregory-Smith & Main, 2015). "Governance failure," in this sense, occurs in the face of inadequate reactive measures to opportunism and corruption, greed and short-termism (Sacchetti, 2015). The "good governance" approach focuses on the binding role of institutions, but still focuses on opportunism. Individual needs and motivations are mostly considered exogenous to the explanatory framework, whereas we argue that an approach that takes the satisfaction of needs as the most fundamental function of governance downgrades opportunism to the role of a pure risk factor.

In a later work, Williamson (2000) developed a multilevel framework for analyzing the economic institutions that constitute organizational governance. In this work, Williamson identifies four interacting institutional levels: (1) informal institutions defined by cultural norms and beliefs; (2) formal institutions that define ownership; (3) contracts that align governance structures and transactions; and (4) rules related to resource allocation, such as market mechanism and employee incentives. Established values and beliefs, at the first level, are reflected in the legal framework at the second level. This defines the basic institutional structure of economic organization and requires individuals' compliance with the legal constraints that establish control rights and define resource allocation. Variations occur at the third and fourth levels, where organizations can choose, through different mechanisms (e.g., exclusive or inclusive, formal and informal or tacit), how to specify the governance rules, i.e., the self-production of working rules and the evolution of organizational routines, and the type of incentives offered to individuals (Ostrom, 1990). These dimensions of need satisfaction are also close to Herzberg's (1968) conception of hygiene factors as (de)motivators of employees. The most basic rules are also directed at precluding opportunistic behavior and ensuring a high degree of compliance with collectively defined goals, while inclusion and autonomy in the production process are more conducive to satisfying higher-level needs.

Well-Being and Need Satisfaction in the Organization

Maslow's human psychology and his definition of a hierarchy of diverse needs, along with the seminal work of other authors such as McGregor's (1960) X and Y theory, who have long argued that organizations can be places of human development. Montuori and Purser (2014) have recently observed that management has missed the need satisfaction and self-actualization side of organizations and that organizations should not oppose the individual and his or her well-being. The point of contention is the pursuit of organizational solutions that truly seek engagement and nonauthoritarian relationships between managers and workers, for modes of engagement that release creative and mutually beneficial cooperation, rather than the exercise of supervisory power by superiors over subordinates (Sacchetti and Sugden, 2009).

Maslow's contributions have fundamentally influenced management studies, especially with regard to occupational well-being. The project of this article is to make them also applicable to the governance of industrial relations within organizational boundaries, that is, how governance supports the satisfaction of producers' psychological needs. From this perspective, the working rules that make up governance structures, along with the attached organizational routines, emerge and evolve over time to ensure that needs are met (Wahba & Gridwell, 1972; Tietze & Shakeshaft, 1982; Gopinath, 2020).

In addition to Maslow's human psychology approach, the management literature has dealt with various decision-making regimes and models, and the cross-cultural approach developed by Hofstede and co-authors is particularly important. In this literature, the initial studies go back to Elton Mayo (1933). In most cases, work-related well-being is operationalized as job satisfaction (Clegg & Wall, 1981). Although employee well-being is related to both physical and mental well-being, research on psychological well-being began to develop in the last decades of the 20th century (Vanhala & Tuomi, 2003). For example, several studies point to job insecurity as a major negative factor in health and well-being in the workplace (Borg, Kristensen & Burr, 2000; McDonough, 2000; Guest, 2002; Tortia, 2022). Human resources (HR) research has shown that HR practices can have positive effects on employee well-being when they create an equitable organizational and procedural environment (Spector, 1987; Blau, 1999; Tortia, 2008). In addition, Browne's (2000) study showed that most HRM practices are positively correlated with organizational effectiveness and job satisfaction, while they are negatively correlated with stress, as well as internal career opportunities.

The job characteristics model developed by Hackman and Oldham (1980) studies how job characteristics influence employee well-being. In this literature, direct perception of employee involvement in organizational practices is an important predictor of health and well-being, especially with regard to control over the work environment, while low levels of control have been found to be psychologically damaging (Spector, 1986; Mullarkey et al 1997). With regard to burnout, performance appraisal and merit pay systems have been found to contribute to exhaustion and employee malaise (Gabris & Ihrke 2001).

Cultural Differences in Organizations

Management literature has introduced the study of different managerial models in different national and organizational contexts in relation to Hofstede's (1991) and Schwartz's (1990) research on cross-cultural differences. Hofstede (1991) focused on the empirical identification (through factor analysis of survey data and in-depth interviews) of several cultural dimensions or constructs that show persistence in each national culture. These constructs are significantly different among nations and evolve over time, but in a regular manner (the different evolutionary patterns do not intersect). The basic cultural constructs have been identified as power distance, individualism-collectivism, masculinity-femininity, and uncertainty avoidance, to which two other constructs have been added in later work: long-term versus short-term orientation and indulgence versus restraint (Hofstede & Bond, 1988; Minkov, 2009; Minkov & Hofstede, 2011). The same approach has been contextualized by Hofstede and colleagues in relation to different organizational cultures and management models in the same or a limited number of countries (Minkov & Hofstede, 2011). In this case, factors representing the values, HRM practices, and promotion/dismissal characteristics of organizations were identified (Hofstede et al., 1990). In the needs theory presented in this work, special attention is paid to the categorization of organizational values, as the main dimensions identified by Hofstede relate to the need for work security, which is close to the need for security in Maslow's theory of human motivation. In addition, the importance given to the reasons for promotion and dismissal in Hofstede's framework suggests the existence of higher-level needs related to promotion, but also lower-level needs that have to do with security at work. The same authors also introduce organizational meta-dimensions in which practices, values and promotion/dismissal are combined. Among the three main meta-dimensions, there is a strong centrality of a work-related factorial cluster (professionalism), along with a cluster describing "closeness" or "retention" in the system. These two clusters, again, testify to the importance of security and uncertainty avoidance, as the accumulation of adequate resources (both human and material) and the creation of appropriate structures to govern production processes are instrumental in satisfying basic needs (Hofstede et al., 1990). While Hofstede (1998) criticized Maslow's and Herzberg's theories as being culturally constrained to Anglo-Saxon countries, where individualism (esteem) and masculinity (low uncertainty avoidance) prevail over collectivism and femininity (belonging), our framework, at present, focuses only on the importance of basic needs (survival and security) as compared to higher-level needs (belonging, esteem and self-actualization). Further insights into the difference between individualism and collectivism and between femininity and masculinity are left for future research.

As for Schwartz (1990, 1994), it is worth noting the focus on those cultural values that emphasize the preservation of social systems rather than individualism and autonomy. These values primarily benefit the community and relate to self-transcendence. Complementary, this approach also emphasizes a dimension of egalitarian compromise and harmony, as opposed to hierarchy, which requires the sacrifice of personal interests to maintain the social and material environment (Gouveia & Ros, 2000). As it will be better explained in later sections, these dimensions (system stability and egalitarianism) are highly compatible with the approach followed in this paper.

Social Embeddedness

The discussion of governance in light of human welfare takes place against the backdrop of the embeddedness of organization into social ties. While the classics of institutionalism anticipated the importance of social relations in influencing individual and corporate behavior, the concept of (dis)embedding the market economy from the broader social context was first theorized by Karl Polanyi, according to whom: "... Instead of incorporating the economy into social relations, social relations are incorporated into the economic system" (1944: 57). In Polanyi, the autonomy of the market from society was seen as an exception in the history of economic relations that belongs only to the capitalist system of production and creates tension and friction between the goals of society and the economic value of fictitious commodities such as money. Similarly, this kind of dyscrasia has also been theorized by leading authors in social systems theory, who emphasize the complexity-reducing characteristics and insensitivity of social systems, such as organizations and markets, to broader social and human needs that exist outside the organization but are not taken into account by their internal structure and governance (Luhmann, 1995; Valentinov, 2013). Relatedly, the structuralist approach of Granovetter's (1985) focuses on social relations and networks within economic systems, showing that purely economic outcomes depend not only on the forces of market competition, technology, and ownership rights as advocated by orthodox economics, but also on the configuration of "networks of weak social ties" among co-motivated and co-interested actors. Different configurations of relationships, institutional and organizational arrangements can lead to different outcomes, for example production of social value and welfare, not just economic value (Granovetter, 1973).

Network analysis developed primarily from Granovetter's work and focused on the network of social relations that constrain and enhance economic action, including in organizations and firms (Krippner, 2001). Organizations have been seen as actors operating in networks of similar and complementary activities, embedded in local systems characterized by homogeneous culture and institutions, and developing embedded ecosystems of technology and innovation (Cangiani, 2011; Tsouri & Pegoretti, 2020).

Firms in markets have been studied as systems "constructed" within a historically determined socio-institutional environment (Gertler, 2001). In the business systems literature, firms are defined as coordinating and controlling systems that are always socially embedded in their national and macro-regulatory environment (Whitley, 1999). Governance enters this framework as the main institutional basis of organizations (Tortia & Valentinov, 2018). In Dacin, Ventresca and Beal (1999) importance is attached to:

... the political and cultural constructions of governance rules and routines, logics of actor and ordering principles, and market elements that give shape to economic activity, organization, and management. ... recalls the virtues of the old institutionalism in economics, including its concern with history and process, embeddedness in social structures, and political dynamics in explaining forms and routines of economic activity (1999: 333).

This paper considers governance as an embedded structure that adapts to and interacts with external socio-economic conditions, especially in relation to the satisfaction of needs, since the goal is primarily the collection of sufficient resources, the creation of stable employment conditions, and the equitable distribution of the added value. The construction of governance is part of a process of increasing internal complexity of the system in which structures and routines are at least partly self-produced to protect, stabilize and direct internal processes toward organizational goals (Ostrom, 1990; Valentinov, 2013; Tortia, 2022). The connection with Williamson's approach to governance is evident. In his 2000 article, he clearly states that the institutional layers that make up the internal structure of the business organization are embedded in the background of social institutions: "The top level is the level of social embeddedness. This is where norms, customs, traditions, etc. are found. Religion plays an important role at this level." (2000: 596). Regarding Maslow's hierarchy of needs, Hofstede's critique (1980, 1998; see also Jacob, 2005) points out that Anglo-Saxon countries are characterized by an individualistic and masculine culture that emphasizes the prevalence of self-esteem and self-actualization. Other authors, however, have been concerned with adapting Maslow's hierarchy to more collectivist cultures, such as China. Gambrel and Cianci (2003) state that a hierarchy of needs based on a collectivist culture may differ significantly from Maslow's in terms of the nature, specification, and order of different needs. However, the basic logic and implications of the pyramid would be preserved. In particular, the need for belonging is likely to be more important than the need for esteem, while self-actualization will be achieved by satisfying the developmental needs of society.

INSTITUTIONS AND NEEDS IN A THEORY OF GOVERNANCE

Legal and internal rules identify the criteria for managing assets and distributing returns. Internal rules, in particular, define the organization's governance model. Governance defines who can participate in decision-making regarding goals and strategic direction, coordination, and resource allocation. It also has a constraining role, implemented through control technologies and the appointment of staff to monitor and preclude behavior that would hinder goal alignment and efficiency.

New Institutionalism and the Theory of Individual Needs

In new-institutionalist theory, the survival and prosperity of organizations are associated with efficiency. Accordingly, the enabling and binding functions of governance have to do with economizing on transaction costs. To justify this function, new-institutionalists start from the observation that organizations procure various types of assets (such as machinery, inventories, knowledge), while contracts are used to define rights to assets. Because writing contracts is costly, new-institutionalism argues that ownership, which defines who owns the residual rights of control and appropriation, is preferable to contracting when the costs of contracting are high and contracts are not suitable instruments to protect the asset owner's interests (e.g., because of information asymmetry, incompleteness of the contract, and the risk of opportunism, especially in the presence of asset specificity, as in Williamson, 1975; Hansmann, 1988, 1996). Rules are thus justified by their ability to assign strategic control over assets (ownership) to those stakeholder groups who have the greatest interest in containing opportunism. Coordination of resources occurs through a command and control structure, and incentives are defined under the assumption that individuals respond mechanically to monetary rewards or punishments. In this way, the role of individual motivations is mostly limited to extrinsic and monetary rewards, while intrinsic and social motivations are excluded from the explanatory framework (Grant & Berg, 2012).

Human psychology, with the works of Maslow, initiated a different scientific paradigm that has played a key role in the study of human motivation both inside and outside the organization. This paradigm has achieved prominence in the field of management, particularly in the works of Herzberg (1987) and McClellan (1987). The analysis of what motivates individual action begins with the study of what human beings value, desire and need. For Maslow, these desires are only partly culturally determined. In fact, each individual's attitudes are also defined by his or her biology, from which innate or intrinsic predispositions are derived. Maslow's work emphasizes that when individuals, in interaction with the social and organizational context, fail to realize their inner inclinations, they will be frustrated and unhappy. Their well-being may be compromised and they may react by decreasing their active participation, cooperating superficially or even rebelling and obstructing externally imposed goals (Wahba and Bridwell, 1976; Neher, 1991).

The fulfilment of both basic and higher-level needs require appropriate contextual conditions, which may be material or psychological and intangible. Individual attainable potential represents the inner self, which must be discovered, enabled and cultivated over time. As Maslow specifies, discovery and creativity are primary functions, because without discovering and reinterpreting what we desire, it would be difficult to begin taking steps toward our self-actualization (Maslow, 1998). In contrast, the satisfaction of primary needs and the location of resources, especially strategic resources, require a greater degree of control and regulation by social and economic institutions in which organizations are embedded and with which exchanges take place.

Some clarification is needed on the nature of needs, both basic and higher-level needs. First, desires and needs are not linked by simple equivalence. To explain this, consider John Dewey's theory of moral inquiry, which suggests that the fact that something is "desired" does not also make it "desirable." Dewey suggests that the moral quality of a desire is debatable (Dewey, 1930). Carrying this insight into needs theory, the thesis is that whether a desired object becomes desirable is a matter of functionality to human needs. The functionality of a desire with respect to need satisfaction must be discovered empirically or inferred through some nomological law of psychology. It is through life experience, or our ability to critically evaluate the consequences of actions taken toward needs satisfaction, that we learn which of our desires are desirable, valuable or necessary at a particular time. In this sense, this paper considers a need to be a desired object with moral qualities, or in other words a desire functional to the pursuit of need fulfillment. Second, the idea of need satisfaction should not be misunderstood as selfishness. Among the human needs identified by Maslow are those of belonging, of love and affection, of fairness and justice, of being accepted and feeling part of a community. This suggests that individual self-actualization occurs only if it happens "with" and "for" others through social relationships.

This work argues that trust can be generated by a sense of belonging and self-esteem (exclusion of opportunistic behavior) in repeated interactions within organizations. Cooperation can be achieved through values (self-esteem and altruism) that are morally projected onto all other participants through positive reciprocity, and supported over time by inclusive rules of governance. These elements are absent or play a marginal role in orthodox organizational theory. This absence can be an obstacle in explaining the real phenomena of commitment to a cause, trust and spontaneous cooperation.

In Maslow, the movement from the satisfaction of primary needs toward self-actualization is inevitable because primary needs must be satisfied first, but at the same time the individual cannot stop at primary needs. Take the example of the need for security, such as job security (the second layer of Maslow's pyramid). Although survival (first layer) comes first and is the most "prepotent" need in terms of acquiring a salary to meet survival needs, security is also crucial, as its satisfaction is directed at reducing the risks and negative impacts of unforeseen events and threats, e.g., layoff or being fired, which in principle can also endanger survival. Corporate governance can participate crucially in decisions about security needs. As for higher-order needs leading to self-actualization, they mainly have to do with psychological health and well-being, which can reveal the ability of governance and routines to contribute to positive outcomes.

Despite proposing innovative solutions, the claims of human psychology have not been supported by the study of alternative governance models. Management has adopted a rhetoric of involvement, developing techniques and practices that have not critically discussed the nature of the enterprise. Managerial techniques have been used as tools to increase productivity rather than stimulate critical thinking and creativity, thus trivializing the idea of humanistic psychology. It is not surprising, then, that these "manipulative practices" in HRM have often failed to achieve the expected results (Montuori & Purser, 2014). On the other hand, the "needs dimension" is addressed in different ways governance theory and its explicit introduction is inescapable in both inclusive and exclusive governance forms.

The reason for this, in our view, is the existence of institutional failure: a failure that human psychology has only sensed and that management theory has addressed in a limited way, for example in the writings of McGregor (1960). The use of authority and exclusive decision-making are incompatible with greater democracy, cooperation, use of creativity, and ultimately self-actualization. They are also inconsistent with the most basic needs when good material conditions, decent wages and a system of rules and use of resources that reduce the risks faced by workers are not introduced. In Italy, the case of the industrial company Olivetti has been studied by several generations of scholars as one of the positive examples of a company that not only sought competitive success, but was able to build its own internal system of corporate welfare. The Mondragon group of worker cooperatives, in the Basque region of Spain, is a second such example in which workers gained membership and control rights and a reasonably high degree of involvement in decision-making. A third example is the employee-owned retail chain of the John Lewis Partnership in the United Kingdom. These cases are rare but not unique (Taylor, 1977; Bar-Haim, 2002; Rodríguez-Ruiz, 2014).

In the more standard case of the traditional hierarchical organization, the emancipatory role of management suggested by Maslow and McGregor may be impractical because of the fundamental conception of governance. When human psychology is applied to organizations, reference is made to "progressive" organizational developments, but the use of these "empowering" tools depends on the discretion of management, that is to the orientation and will of a restricted and exclusive group of decision makers.

A NEEDS THEORY OF GOVERNANCE

The main elements of a needs theory of governance (NTG), which relates economic institutions to their ability to meet human needs, are outlined and compared with the governance theory of new institutionalism (Table 1). In a NTG, in addition to limited cognition and information asymmetries, the problem of need satisfaction lies in the disconnect between individual needs on the one hand and economic institutions on the other. Governance rules can be tools for interpreting needs and implementing them through a dialogic approach. Compared to new-institutional theory, NTG suggests that improvements in contracts, incentives, information and control are not sufficient conditions to resolve deficits in the attitudes and behavioral outcomes of individuals. Rather, the problem lies in the structure and method used to define organizational goals, direction and control, resource allocation, and decision-making processes (e.g., inclusion or exclusion).

In NTG, the human dimension becomes the end rather than the means in the pursuit of organizational goals, while contractual exchanges with lenders, employees, customers and suppliers are instrumental to human development. Similarly, the organization is conceived as an ecosystem functional to the satisfaction of human needs. As anticipated, the underlying logic of this theoretical proposition rests on the hypothesis that the satisfaction of needs fosters increased well-being and, through this route, can effectively contribute to increased economic and social value added and improved competitive position. Several empirical tests have already shown that increased well-being, especially in terms of satisfaction, and also the strengthening of intrinsic motivation, are positively correlated with variables indicating individual and organizational outcomes (Tortia et al., 2020). With this in mind, we strive to make explicit the hypotheses regarding organizational behavior and need satisfaction that have been largely left implicit so far.

The universality of the needs that individuals seek to satisfy requires collective action, common rules, and organizational routines as interlocking coordination mechanisms. Common goals and collective action correspond to the interconnection between individuals, and must be built into the structure of the organization through an evolutionary process of institutional design, as in Ostrom (1990) and Ostrom and Basurto (2011). A NTG does not atomize the individual, but views the individual as part of a collective, or as part of a public sphere of choice in which need satisfaction is pursued not at the expense of, but with and for others (Sacchetti & Borzaga, 2021). Consistent with Maslow and McGregor's Theory Y, the well-being of the creative and cooperative individual is the primary concern.

Once discovered, each need must be supported by the institutional context, otherwise it will come into conflict with the context itself, harming both the frustrated individual and the organization as a whole. In other words, the resilience of individual motivations requires that individual needs be supported by appropriate organizational processes (Tortia et al., 2020). The broader the spectrum of needs recognized by the governance of the organization, the greater the ability of individuals to achieve need satisfaction. The greater the match, the greater the individual's ability to engage in the process or set of activities that can lead to the desired ends.

The central idea of NTG is that individual needs interact with different institutional layers and, specifically, with governance structures and rules. When the interaction satisfies individual needs in accordance with organizational goals, the results promote well-being, thereby releasing motivational energy to promote new activities. The interaction between needs and institutions is expected to be greater when individuals participate, through a dialogic process, in defining the goals and institutional solutions deemed appropriate to achieve those goals. Therefore, institutions that foster the inclusion of individuals in the dialogic process are expected to contribute more to need satisfaction than hierarchical and exclusive institutions (Sacchetti, 2015).

The second main proposition states that while the new institutional economics assumes imperfect rationality, selfish preferences, monetary needs and rewards, and opportunism as the fundamental characteristics of human and organizational behavior, NTG considers imperfect rationality, multiple needs, and collective action based on cooperation and reciprocity as the main mechanisms that protect the organization from opportunistic behavior and empower people to achieve value goals as required by need satisfaction.

Table 1. The needs theory of governance and organizational economics compared

Components	Needs Theory of Governance	New Institutional Economics
1. Main Thesis	Needs fulfilment at work is an outcome of governance.	Efficiency is an outcome of governance.
2. Dependent variable	• First material needs (survival and security), then higher level needs (belonging, esteem, self-actualization) • Economic sustainability (instrumental)	Transaction costs, cost minimization
3. Units	• Individuals/Organizations. • Interconnectedness between the inner (individual) and outer (organizational) dimension is expressed prevalently by means of cooperation, ultimately aiming at shared organizational aims and self-actualization.	• Organizations/individuals. • Interconnectedness between the inner and outer is expressed in terms of incentives and control, ultimately aiming at the pursuit of organizational goals defined exclusively, risk reduction and cost efficiency.
4. Organizational objective(s)	Organizational objectives based on needs satisfaction, consistently with economic sustainability.	Organizational objectives are mainly focused on minimization of transaction costs/maximization of monetary rewards.
5. Individual needs	• Multiple, evolving, related to self-interest and other-regarding preferences. • Basic and higher level needs	Monetary and material, material well-being, related to self-interest.
6. Behavioral assumptions	• Common aims and mutual benefit. • Intrinsic motivations • Complexity of motivations (survival, security, belonging, esteem, self-actualization) • Individuals are well-meant and cooperate towards need satisfaction. • Opportunism not assumed a-priori, but explained and overcome.	• Heterogeneity of aims and contrasting interests. • Monetary and extrinsic motivations • Individuals will behave opportunistically if they can.
7. Well-being	• Well-being both monetary (material) and psychological; • Work generates both disutility (strain and exhaustion) and utility (personal and professional growth, pride, social recognition).	• Well-being generated by monetary and extrinsic incentives; • Work (effort) generates disutility.
8. Rules and incentives	• Shared, self-defined. • Prevalence of rules that enable needs satisfaction (inclusive governance bodies, participation and deliberation among cooperators)	• Prevalence of rules that activate regressive forces (exclusive governing bodies, hierarchical organizational relationships, binding control mechanisms to block potential defectors). • Externally determined (dictated to the individual).

Continued on following page

Table 1. Continued

Components	Needs Theory of Governance	New Institutional Economics
9. Empowerment	Important, endogenous, tending to higher needs, self-actualizing.	Not important, or not to be trusted.
10. Strategic control	Strategic control is shared among peers, transformative and dialogic processes of decision-making.	Concentration of strategic control in a restricted group of decision-makers.
11. Prevalent coordination method	Deliberation	Authority
12. Social embeddedness	• Markets and organization are socially embedded. • It interacts with the external social environment. • Internal complexity and self-production of rules (governance), functional to needs satisfaction.	• Markets and organization can be both embedded or dis-embedded depending on dominant culture and ideology (e.g. neo-liberalism vs collectivism or communitarianism) • Governance rules are functional to achieving efficiency and cost minimization.

If the organization does not act at the expense of individual need satisfaction, we expect individuals not to act at the expense of the organization (Akerlof, 1982). In terms of organizational survival, a non-secondary consequence of the misalignment between need satisfaction and organizational governance would be the emergence of X-inefficiency (Leibenstein, 1966), for example in terms of reduced member involvement and commitment (citizenship behavior), or the emergence of behaviors that oppose organizational strategies. Popular remedies proposed in both the orthodox and institutionalist literature range from increasing hierarchy to tightening control and pay for performance (Prendergast, 1999). All of these remedies risk increasing control and other organizational costs without delivering the expected efficiency (Frey and Osterloh, 1999; Akerlof & Kranton, 2000). In contrast, when rules are co-decided and cooperation is the norm (while opportunism is the exception), coordination is based on dialogic processes rather than monitoring and control (Leibenstein, 1978). This is because rules based on cooperation, including incentives, favor the search for understanding and consensus even in the presence of divergent interests over the use of authority and resources. The command-and-control model of governance is also more likely to generate strong biases on individual willingness and ability to use voice and creativity, thus further reducing need satisfaction and self-actualization. The negative impact of a model that incentivizes individuals to respond to authority rather than to use creative intelligence and cooperation would reinforce the need controlling practices and generate a vicious cycle of dissatisfaction and feelings of "not counting", while a context ripe for the development of a dialogic process disappears (Deci and Ryan, 2000).

John Commons (1931) argued for the empowering role of institutions, being "collective action in control, liberation and expansion of individual action". In this sense, governance structures and working rules manifest their dual role of limiting opportunistic behavior, on the one hand, and enabling the discovery of multiple needs and solutions, on the other. It follows that rather than being a tool of coercion used by management, incentive mixes represent an emergent property of complex organizations, the function of which is to improve consistency between organizational goals and multiple individual needs (Bacchiega & Borzaga, 2001). A simple example at hand is the role of wages in labor relations. From the company's point of view, wages reflect the scarcity of resources and the need to pay the worker according to his or her productivity, which contributes to the growth of the organization. From the worker's perspective, as suggested by Maslow (1998), motivations cannot be reduced solely to the payment of a monthly paycheck. However, when the satisfaction of needs is the ultimate goal of the organization, there is no doubt that monetary pay is essential for the basic needs of survival and the achievement of material well-being. On the other hand, monetary pay also promotes the satisfaction of higher-order needs, such as personal gratification, professional growth, and recognition of one's contribution, thus contributing to individual autonomy and self-actualization (Rhoades, Eisenberger, & Armeli, 2001; Guest, 2002).

However, despite the dual function of monetary incentives, higher-order needs also call for different solutions. While new-institutionalist approaches argue that monetary incentives are the main drivers of productive efficiency, evidence suggests that monetary incentives should be appropriately balanced with nonmonetary incentives, which are likely to better match intrinsic motivations for work and self-fulfillment (Deci and Ryan, 2000). Since need satisfaction and self-actualization may be desirable not only from the perspective of human psychology, but also beneficial to organizational survival, the third proposition of NTG asserts that Williamson's (2000) layered institutional model aims to emphasize cost efficiency (the transaction cost-minimizing characteristics of control rights and governance) and extrinsic incentives. On the contrary, NTG aims to highlight the need satisfaction potential of control rights, governance and organizational practices.

INSTITUTIONAL LAYERS AND SELF-ACTUALIZATION

The overarching message emerging from the foregoing sections relates to economic institutions and their impact on individual well-being and behavioral outcomes (both individual and collective). It has emphasized the idea that there are links between the fulfillment of needs and the governance of organizations. Some important illustrations of how this connection can be understood and implemented in practice come from the much-discussed and varied forms of shared capitalism and employee-owned businesses (Erdal, 2011). Similarly, Ostrom's (1990) studies of the effects of governance rules on the sustainable use of common resources and their economic impact on the people who live off their use developed within the new institutionalist paradigm, but are not unrelated to the recognition of the role of intrinsic motivations and other-regarding preferences (Ostrom, 2002).

The inverted pyramid in Figure 1 identifies the benchmark for assessing the combined action of control rights, governance structure and rules in enabling the full expression of individuals' inner needs. It emphasizes that the satisfaction of needs requires appropriate institutional preconditions, namely, the existence of a governance structure and rules that facilitate continuous adjustment and mediation between organizational goals and individual needs. While in Williamson (2000) the analysis of institutional levels focuses on transaction cost minimization and efficiency, our NTG suggests that those same levels can be interpreted predominantly as responses to stratified needs and ultimately self-actualization, similar to Maslow's ordering of human needs. Our thesis is that the basic needs of Maslow's theory (survival and security) loosely correspond to the most basic layers of Williamson's framework (control rights, resource allocation and formal governance), while the highest Maslowian needs (belonging, esteem and self-actualization) correspond to the outermost layers of Williamson's framework (managerial patterns and labor relations). At the same time, Williamson's basic institutional layers also represent the precondition for the proper functioning of the higher institutional layers in terms of the continuous organization of production and interaction with the external environment. In the latter case, higher-order needs are achieved through self-esteem and self-actualization. The pursuit of organizational goals, that is, production and exchange, is thus intertwined with the self-actualization of the actors involved (Sacchetti, 2015). Indeed, the satisfaction of needs as self-actualization, for example in terms of the use of creative intelligence, is likely to occur primarily in the sphere of production and work organization, since, as Loasby (2006) notes, this level is intertwined with the creation and use of knowledge. Needs theory, in this sense, changes the main "function" of productive institutions from efficiency to need satisfaction. While the satisfaction of basic needs for survival and security requires the allocation of adequate resources, their protection and equitable distribution among all stakeholders through control rights and formal governance, other institutional levels (work process and technology) are closer to the satisfaction of higher-level needs. For example, involvement in decision-making and cooperative interpersonal relationships can support a sense of belonging, deliberation and autonomy have to do with self-esteem, creativity in process and product innovation with self-actualization.

Interaction with the external environment can be particularly challenging, especially in the presence of unexpected and negative shocks or stimuli. When governance is built around meeting needs, external shocks and threats are expected to be addressed with *greater* rather than less involvement and deliberation. Existing organizational routines are activated or new ones are created that aim to increase adaptation by improving the connection between the necessity to achieve economic sustainability, while at the same time not reducing the organization's ability to meet needs. This type of effort is not without difficulties, or even limitations, but it is the best possible model to follow in the presence of unforeseen events. For example, during a pandemic, the organization would strive to restore production as soon as possible so as not to disrupt the supply of a steady flow of goods and services for its customers and to continue paying salaries to its employees. To this end, remote work can be a necessary tool that, however, has the added benefit of increasing employee autonomy and flexibility in the use of work time. New routines are created, including new remote-control systems, and the introduction of new (digital) technologies, to reconcile autonomy and independence with efficient production. On the other hand, when the constraints imposed by a blockade become weaker, the need arises to recover an appropriate relational context in which members can meet, work together, exchange ideas and deliberate. Sufficient security measures are introduced to protect the entire community from the emergence of new infections. It is unlikely that the organization will return to a pre-pandemic arrangement, as the lockdown has forced the introduction of new and more efficient mechanisms for controlling and organizing remote work, along with the adoption of advanced technologies. The specific way in which distinctly different and potentially opposing organizational patterns and goals are reconciled is left to the free process of investigation and discovery by each individual organization.

Figure 1.

FIGURE 1

Institutional layers and self-actualization in cooperative firms

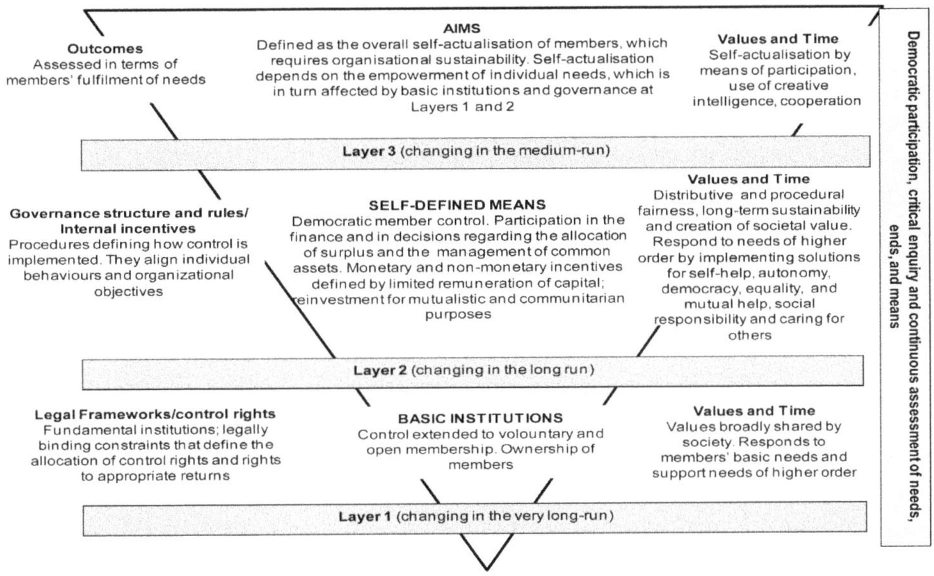

In Figure 1, as in Williamson (2000), the different institutional layers interact through specific connectors: rules, individual norms of behavior and strategies. Level 1 of the pyramid represents basic institutions, such as control and appropriation rights, which usually undergo a high degree of legal formalization (level 1). The process of evolution of control rights is likely to occur in the long run. At this level, control rights seem to interpret the need for "survival" of the organization and its stakeholders, the strongest need in Maslow's theory. This institutional layer makes individuals value asset ownership as a way to increase appropriable economic value and achieve material well-being. It can be interpreted as a precondition for the satisfaction of higher-order needs, as material well-being can provide sufficient resources to achieve self-esteem and self-actualization. On the other hand, material well-being is likely to be a necessary but not sufficient condition for achieving higher-order needs. Control rights are binding in defining who has access to decision-making and scarce resources; however, they do not unambiguously define how resources are managed, what and how outcomes are distributed and used.

Resource allocation and distribution patterns relate to the governance structure and work rules, defined at Level 2. Formal governance (e.g., board of directors and supervisory bodies) links control rights at Level 1 with the organization's operational and ultimate goals at Level 3. At Level 2, we observe the means by which the organization's purpose is pursued. In the case of inclusive forms of governance, organizational goals coincide with those defined by self-organizing members (Ostrom, 1990). Similarly, governance rules are at least partially defined on an ongoing basis by members themselves as a way of reflecting their needs and evolving based on their experience and critical evaluation of results (Ostrom & Basurto, 2011). Formal governance and self-regulation may correspond to Maslow's second layer of needs, as they are primarily geared toward ensuring the smooth functioning of the organization, stability and security. The needs for security and belonging can be exemplified by the sustainability of natural resources in self-managed commons, or job stability in employment relations; low-risk financial investments for households and small businesses in mutual credit banks and credit unions. Higher-level needs can be met through inclusive governance (in conventional enterprises) or democratic governance (in cooperative enterprises). Inclusion and active participation provide prerequisites for critical evaluation of organizational processes by stakeholders, creative thinking and self-actualization. The binding nature of rules is not intended to undermine individual potential, but to ensure that an individual's right to participate and share results is respected and compatible with the rights of other participants. Mutual recognition of individual rights leads to increased freedom and empowerment. Rules that inhibit inclusion, from this point of view, would be perceived as unfair and would have the unintended effect of undermining intrinsic motivation, feeling of belongingness, and self-esteem, thus violating a fundamental condition for self-actualization. Self-actualization, the highest goal on Maslow's hierarchy, occurs when individuals can stimulate and use their creative intelligence for the benefit of themselves and others. The third layer of the inverted pyramid in Figure 1 represents an organizational domain that lends itself to self-realization in the context of production through creativity and critical thinking and is co-extensive with the outermost organizational layer of Williamson's (2000) framework.

FUTURE RESEARCH DIRECTIONS

Future research directions will require the progressive integration of the need's perspective into governance theory. Given the complexity of this undertaking, it is expected to be long and painstaking. The perspective is clearly an analogy between the biological and psychological nature of organisms and the institutional nature of organizations. The way in which organizations satisfy basic needs (survival and security) is easy to identify. Economic added value is produced primarily to satisfy basic needs, and internal regulations related to important issues such as job stability and corporate welfare are developed to enhance the economic and social security of participants. On the other hand, as in Maslow, satisfaction of basic needs is likely to influence and support higher-level needs, since in the absence of production of economic value added and protection from possible negative events such as dismissal or the onset of occupational illness, self-esteem and self-actualization are likely to be damaged or diminished. The exact or main ways in which governance and management models can support the satisfaction of higher-level needs are the subject of discussion, which is ongoing anyway (Ivtzan, 2013; Gopinath, 2020; Bell & Taylor, 2004). Several fields are open to new investigation, e.g., the use and creation of new technologies and work environments that foster greater engagement and satisfaction, but also managerial practices and participatory management, among others.

CONCLUSION

A need theory of governance has been developed with the aim of connecting and combining human psychology and economic institutions. Needs theory has been used as a tool for critical, interpretive and descriptive analysis to discuss governance solutions characterized by inclusion and deliberation. Our findings emphasize that when governance is explained by focusing on the needs of individuals, opportunism, as described in most orthodox economic theories, ceases to be a dominant dimension of human behavior and is left the role of a behavioral hazard to be kept in check. Needs and the attached motivations become the fundamental driver of governance choices. Greater well-being is expected to contribute positively to the achievement of goals, including but not limited to competitiveness and performance. The governance structure and routines that contribute to these outcomes must balance two characteristics: the liberating and the constraining.

The basic elements of this framework consider the interconnections between needs and institutional layers, between the individual and his or her ecosystem. In a nonauthoritarian context, governance structures are designed to promote dialogic processes of inquiry at all levels of productive activities, over time. In addition, institutional design leaves room for the expression of specific motivations and goals and allows members to creatively shape the governance of the organization while preventing opportunistic behavior and ensuring compliance with collectively defined goals. Finally, it is important to mention that this needs theory of governance requires organizations to be socially embedded, since needs and motivations exist before members enter the organization and are "subsumed" in its operation and development. The motivation of the involved actors and the ways in which members and stakeholders achieve need satisfaction are in turn influenced by the institutional, cultural and historical context. Interaction with the external societal environment is necessary, since the satisfaction of needs cannot be achieved without stakeholders being able to exchange and express themselves outside organizational boundaries. At the same time, the autopoietic self-production of rules, routines and internal structure is instrumental in achieving internal complexity, which is necessary to sustain need satisfaction.

REFERENCES

Akerlof, G. A. (1982). Labor contracts as partial gift exchange. *The Quarterly Journal of Economics*, *97*(4), 543–569. doi:10.2307/1885099

Akerlof, G. A., & Kranton, R. A. (2000). Economics and identity. *The Quarterly Journal of Economics*, *115*(3), 715–753. doi:10.1162/003355300554881

Bacchiega, A., & Borzaga, C. (2001). Social enterprises as incentive structures. An economic analysis. In C. Borzaga & J. Defourny (Eds.), *The emergence of social enterprises (pp* (pp. 273–295). Routledge.

Bar-Haim, A. (2002). *Participation programs in work organizations: past, present, and scenarios for the future*. Praeger.

Bell, E., & Taylor, S. (2004). 'From outward bound to inward bound': The prophetic voices and discursive practices of spiritual management development. *Human Relations*, *57*(4), 439–466. doi:10.1177/0018726704043895

Ben-Ner, A., & Jones, D. C. (1995). Employee participation, ownership and productivity: A theoretical framework. *Industrial Relations*, *34*(4), 532–554. doi:10.1111/j.1468-232X.1995.tb00387.x

Blau, G. (1999). Testing the longitudinal impact of work variables and performance appraisal satisfaction on subsequent overall job satisfaction. *Human Relations*, *52*(8), 1099–1113. doi:10.1177/001872679905200806

Borg, V., Kristensen, T. S., & Burr, H. (2000). Work environment and changes in self-rated health: A five-year follow-up study. *Stress Medicine*, *16*(1), 37–47. doi:10.1002/(SICI)1099-1700(200001)16:1<37::AID-SMI830>3.0.CO;2-O

Browne, J. H. (2000). Benchmarking HRM practices in healthy work organisations. *American Business Review*, *18*(2), 54–61.

Cangiani, M. (2011). Karl Polanyi's institutional theory: Market society and its "disembedded" economy. *Journal of Economic Issues*, *45*(1), 177–198. doi:10.2753/JEI0021-3624450110

Clegg, C., & Wall, T. D. (1981). A note on some new scales for measuring aspects of psychological wellbeing at work. *Journal of Occupational Psychology, 54*(3), 221–225. doi:10.1111/j.2044-8325.1981.tb00062.x

Commons, J. R. (1931). Institutional economics. *The American Economic Review, 21*(4), 648–657.

Dacin, M. T., Ventresca, M. J., & Beal, B. D. (1999). The embeddedness of organizations: Dialogue & directions. *Journal of Management, 25*(3), 317–356. doi:10.1177/014920639902500304

Davis, J. H., Schoorman, F. D., & Donaldson, L. (1997). Toward a stewardship theory of management. *Academy of Management Review, 22*(1), 20–47. doi:10.2307/259223

Deci, E. L., & Ryan, R. M. (2000). Self-determination theory and the facilitation of intrinsic motivation, social development and well-being. *The American Psychologist, 55*(1), 68–78. doi:10.1037/0003-066X.55.1.68 PMID:11392867

Dewey, J. (1930). *The quest for certainty. A study of the relations of knowledge and action.* Allen and Unwin.

Erdal, E. (2011). *Beyond the corporation: Humanity working*. The Bodley Head.

Foss, N. J., & Weber, L. (2016). Moving opportunism to the back seat: Bounded rationality, costly conflict, and hierarchical forms. *Academy of Management Review, 41*(1), 61–69. doi:10.5465/amr.2014.0105

Frey, B. S. (1997). *Not just for the money. An economic theory of personal motivation*. Edward Elgar.

Frey, B. S., & Osterloh, M. (1999). Yes, managers should be paid like bureaucrats. *Journal of Management Inquiry, 14*(1), 96–111. doi:10.1177/1056492604273757

Gabris, G. T., & Ihrke, D. M. (2001). Does performance appraisal contribute to heightened levels of employee burnout? The results of one study. *Public Personnel Management, 30*(2), 157–172. doi:10.1177/009102600103000203

Gertler, M. S. (2001). Best practice? Geography, learning, and the institutional limits to stro convergence. *Journal of Economic Geography, 1*(1), 5–26. doi:10.1093/jeg/1.1.5

Gopinah, R. (2020). Prominence of Self-Actualization in Organization. *International Journal of Advanced Science and Technology, 29*(3), 11591–11602.

Gouveia, V. V., & Ros, M. (2000). Hofstede and Schwartz's models for classifying individualism at the cultural level: Their relation to macro-social and macro-economic variables. *Psicothema, 12*(Suppl), 25–33.

Granovetter, M. (1973). The strength of weak ties. *American Journal of Sociology*, *78*(6), 1360–1380. doi:10.1086/225469

Granovetter, M. (1985). Economic action and social structure: The problem of embeddedness. *American Journal of Sociology*, *91*(3), 481–510. doi:10.1086/228311

Grant, A. M., & Berg, J. M. (2012). Prosocial motivation. In K. S. Cameron & G. M. Spreitzer (Eds.), *The Oxford handbook of positive organizational scholarship* (pp. 28–44). Oxford University Press.

Gregory-Smith, I., & Main, B. (2015). Heads I win, tails you lose? A career analysis of executive pay and corporate performance. *Cambridge Journal of Economics*, *39*(5), 1373–1398. doi:10.1093/cje/beu049

Guest, D. (2002). Human resource management, corporate performance and employee wellbeing: Building the worker into HRM. *The Journal of Industrial Relations*, *4*(3), 335–358. doi:10.1111/1472-9296.00053

Hackman, J. R., & Oldham, G. R. (1980). *Work redesign*. Addition-Wesley.

Hansmann, H. (1988). Ownership of the firm. *Journal of Law Economics and Organization*, *4*(2), 267–304.

Hansmann, H. (1996). *The Ownership of Enterprise*. Belknap Press Harvard University.

Herzberg, F. (1968). One more time. How do you motivate employees. *Harvard Business Review*, *81*(1), 87–96. PMID:12545925

Hodgson, G. M. (2004). Opportunism is not the only reason why firms exist: Why an explanatory emphasis on opportunism may mislead management strategy. *Industrial and Corporate Change*, *13*(2), 401–418. doi:10.1093/icc/dth016

Hofstede, G. (1980). Motivation, leadership, and organization: Do American theories apply abroad? *Organizational Dynamics*, *9*(1), 42–63. doi:10.1016/0090-2616(80)90013-3

Hofstede, G. (1991). *Cultures and organizations: software of the mind*. McGraw-Hill.

Hofstede, G. (1998). Think locally, act globally: Cultural constraints in personnel management. *MIR*, *38*(2), 7–26. doi:10.1007/978-3-322-90989-3_2

Hofstede, G., & Bond, M. H. (1988). The Confucian connection: From cultural roots to economic growth. *Organizational Dynamics*, *16*(4), 5–21. doi:10.1016/0090-2616(88)90009-5

Hofstede, G., Neuijen, B., Daval Ohayv, D., & Sanders, G. (1990). Measuring organizational cultures: A qualitative and quantitative study across twenty cases. *Administrative Science Quarterly*, *35*(2), 286–316. doi:10.2307/2393392

Ivtzan, I., Gardner, H. E., Bernard, I., Sekhon, M., & Hart, R. (2013). Wellbeing through self-fulfilment: Examining developmental aspects of self-actualization. *The Humanistic Psychologist*, *41*(2), 119–132. doi:10.1080/08873267.2012.712076

Jensen, M., & Meckling, W. (1976). Theory of the firm: Managerial behavior, agency costs and ownership structure. *Journal of Financial Economics*, *3*(4), 305–360. doi:10.1016/0304-405X(76)90026-X

Krippner, G. R. (2001). The elusive market: Embeddedness and the paradigm of economic sociology. *Theory and Society*, *30*(6), 775–810. doi:10.1023/A:1013330324198

Leibenstein, H. (1966). Allocative VS "X-efficiency. *The American Economic Review*, *56*(3), 392–415.

Leibenstein, H. (1978). *General X-efficiency theory and economic development.* Oxford University Press.

Loasby, B. (2006). Industrial organization. In T. Raffaelli, G. Becattini, & M. Dardi (Eds.), *The Elgar Companion to Alfred Marshall* (pp. 371–378). Edward Elgar.

Luhmann, N. (1995). *Social systems*. Stanford University Press.

Maslow, A. H. (1943). A Theory of human motivation. *Psychological Review*, *50*(4), 370–396. doi:10.1037/h0054346

Maslow, A. H. (1962). *Towards a psychology of being*. D. Van Nostrand. doi:10.1037/10793-000

Maslow, A. H. (1998). Maslow on management. New York, NY: Wiley.

Mayo, E. (1933). *The human problems of an industrial civilization*. Macmillan.

McDonough, P. (2000). Job insecurity and health. *International Journal of Health Services*, *30*(3), 453–476. doi:10.2190/BPFG-X3ME-LHTA-6RPV PMID:11109176

McGregor, D. M. (1960). *The human side of enterprise*. McGraw-Hill.

Minkov, M. (2009). Predictors of differences in subjective well-being across 97 nations. *Cross-Cultural Research*, *43*(2), 152–179. doi:10.1177/1069397109332239

Minkov, M., & Hofstede, G. (2011). The evolution of Hofstede's doctrine. *Cross Cultural Management*, *18*(1), 10–20. doi:10.1108/13527601111104269

Montuori, A., & Purser, R. (2014). Humanistic psychology in the workplace. In K. J. Schneider, J. F. Pierson, & J. F. T. Bugental (Eds.), *The handbook of humanistic psychology: Theory, research, and practice* (pp. 723–734). Russel Sage.

Mullarkey, S., Jackson, P. R., Wall, T. D., Wilson, J. R., & Grey-Taylor, S. M. (1997). The impact of technology characteristics and job control on worker mental health. *Journal of Organizational Behavior, 18*(5), 471–489. doi:10.1002/(SICI)1099-1379(199709)18:5<471::AID-JOB810>3.0.CO;2-V

Neher, A. (1991). Maslow's theory of motivations. *Journal of Humanistic Psychology, 31*(3), 89–112. doi:10.1177/0022167891313010

Ostrom, E. (1990). *Governing the commons. The evolution of institutions for collective action.* Cambridge University Press. doi:10.1017/CBO9780511807763

Ostrom, E. (2002). Crowding out citizenship. *Scandinavian Political Studies, 23*(1), 3–16. doi:10.1111/1467-9477.00028

Ostrom, E., & Basurto, X. (2011). Crafting analytical tools to study institutional change. *Journal of Institutional Economics, 7*(3), 317–343. doi:10.1017/S1744137410000305

Polanyi, K. (1944). *The great transformation: the political and economic origins of our time.* Farrar & Rinehart.

Prendergast, C. (1999). The provision of incentives in firms. *Journal of Economic Literature, 37*(1), 7–63. doi:10.1257/jel.37.1.7

Rhoades, L., Eisenberger, R., & Armeli, S. (2001). Affective commitment to the organization: The contribution of perceived organizational support. *The Journal of Applied Psychology, 86*(5), 825–836. doi:10.1037/0021-9010.86.5.825 PMID:11596800

Rodríguez-Ruiz, Ó. (2014). The history of human resource management in Spain: An autocratic legacy beyond the waves of rational and normative control. *Management & Organizational History, 9*(3), 256–271. doi:10.1080/17449359.2013.878251

Sacchetti, S. (2015). Inclusive and exclusive social preferences: A Deweyan framework to explain governance heterogeneity. *Journal of Business Ethics, 126*(3), 473–485. doi:10.100710551-013-1971-0

Sacchetti, S., & Borzaga, C. (2021). The Foundations of the "Public Organisation": Governance failure and the problem of external effects. *The Journal of Management and Governance, 25*(3), 731–758. doi:10.100710997-020-09525-x

Sacchetti, S., & Sugden, R. (2009). The organization of production and its publics: Mental proximity, markets and hierarchies. *Review of Social Economy*, *67*(3), 289–311. doi:10.1080/00346760802621906

Schwartz, S. H. (1990). Individualism-collectivism: Critique and proposed refinements. *Journal of Cross-Cultural Psychology*, *21*(2), 139–157. doi:10.1177/0022022190212001

Spector, P. E. (1986). Perceived control by employees: A meta-analysis of studies concerning autonomy and participation at work. *Human Relations*, *39*(11), 1005–1016. doi:10.1177/001872678603901104

Spector, P. E. (1987). Interactive effects of perceived control and job stressors on affective reactions and health outcomes for clerical workers. *Work and Stress*, *1*(2), 155–162. doi:10.1080/02678378708258497

Taylor, J. C. (1977). Experiments in work system design: Economic and human results. Part II. *Personnel Review*, *6*(4), 21–34. doi:10.1108/eb055345

Tietze, I. N., & Shakeshaft, C. (1982). *Toward a reconstruction of organizational theory: Androcentric bias in A. H. Maslow's* Theory of Human Motivation and Self-Actualization. Paper presented at the Annual Meeting of the American Educational Research Association, New York, NY. https://files.eric.ed.gov/fulltext/ED216440.pdf

Tortia, E. C. (2008). Worker well-being and perceived fairness: Survey-based findings from Italy. *Journal of Socio-Economics*, *37*(5), 2080–2094. doi:10.1016/j.socec.2007.10.005

Tortia, E. C. (2022). Employment protection regimes and dismissal of members in worker cooperatives. *Scandinavian Journal of Management*, *38*(3), 101213. doi:10.1016/j.scaman.2022.101213

Tortia, E. C., & Valentinov, V. (2018). Internal organization and governance. In B. A. Seaman & D. Young (Eds.), Handbook of Research on Nonprofit Economics and Management (2nd ed., pp. 285–299). Edward Elgar. doi:10.4337/9781785363528.00022

Tsouri, M., & Pegoretti, G. (2021). Structure and resilience of local knowledge networks: The case of the ICT network in Trentino. *Industry and Innovation*, *28*(7), 860–879. doi:10.1080/13662716.2020.1775070

Valentinov, V. (2013). Veblen and instrumental value: A systems theory perspective. *Journal of Economic Issues*, *47*(3), 673–688. doi:10.2753/JEI0021-3624470304

Vanhala, S., & Tuomi, K. (2003). Individual, organisational and work-related determinants of employee well-being. *EBS Review*, (Autumn), 70–81.

Veblen, T. (1899). *[1994]. The Theory of the Leisure Class*. Dover Thrift.

Wahba, M. A., & Bridwell, L. G. (1976). Maslow Reconsidered: A review of research on the need hierarchy theory. *Organizational Behavior and Human Performance*, *15*(2), 212–240. doi:10.1016/0030-5073(76)90038-6

Whitley, R. (1999). *Divergent capitalisms: the social structuring and change of business systems*. Oxford University Press.

Williamson, O. E. (1975). *Markets and hierarchies: Analysis and Anti-trust implications: A study in the economics of internal organization*. Free Press.

Williamson, O. E. (2000). The new institutional economics: Taking stock, looking ahead. *Journal of Economic Literature*, *38*(3), 595–613. doi:10.1257/jel.38.3.595

Chapter 4
What Should Work-Life Be Like in a Globally Emancipated Society?
About Really Decent Work and Authentic Social Sustainability in the Future

Raquel Varela
https://orcid.org/0000-0001-6121-1379
New University of Lisbon, Portugal

Roberto della Santa
New University of Lisbon, Portugal

ABSTRACT

The authors seek to critically reflect on the meaning of work in a globally emancipated society. They start by arguing that work is a central issue for human societies, whether to produce socially useful goods, to provide basic needs or as the making, objectification, and safeguarding of ontological humanization of Mankind itself – even if in the field of socialist politics this centrality has been overshadowed by programs mainly focused on the defense of assistentialism, philanthropy, or even charity. To conceive work today, in the current stage of the capitalist society, we have to mobilize several concepts, methods, and areas of knowledge, among which the authors highlight critical sociology, global labor history, and psychodynamics of work. Finally, they argue about what would be the fundamental aspects of work in an emancipated society.

DOI: 10.4018/978-1-6684-2364-6.ch004

INTRODUCTION

Work occupies a central place in societies: in politics, culture and economy. It supports the social production of goods or services; it has a fundamental social value and is preponderant in human socialization. Work ensures access to consumption; it is the source of social rights and political citizenship; it qualifies and situates people in society at large; it seems relevant in solving all environmental and ecological problems. This prominent centrality constituted a complex path of struggle and resistance for the dignity of the worker and against alienation. A rare balance between the individual and the collective, affirming and reaffirming human work as a universal historical value is the aim. Indeed, labor is all these aspects and much more, for the individual and for the humankind. The centrality of work is a fundamental starting point of our own intellectual work (Antunes, 2013; Dejours & Deranty, 2010).

Work is undoubtedly central, but despite all the efforts of dialectical criticism in the last two centuries, it is still necessary to affirm something that is even more immanent and transcendental: work is a vital human life activity. Work is central and decisive in the process of production and reproduction of the social being for the historical form assumed by the humankind over time. Karl Marx – as stated in both his critique of idealist philosophy and his first critique of political economy – took a foundational step by formulating a radically new conception of work. He observed that private property, by opposing to the so-called free human development, created the conditions for the enduring objectification of what he described as alienated work.

The production processes of the means necessary to satisfy human needs have been transformed into a fundamental condition in human life. They became the basis of the process of humanization, or hominization, of long historical duration. Work is inherent to the life of those who have become human beings, so much so that – from the bipedal upright posture to the articulated language and complex thought – everything that defines us as "hominids" – distinct from natural beings – is and must be attributed to the fact that – as Eduardo Galeano wrote in the *Open Veins of Latin America*,

We are what we do, and especially what we do to change who we are (Galeano, 1973, p. 13).

It is because of the categorical invention of work, that it becomes possible for us to transform nature, history and human nature itself. Affirming the centrality of work, therefore, is not an act without consequences.

Once the social production of commodities became widespread, the capitalist socio-metabolic system subsumed the activity of work as a form of 'wage labor'. The decommodification of work, as well as the deprivatization of the means of production beyond the historical overcoming of state apparatuses, were described as an effective possibility for a real community made up of free, collaborative and associated workers. From a critique to the reification of social relations, which appear – in the capitalist system – as relations between things and against the fetish of the State-form it becomes possible to think about the disalienation of work. Not to mention atrocious relations of exploitation assumed in the wage-earning regime itself, naturalized by the notion of 'labor market'.

The dawn of the 21st century brought all these debates back to life. Social sciences turned from the mainstream declaration of the 'end of work', 'post-history' and so on to the now so trendy topic of the 'future of work'.

On the basis of the numerous studies (teachers, doctors, dockers, cabin crew, civil servants, train drivers, metro operators, nurses, journalists and metalworkers from AutoEuropa, among others) the Authors have carried out in the Observatory on Living and Working Conditions, at the New University of Lisbon, in dialogue with social critical theory and the centrality of work, this Chapter conceptualizes labor and work today, in an eventual, non-marketized future.

THE MULTIDIMENSIONAL CENTRALITY OF WORK

The pusillanimous or apologetic denial of the centrality of work, an important and persistent theme in the social and human sciences has become more pronounced in recent decades, coinciding with the genesis of a structural crisis of capital (Varela & Pereira, 2016). The origins can be traced back to 1925, when Karl Mannheim, in his famous work titled *Ideology and Utopia*, claimed that 'classes are merging', since – according to the idea borrowed from the German philosophical tradition – we are living in an 'era of equalization'.

A few years had passed since Mannheim's projection and, precisely in 1929, the Great Depression had turned out to be a serious global systemic crisis, which occurred throughout the 1930s opening a new era of revolutions and counterrevolutions, whose epicenter was, once again, work. The year of 1929 brought an era of famines, decay, and despair – the opposite of the equalization – and was considered the longest, deepest and most widespread depression of the 20th century. The real tendency was that of an equalization of the differential rates of global exploitation, by which the capitalist class – throughout the world – tried to put the labor power of humanity back under an ever more intense form of social subordination. The countering of this tendency climaxed with the Spanish social revolution, the resistance to Nazi-fascism and in the social pact resulting from its defeat in Europe and the core countries that brought – for three decades, dubbed as the golden years of capital – the illusory belief in the effective possibility of reconciling wealth concentration and poverty alleviation.

Later, the crisis of the 1970s, quickly began its historic reversal and absolute impoverishment returned to the core countries. This was accompanied by the relocation of part of heavy production to Asia, the entry of the Chinese for super-expensive, or hyper-unprotected, labor into the world market, the spread of precariousness (and subcontracting) in Europe, and the exponential increase of social inequality. The various intellectual mystifications no longer succeed in dismissing the social question as the anachronistic 19th century concerns. The need to challenge the hierarchical and structural subjugation of work to capital remains the great issue of our time, namely in the effective establishment of an authentic substantive democracy in the world of work. To think and act on this summit issue – in theory and in methodology as well as in the social and political sphere – is unthinkable without convincingly reaffirming the centrality of work in all aspects of life: ontological, epistemological, economic, social, cultural and political, everyday life and historical span, individual and collective, as means and ends, in quantity and quality, in the past or in the future.

To reaffirm the centrality of labor, however, it is necessary to list the various – humanly objective – constitutive dimensions of a social being.

Neoliberal globalization is an overarching social phenomenon that has connected commodities, investments, and the workforce on a global scale. This process has remade the world – quantitatively and qualitatively – and has acquired a new momentum in the last five decades with the massive population migrations and relocation of companies around the globe. Urbanization and wage employment of millions of workers from the Global South were making this process, which occurred in an unequal and combined movement, joining the same massive global supply chain across different territories, nationalities, regions, cultures, differences in training and qualification of the workforce, access to transport and services, and diverse wage levels, living and working conditions.

What are the key factors in shaping the current productive restructuring on a global scale? What is the relationship between the labor force and the peripheries, semi-peripheries and the living center of the inter-state system? There was a worldwide boost in both the movement of commodities (including consumer goods) and in the social labor force in the world after the 1970s. Since then, the metropolises prevail in a very preponderant way over the countryside, and most of the world's population works for the markets, in their various social forms, and heterogeneous social labor relations, which has rearranged the inter-state world system.

The amplified reproduction of the contradiction between accumulation and legitimation has increased both the financialization of capital, the dispossession of labor without the creation of actual jobs. Also, it has given rise to a new chauvinist discourse, political *bonapartisation* and systemic corruption on an unprecedented scale. It must be recalled that the growing degradation of labor supported by the government's encouragement of subordinate entrepreneurship, labor immigration and cheap labor is nothing but a way to turn wine into water, i.e., it tends to aggravate the deleterious effects of the clash between the pole of accumulation and the pole of legitimation. In a context of global erosion of labor income, popular illusions about individual solutions to the crisis will inevitably fade in the face of the brutal recession on the horizon.

The so-called capitalism 4.0 simply cannot replace the old promises of the post-war Keynesian consensus, or the 'social pact' of the golden years of social insertion via labor – subsequently to wage citizenship – precisely because it cannot reproduce the proletarian condition without marginalizing large fringes of workers from access to the most elementary social rights, including the right to labor itself. The 'Fordisation' of service work – see the conveyor belt extending from hospitals to schools, and the chronic proletarianization and deskilling that prevails, along with the new waves of labor phantomization reveal the universalization of the logic of competition within the very ranks of those 'from below' espoused to the pole of accumulation and, at the same time, structurally divorced from the pole of legitimation 'from above'. In this sense, it is not difficult to see how the economic crisis feeds the political crisis, or the supposed 'sacred salvations' for the crisis are its 'unholy damnation'.

The pandemic and the response to it, emphasized the irrationality of the dominant socio-metabolic system and draws our attention once again to the centrality of work. We must reflect on the value of all human labor, on the values on which it must be based, on its rigid social or international divisions. The precariousness of life and the non-regulation of labor are violent and unilateral forms of control over workers, thus favoring selfishness, utilitarianism, and scandalous, unjust and sterile concentrations of social wealth. The debate on capitalism is here to stay. To avoid its controversy, it is not astute.

Alongside the centrality of work, we must highlight two trends of theoretical and methodological significance in labor studies, namely: critical social theory as a founding horizon over the traditional mode of knowledge production, and the primacy of praxis – e.g., the theory-practice inseparability nexus conceived in the old dialectical tradition.

In the last decades, the public sphere has been drained of debate on strategic imagination, utopian horizons and alternative solutions for social transformation, and intellectual discussion on politics, which gravitated mainly towards the validation of mitigating public policies, palace conflicts for power or techno-bureaucratic micro-guerrillas from governance. The classic distinction between grand politics, of the transformation of the state, and small politics, of the indiscretions of the corridors vanished. It is precisely when reality demands the will and intellect of times of transition that we find a metamorphosis of those who presented themselves as radical critics of order, and have now been reconverted into the routine representation of order in the face of all criticism.

The impact of the digital reconversion on the social organization of labor is as (or more) important than that of the preceding industrial revolution that gave rise to the welfare state. if we look at the psychic and physical connections of entire generations who have already experienced these great transformations in the world of work and life, we realise that the corporeal *sensorium* itself – that is, the material-sensible apparatus of every human organism as a whole – has undergone radical, unexpected changes in the course of history.

Isn't it reasonable to suppose that the gap between the country and the city is as abyssal for work and social life as the gap from pencil and pen to digital platforms or screens?

Technological mutations of such magnitude are necessarily accompanied by institutional restructuring. The social and labor crisis is accompanied by an unprecedented ecological crisis and raises the issue of sustainability to a new level.

The vertiginous growth of social inequalities, the abandonment of subordinate social classes to job insecurity and sub-proletarianization, the mass migrations of populations expelled – by misery, wars or global devastation – arouse anger and violence and the return of nationalism and xenophobia. In most countries, especially those with a record of structural adjustment, the latent hatred aroused by social injustice provokes the resurgence of political bonapartism and the divisions between 'them' and 'us'. The introduction to the ILO Constitution itself and the Declaration of Philadelphia (International Labour Organization, 1944) already asserted that 'lasting peace will come only from social justice.' The national historical particularities of the Global South allow us to foresee the future of the global North, in an inversion of the progressive ideology.

LABOR AND WORK AS AN ARENA OF PSYCHIC AND PHYSIC SUFFERING

Socio-economic coercion on workers has risen to an unbearable level, in view of the advance of the social forces of production in recent decades. The organization of labor, through new methods and techniques of labor management, is increasing the individualism of workers and, as a result, their social isolation. The so-called pathology of loneliness reigns, meaning that workplaces today are marked by cold, hostile, and meaningless environments. This greatly weakens the mental health of workers and increases the roots of work-related illnesses. Fierce competition has spread from the company floor to the workers themselves. The often-unattainable goals and objectives imposed by the organization do not, consider the difficulties encountered by workers in real work. By destroying teams, workers' groups and collectives, the solidity of cooperation, trust and solidarity between workers vanishes into thin air, decisive factors in any sector, be it metal workers or specialist nurses. Certain practices of injustice are already banalized, and such factors potentiate alienation, estrangement, anxiety, depression and, in extreme cases, work-related suicide. Contemporary work has already become an authentic stage for psychic suffering.

Back in 1870 a Report on the *Conditions of Working Classes in Foreign Countries* was presented in the English Parliament to Queen Victoria on the labor conditions faced by the ruling imperialism in each country – from the Iberian Peninsula to the Ottoman Empire, from the USA to Greece. The section on Portugal already effusively recommended indigenous workers because: 'they don't drink too much on Sundays – and therefore work well on Mondays' and 'they are content with little'. Already in 1880, La Revue Socialiste published a very different report. A bearded gentleman, who would become globally recognized, had submitted a set of 101 questions on the living and working conditions of working men and women in France, since the various public authorities and official bodies, made enquiries into everything and anything (agriculture, finance, commerce) without ever being interested in how those who worked lived. The name of this social scientist was Karl Heinrich Marx.

With a long intellectual tradition, since the end of the 19th century – the 'workers' study', or '*enquete ouvriere*' – up to the present day (from the Johnson-Forest Tendency of C.L.R. James in the USA to the autonomist operaism of the *Quaderni Rossi* in Italy via France, *Socialisme* o Barbarie of C. Castoriadis), combines the production of knowledge, living contact with workers and a revaluation of what the statistics officiate conceal, constituting a powerful tool for interpretation and social transformation. The results of the study conducted by the team of the *Observatory for Working and Living Conditions* in Portugal has revealed that the situation of the working class is at present day not auspicious: semi-periphery, cheap labor, and national decline, with about half or more of the workforce in burnout, sometimes more than half in emotional exhaustion, with labor harassment rates between 15% and 40%, in debt (70% on average), with work conflicts standing out as a determinant of sickness at work.

Globalization has restructured the world dynamics around what is a regressive reconfiguration of national societies, marketization and precarization of labor relations, degradation, and destruction of the whole social metabolism of human and nature. Furthermore, it has caused an obscene financialization, economic dislocation, an exponential increase in forced labor immigration flows, the indebtedness and disintegration of families, the intensification of the exploitation or spoliation of living labor, the brutal alteration of rural-city relations due to the international capitalist mode of production. To top it all, a tremendous crisis of hegemony of those 'from above' emerged combined with an unprecedented crisis of direction of those 'below'. What has occurred is not a natural catastrophe, but rather a social tragedy, which could have been avoidable before and, fortunately, surmountable today. But to really overcome this organic crisis, it is indispensable that a radical social critique takes its time and place. Therefore, renewed forms of science are necessary, and it is in this context that the program of global social enquiry, a plan of collective research for the dilemmas of the 21st century shall be presented.

Burnout is defined as a state of chronic fatigue, depression and frustration caused by devotion to a cause which does not produce expected rewards and eventually leads to a reduction in work engagement (Freudenberger, 1980), highlighting the internal pressure which describes its victims. These symptoms drive the individual to solicitude and self-giving by a subjective need, considered excessive or unrealistic. In this perspective, decompensation results from the subject's incapacity to contain himself. This is common sense and widely spread among health professionals and in many – and varied – workplaces: a model of internal demand, unstoppable impulse, or additive logic.

The burnout syndrome is also linked to the 'specific demands' of the caring professions, the so-called "human services." In fact, it is thought that the very nature of the helping relationship would play a role in the genesis of the disorders: the repeated confrontation with the suffering of others, the impossibility of responding satisfactorily to requests for help, and the inevitable and repeated failures to deal with the suffering of patients or vulnerable users would then seem decisive and would explain in part the symptomatologic picture. In other terms, the cynicism and apathy of the relationship, some emotional distancing or professional unrealization could be considered as symptomatic manifestations of the impediments of the very work of reproduction and logics of 'care' (Molinier, 2013).

Finally, many of the national and international studies on the subject are devoted to the identification of the so-called risk factors. Yet supported by a peculiar theory of stress and limited to a psychometric conception, we find a multitude of situations, personality traits, organizational or professional constraints, relational configurations etc. at the origin of the social phenomenon of burnout. Over half a century, the number of etiological factors described have increased considerably, leading to an extension of the field of the syndrome, for which it is already difficult today to identify any specific or uniform causes. To call evil by its name:

1. work intensification and work overload – i.e. the profligacy of capital and its pathogenic effects on occupational health – must return to centre stage and re-emerge as, after all, central social determinants of psychic decompensation;

2. the strategic focus on the key idea of a new dialectical aetiology, with the forefront of the stage occupied by the conflictual encounter between psychic functions and social dynamics, in the best tradition of critical and reflexive social theory, on the contact points between disorders of the individual and public issues of society,
3. a methodological critique, radically antipositivist, of the different models of analysis and interpretations to some extent heir to the scientific legacy of so-called psychometrics; especially when they are used in a way that is absolutely devoid of the antidialectical assumptions that embody their peculiar conceptions of life, of man, of the world and of knowledge.

Beyond nosological or semiotic conceptualisations, the categories of alienation, estrangement and reification are irreplaceable canons of interpretation of the theme. Recent studies, on the alienation bias, unfortunately lack all media attention. We will focus on the biases of alienation [Entäusserung] or estrangement [Entfremdung] as typically carved by classic philosophy.

FROM THE DEHUMANIZATION BY CAPITAL TO HUMANIZATION THROUGH WORK

The theme of alienation – in the face of the precariousness of living conditions and the generalization of teleworking during the pandemic – has once again brought into discussion the effects of the social production process on the world of work in its multiple aspects. The phenomenon of the 'big quit' – that is, the mass resignation from underpaid, unsafe, unhealthy and unhygienic jobs in the United States – is also part of this new devastating panorama, to which is added a new wave of strikes known as 'Striketober', among other unprecedented phenomena of the working class worldwide.

Perhaps rather than starting with Hegel, Feuerbach or even the young Lukács, it is worth taking as a point of departure the first systematic study of the subject in history, namely the worldwide notorious *Economic-Philosophical* Parisian *Manuscripts* by Karl H. Marx (Marx, 1844 (1975)).

Workers do not recognize themselves in their own productive action. Their activity represents a moment that internalizes alienation, which is present in the very process of wage labor as it is. Alienation appears initially in connection to the products of work, which corresponds to its first manifestation. Nevertheless, this condition of alienation is expressed not only by the result of the production process, but also in the act of production itself – within the productive activity. This double manifestation hinders the vital activity of work, and transforms the generic being of man, both his nature and his spiritual properties, i.e., into a being alien to him, a mere means to his individual existence, and not an end in itself.

Marx thus arrives at this critical assertion, namely that the worker only feels at one with himself outside his work, and in his work activity he feels outside himself. He feels at home when he is not working, and when he is working he does not feel at home. His work, therefore, is not voluntary but coerced; it is forced work. Instead of carrying out a vital activity to satisfy needs and desires, labor becomes a mere means of satisfying needs that are external to it.

The risks of the dehumanization of labor are brutal in this new era. A new psychic nexus has now been added to the dominance of the physical nexus of the worker. The living work of people is reconceived on the basis of the protoform of the dead work of computers, i.e. as the execution design of an immovable programming. Transformed into new appendages of computational networks designed to handle – twenty-four hours a day – seven days a week, increasing quantum of decreasing qualis, they are now individually assessed on the basis of performance indicators isolated from their experience and from the tasks to be accomplished (Dejours, 2012). Hence the spectacular increase in psychic suffering at work, is already perceived throughout the world. Informational management, with all the elements of wage subsumption but without its old guarantees, brings with it a whole new cohort of demeaning and subjection, or voluntary servitude (Antunes, 2013; Dejours & Deranty, 2010).

The new era could emancipate all non-calculable and non-programmable activities, praxis or poesis into tasks that presuppose freedom, creativity and attention to the other, but this would require relationships of direction rather than domination, i.e. the principle of the authority of the argument rather than the argument of authority degenerated into power: common co-responsibility instead of a single chain of command.

The social organisation of labor depends on producers – and not only consumers – opting for durable and sustainable production, both as regards means and ends: for what and for whom? The commodification of life spheres as a not-so-new hegemon of our epoch starts from the absolute generalisation of the concept of capital, including that of 'human capital'. In his lecture de *clôture* at the Collège de France, Alain Supiot pleaded that:

Let us not forget that the first inventor (of the idea of 'human capital') was Stalin, and that the only strict meaning one can give to it (it) is in the assets of the slave owners' account books. (Supiot, 2019, p.8., 'The most precious capital is man' and 'For a Bolshevik formation' 4/5/1935, Speeches in the Kremlin, Stalin apud Supiot).

If we do not make the most merciless criticism of the Stalinist dictatorship and Eastern societies, the expression 'labor makes free' will be an exclusive appanage of the Auschwitz thresholds.

It is no easy task to interpret such a complex, multi-dimensional and elusive universe. To understand such interpenetrations of complicated phenomena – events and processes, facts or categories, realities or representations – requires us to deal with robust transdisciplinary and multi-professional investigations into global studies in the context of various academic systems. How – as the metamorphosis of global capital increasingly integrates everyone – can we resist the pressures that drive us towards 'methodological nationalism' and fragmented studies? What would be their symmetrical equivocation, an Olympian, 'universalist' abstraction from empirical particularity?

THE NEXUS BETWEEN THE 'WORST ARCHITECT' AND THE 'BEST BEE'

The distinction made by Marx at various points in his vast work between the 'worst architect and the best bee' is famous. The first performs the social pre-ideation of the work he is going to do, while the bee 'labors', so to speak, instinctively.

This human-societal know-how has made the history of the social being a truly monumental achievement, rich and full of adventures and misadventures, challenges and dilemmas, of advances and setbacks.

The spectre of man's self-determination over himself, the other and the environment has found its place there. It is from this momentum, the widening of natural barriers, that freedom is founded. Labor became a moment of socio-metabolic mediation between humanity and nature, thus social being and natural being, and the starting point for the constitution of the social being. The assertion is supported by Marx, Lukács, Vygotsky and many other classical thinkers, but despite the crude expository mode, it is even more conspicuous from Friedrich Engels' The Dialectics of Nature (Engels, 1934) or, specifically, The Part Played by Labor in the Transition from Ape to Man (German: Anteil der Arbeit an der Menschwerdung des Affen, 1876), a work that had its scientific reputation somewhat disturbed for years.

The true recovery as a scientific piece would come not from social historians and/or political economists, but from natural scientists.

In 1975, Stephen Jay Gould, writing in Natural History, openly celebrated the evolutionary theory in Engels' work, who emphasised the role of labor, describing it as the most advanced notion of human evolution (Gould, 2011 in: Kangal, 2020, p. 18-19) Gould extended his argument, by pointing out that all theories of human evolution were theories of "gene-culture coevolution" and the best case for that was Engels' (1876) essay where he demonstrates the intimate relationship between human labor and nature, a nexus that, if disrupted, would be devastating for humanity, as well as for the other species on the planet. For Gould, our advantage over the environment comes from the fact that we already have the benefit of previous labor ideation, precisely that which allows us not only to live in society but to 'produce society itself', as Maurice Goudelier would say.

Marx demonstrated that labor is fundamental in the life of men because it is the condition for their social existence. While individuals transform their external nature, they also alter their own human nature in a process of reciprocal transformation that turns social labor into a central axis of self-development and of human-social sociability. However, labor is founded on a double, rather contradictory, character. On the one hand, it is a founding moment of human life's process of humanization or hominization; on the other hand, capitalist society has transformed it into wage labor. That which was the founding end of social being now becomes a means of subsistence. Labor power then becomes a commodity, albeit a special one, whose purpose is to create new commodities and thus valorize capital. It becomes a means and not the first necessity of human self-realization.

It is worth a short paragraph to return to the usefulness of labor – which fulfills us – and the abstraction of labor, which alienates us. There were commodities in other societies, but it is in capitalist society that commodity is the dominant form. A sack of wheat has a material content, whether in feudalism or capitalism, its social form differs (it is tithe or tribute in feudalism, and commodity in capitalism). In feudalism it is produced to pay tribute or tithes; in capitalism, in an association of free men (socialism), it is a sack of wheat produced to satisfy human needs. The product of labor takes the form of a commodity in capitalism, it is produced for accumulation and not to satisfy needs, which generates useless production, waste of energy in production methods like surveillance and quality control, simplified mass production, which removes creativity and inserts the separation between manual and intellectual labor. All of this generates the feeling of useless labor. In capitalism it is the abstraction of use-values that enables commodity exchanges. What is left when we abstract all useful properties? Not a particular labor, a chair, a sack of wheat, but abstract human labor. It is evident that all societies need to divide labor, the question is how is this done? This degree of alienation has reached new heights with neoliberalism and the proletarianisation of liberal professions, which have now been Fordised:

In France there is an absolutely tragic deterioration in the relationship between teachers and students, because the volume of work that falls on teachers today is administrative work, management work. They produce data to enter it into the computer, to be able to provide the data that managers need all the time to direct and dominate teachers. It is the administrators who dominate the teachers. It is the administrators who direct the work of the doctors. It's unbelievable! And the doctors and nurses spend more and more time of their working day entering data, because the managers are incapable of producing themselves the data on the effective work of the nurses, doctors, assistants, psychologists and physiotherapists. Therefore, they force the physiotherapist, the psychologist, the nurse and the doctor to produce data and enter them into the computer. And if they don't enter that data they can't even prescribe medicine to a patient in hospital. It's diabolical! And all these people are obviously suffering, because that's not why they became nurses, that's not why they became doctors. This ethical suffering takes on monstrous proportions today and is particularly dangerous. It is dangerous because if I accept to participate in acts that my moral sense disapproves, then there is the risk that, at the expense of betraying others, at the expense of betraying the patient, at the expense of betraying medical ethics, I end up betraying myself. And the betrayal of oneself can very quickly degenerate into self-hatred, into contempt for oneself. This is how suicides appear in the workplace. Ethical suffering is the key element in understanding the emergence of suicides in the workplace (Dejours, 2021, p. 97).

With the advent of the capitalist system, there was an essential transformation that altered and complexified human labor. This dual character present in the labor process that simultaneously invents and subordinates, emancipates and alienates, humanizes and alienates, offers autonomy but subordinates, liberates and at the same time also enslaves, has been treated in various ways in Marxist writings from the Economic-Philosophical Manuscripts to Capital (Marx 1844, 1867). From the theory of alienation to the fetishism of commodities, when highlighting the real subsumption of labor to capital or reification, the categories do not fail to problematize the critique of the political economy of capital or the emancipation of labor-being; from 'estrangement' – in the Grundrisse – to 'surplus value' in the Critique of Political Economy, which is to say, from its first exploratory drafts to the magnum opus Capital.

THE "REAL OF WORK"

The psychodynamics of work offers a theoretical and practical tool to improve the relationship between man and labor and hence respond to the social issues generated by labor problems, from the nexus between work organization and psychic functions. The new forms of management of the social organization of work cause social pathologies. Born from the encounter between ergonomics and psychoanalysis in France, at the end of the 1970s, the psychodynamics of work scholarship investigates workers' defense strategies against these harmful situations at work. This strand seeks to explain and understand the malefices of work on the processes of psychosocial decompensation and health. The psychodynamics of work is an intervention aiming at transformation of the work organization by the tool of collective elaboration, with the involvement and upon the request of the workers' representatives (Ganem, 2011). Psychodynamics of work is based on a fundamental assumption, that workers' actions always have an unpredictable component, therefore work processes cannot be fully planned. Activity ergonomics studies have shown that there is always a discrepancy between what we call the preset work, i.e. the goals and tasks assigned to the operators and the actual activity, i.e. what the workers actually end up doing.

This sensitive divergence was very often attributed to the irresponsibility and incompetence of the workers, or to shortcomings in the organization of work. It is commonly assumed that if the work is 'well-defined' and/or organized, and if workers scrupulously carry out the instructions, the production process can run smoothly. However, the various studies carried out in the field of 'labor science' have refuted this thesis. No matter how well designed, parameterized or defined it may be, no organization can anticipate all unforeseen events. There are and always will be accidents, which cannot be anticipated by work organization. In the psychodynamics of work (Dejours, 2012) this set of imponderables is called 'real work', which refers to everything that is beyond mastery, and technical and scientific know-how.

Ergonomic analysis of work precisely describes the activity carried out in the action of work precisely, based on observation. However, a considerable part of work is not directly observable, such as the workers' thoughts. To access the hidden dimension of work, particular approaches are needed, such as the analysis of the communication act of those who work.

One needs to improvise to overcome the vicissitudes of real daily working life. Therefore, work is fundamentally the action of inventing new ways to circumvent the prescription (Demaegdt and Rolo, 2013) . Labor is defined as what the individual must give in order to achieve the objectives assigned. One must add of their self to solve what had not been contemplated by the official planning. Therefore a universal and decontextualized typology of socio-human work cannot be simply deduced from previous studies or theoretical models. Any work context is unique and singular. Any research in the field of human labor must consider the 'work enigma', thus understand the operational modes developed by the worker to mitigate the discrepancy of prescribed and actual work.

WORKLIFE IN A GLOBALLY EMANCIPATED SOCIETY

Labor is our main marker of human nature and the origin of social happiness – the Alpha and Omega of human history. Since the defeat of the revolutions of the 1970s, the hegemonic ideas about labor envision it as torture, something painful and as something necessary to survive. With the absence of labor, survival shall be guaranteed by the defense of social assistance to guarantee minimum (degrading, in fact) physiological survival. Indeed, this idea is so strong that most social-democratic programs today, and the smaller political formations to the left of them (even the so-called 'revolutionary left'), have been advocating unemployment benefits rather than full employment for all.

For most people, in the capitalist system, as we have seen, work is tiring, disconnected from thought, repetitive, and represents a place of competition, harassment, injustice, self-alienation, resulting in demotivation and desocialization of the individual. There is only one thing worse than a bad job, not having a job. Because work is the root of everything in us, of language and thought, of doing and knowing how to do, through the well-being or unease it causes in our family, social and affective relationships.

In a word, work is the central force of human societies as such. But since the 1980s, with the triumph of neoliberalism, which, let's not forget, was embraced by social-democratic and socialist parties, labor has been losing its central place. The worst of these is the widespread feeling of subjection of these new non-subjects.

Work must be a field of struggle for individuals who are aware of their rights and the need for their action, and not a field of subjection for victims who don't consider themselves worthy of creative, dignified, exciting work. Who do not depend on passive state assistance, as they go from being subjects to victims, without historical strength? Where today we see torture, quoting the Greeks after Aristotle, we can and should see pleasure, quoting the Greeks after Epicurus.

The great challenge for humanity is to put an end to the hard work. Only when machines built by workers shall be put at the service of giving everyone in the world the right to creative work, without separation between thinking and executing, will reconcile Human with themself.

The debate on socialism has been misleading, since we have always limited ourselves to criticizing capitalism, and rarely asked ourselves how we envisage other types of societies, or how we envisage a socialist society (Foster, 2017; Grespan, 2021).

Socialist, utopian and ecological thinkers have always been divided over the meaning of work in a future society. This debate goes back to classical antiquity, when Epicureans claimed pleasure in work in a creative sense, and Aristotle and his followers shared the idea of labor as torture (the Latin word 'tripallium' meaning a torture instrument is the root of words meaning 'labor' in several Latin languages: 'travail' in French, or 'trabalho' in Portugese, etc.). This debate went beyond the 19th century, and mobilized with the ideologies of anarchists, collectivists as well as other currents, questioning whether the future of labor should be the domination of creative work over the alienated, or whether the center of struggles should be the abolition of labor and the right to leisure, expressed in the work of Paul B. Lafarge, and the anarchist Bob Black. The two novels that marked this dispute, were of two vibrant literary works of utopian art, *Looking Backwards (1888)* of Edward Bellamy and *News from Nowhere* (1890) by William Morris. In *Looking Backwards*, the future of labor is a workless utopia, automation would have eliminated almost all work and humanity could devote itself to the pleasures of art and leisure, separated from working life. In *News from Nowhere*, labor remains the fundamental activity of all human beings, but transforms into creative and autonomous labor, oriented towards creative imagination, as a consequence the bourgeoisie and toil had been eliminated. Morris made his central argument that during the medieval period, particularly in England, the period of the 'victory of the master craftsmen' culminated in the Fourteenth Century. Although the beginning of the Fourteenth Century is often associated with the Black Death, Morris argued that more significant than this, and in absolute surpassing this, was the growth of freer and more egalitarian labor relations. This was the period when the development of the class of free 'yeomanry' in rural areas, and democratic, relatively egalitarian guilds of free master craftsmen in the cities, were at their highest peak.

The work performed by man involves the articulation between teleology and causality. The first refers to the moment of pre-ideation, in which the individual establishes what he intends to produce, and which are the best materials to carry out the manufacture of the object; the second refers to the objective world so that man can transform the portion of reality so that the construction of his objects is possible.

The synthesis between teleology and causality is objectification, which produces exteriorization, that is, always the new: the new object and the new man. Having already exposed some of the internal nexuses that make up the category of labor, we can turn to the role of labor as the founding category of social being. We can cite the example of the pen: an individual is faced with the difficulty of writing with the pen, so he idealizes an instrument that writes and brings in its interior the ink (teleology). After the ideation, the individual needed to observe the objects that are used in writing, and also the disposed materials that would be useful to produce the pen. After doing all these analyses, the individual manages to produce the pen – an objectification useful for the community and generalized for all individuals.

Also along these lines a very strong current in psychology was developed in the Soviet Union with authors like Vygotsky, Leontiev and Luria (Eilam, 2003).

This approach underlined the role of labor in development of the so-called higher psychological functions (Vygotsky, 1978).

Man, only began to develop the processes leading to the formation of the so-called higher psychic functions from the moment when, through labor, he began to produce instruments. This was a fundamental process for the development of consciousness and, of course, of language and signs, which contributed to the complexification – and to the mastery – of those functions that are exclusively human, such as, for example, logical memory, voluntary attention, creative imagination, provisional will and conceptual thought.

The difference between the elementary psychological processes and the so-called higher processes refers to the question that the elementary processes – language, writing, calculation, drawing – are controlled by the external cultural environment and the higher or complex processes obey an internal self-regulation, thus the development of the 'special higher psychic functions', 'which in traditional psychology are called voluntary attention, logical memory, formation of concepts, etc.' (Vygotsky, 2000, p. 29)

What is important to understand in this long process of human becoming human –is how exterior social relations are introjected as interior psychic processes. The objective tool is gradually transformed into a subjective sign. Finally, a superior psychic process becomes a complex cultural form. The expanded concept of work is linked to the development of the species-being across millennia as the development of the early childhood.

An essential condition for creating a humane society and move from the animal realm of necessity, such as pure daily survival, biological reproduction of ourselves as labor power, eating, clothing, housing, procreation toward a realm where music can be played by all, even if we are not all musicians.

Where science and great discoveries are ensured by the productive contribution of all and will be available to all. Where theatre will be part of our neighborhood gardens, which are not silent and empty dormitories. Where children will play in the street, in the squares once crowded with cars. Where we will travel by fast, safe and quality public transport Where, finally, we will free ourselves from the chains of over-living, creating a spectrum of abundance for all that allows art, poetry, creation, science to flourish, along the explosion of individual talents.

The most pertaining question is how to achieve this? How to organize a dispersed, atomized, precarious and cyclically unemployed workforce? What to do with the unions? Will unions have the capacity for renewal, or will they die along with their bureaucracies in lack of adaptation to the challenges of the new conditions? How can we have power structures parallel to the state that create social solidarity and political strength? Which parties do we need? In the end, the key question is: how to transform individual depressive hopelessness into collective civilizational strength, or into a renewed emancipatory elan?

The best conclusion to this line of thought is a quote from John Bellamy Foster:

In a prospective socialist society characterized by sustainable prosperity that recognizes material limits as its essential principle — In accord with Epicurus's notion that "wealth, if limits are not set for it, is great poverty" — I t is crucial to envision entirely new socially and ecologically reproductive work relations. The received notion that the maximization of leisure, luxury, and consumption is the primary goal of human progress, and that people will refuse to produce if not subject to coercion and driven by greed, loses much of its force in light of the deepening contradictions of our over productive, over consumptive society. The prevailing view goes against what we know anthropologically with respect to many pre-capitalist cultures and falls short of a realistic conception of variable human nature, one that takes into account the historical evolution of human beings as social animals. The motivation to create and to contribute in one's life to the social reproduction of humanity, coupled with the higher norms enforced by collective labor, provide powerful stimuli for continuing free human development. The universal crisis that marks our time necessitates an epoch of uncompromising revolutionary change; one aimed at a harnessing human energy for creative and socially productive work within a world of ecological sustainability and substantive equality. In the end, there is no other way in which to conceive a truly sustainable prosperity (Foster, 2017, p.189).

REFERENCES

Antunes, R. (2013). *The Meanings of Work* (Vol. 43). Academic Press.

Dejours, C. (2012). *From the psychopathology to the psychodynamics of work*. Academic Press.

Dejours, C., & Deranty, J. (2010). The Centrality of Work. *Critical Horizons, 11*(2), 167–180. doi:10.1558/crit.v11i2.167

Demaegdt, C., & Rolo, D. (2013). Psychopathology and psychodynamics of work [Psychopathologie et psychodynamique du travail]. *Pathologie Professionnelle et de l'environnement, 3*(8), 1–11.

Eilam, G. (2003). The Philosophical Foundations of Aleksandr R. Luria's Neuropsychology. *Science in Context, 16*(4), 551–577. doi:10.1017/S0269889703000966

Engels, F. (1934). *Dialectics of Nature*. Progress Publishers.

Foster, J. (2017). The Meaning of Work in a Sustainable Society. *Monthly Review (New York, N.Y.)*, *69*(4), 1. doi:10.14452/MR-069-04-2017-08_1

Freudenberger, H. J. (1980). *Burnout: The High Cost of High Achievement*. Anchor Press.

Galeano, E. (1973). *Open Veins of Latin America. Five Centuries of the Pillage of a Continent* (C. Belfrage, Trans.). Monthly Review Press.

Ganem, V. (2011). Relato de uma experiência de terreno de intervenção em Psicodinâmica do Trabalho [Field experience report on Psychodynamics of Work]. *Laboreal (Porto)*, *7*(1). Advance online publication. doi:10.4000/laboreal.8304

Gould, S. J. (2011). *I Have Landed: The End of a Beginning in Natural History*. Belknap Press: An Imprint of Harvard University Press.

Grespan, J. (2021). *Marx: An Introduction* [Marx: Uma introdução]. Boitempo.

International Labour Organization. (1944). *Declaration of Philadelphia*. ILO.

Kangal, K. (2020). Engels's Emergentist Dialectics. *Monthly Review: An Independent Socialist Magazine*, *72*(6), 18–27. https://stanford.idm.oclc.org/login?url=https://search.ebscohost.com/login.aspx?direct=true&site=eds-live&db=aph&AN=146780847

Marx, K. (n.d.). *Economic Philosophic Manuscripts*. Academic Press.

Molinier, P. (2013). The Work of Care [Le travail du care]. Paris: La Dispute.

Supiot, A. (2019). *Work is not a commodity. Content and meaning of work in the 21st century* [Le travail n'est pas une marchandise.Contenu et sens du travail au xxie siècle]. Collège de France.

Varela, R., & Pereira, L. (2016). Social Security, work and the State in Portugal [Segurança Social, trabalho e Estado em Portugal]. *Temporalis*, *15*, 21. doi:10.22422/2238-1856.2015v15n30p21-52

Vygotsky, L. S. (1978). *Mind in Society*. Harvard University Press. doi:10.2307/j.ctvjf9vz4

Vygotsky, L. S. (2000). *Thought and Language*. MIT Press.

Section 2

The Double Movement and Whole Personhood

Chapter 5
Paradise Lost?
Understanding Social Embeddedness Through Crisis and Violence in the Neapolitan "Land of Fires"

Teresa Panico
University of Naples Federico II, Italy

Elise Lobbedez
Emlyon Business School, France

Stefano Pascucci
Business School, University of Exeter, UK

Teresa Del Giudice
University of Naples Federico II, Italy

ABSTRACT

Since the mid-1990s, three million people living in the metropolitan area of Naples (Italy) have been facing one of the most dramatic socio-ecological crises witnessed in Western Europe. This is a crisis orchestrated by Mafia-like organizations (e.g., the Neapolitan Mafia also known as Camorra) and their interest in the illegal management of waste disposal and incineration in the shadow of a weak state, a phenomenon often referred to as the "Land of Fires." In this chapter, the authors attempt to inductively theorise from this prolonged socio-ecological crisis as an exemplar process of embeddedness of market economies in diffused illegal and violent social and economic relations. They use the Land of Fires to extend the notion of "embedded economy," building on the work of Karl Polanyi. The authors argue that this process of social embeddedness through illegal and violent practices are particularly intense in contexts of socio-ecological crises, where the expropriation of land and destruction of nature is coupled with the disarticulation of the role of the state by criminal organizations.

DOI: 10.4018/978-1-6684-2364-6.ch005

INTRODUCTION

Since the mid-90s, three million people living in the metropolitan area of Naples (Italy) have been facing one of the most catastrophic and dramatic socio-ecological crises witnessed in Western Europe. This is a crisis orchestrated by Mafia-like organizations, e.g. the Neapolitan Mafia also known as Camorra, and private businesses, due to their economic interest in the management of waste disposal and incineration. While a mixed of legal and illegal waste economy emerged, in the shadow of a weak national state, thousands of local citizens have initiated public protest and grassroots movements to oppose to the impact of the crisis on their health and the surrounding environment. This well-documented phenomenon has been labelled the 'Land of Fires' (LoF) (D'Alisa et al., 2017; Berruti and Palestino, 2020), in relation to the diffused practice of burning of waste and rubbish in the streets and farmlands. However, what the LoF defines is a wider human and economic geography of continued socio-ecological and political struggles, due to the presence of an illegal and violent regime (D'Alisa et al., 2010; D'Alisa et al., 2017). This regime emerged in the general void of legality and accountability of the public authorities and private businesses in charge of managing waste (Iengo and Armiero, 2017; Cavotta et al., 2021), and more in general the absence of the (Italian) state in 'regulating' violence in this region (Armiero and D'Alisa, 2013; Berruti and Palestino, 2020). This crisis also reflects the complexity and ambiguity of institutional dynamics beyond this specific geography, where the expansion of so-called market economies generates illegal political, economic and social practices, with which they have deeply intertwined over time (D'Alisa et al., 2017). In this context, illegal waste management activities have become one of the many 'markets' for the Neapolitan Camorra, and other forms of organised crime (D'Amato et al., 2015; Lucchini and Membretti, 2016). At the same time, despite the continued crisis, and the extreme socio-ecological conditions, collective actions (e.g. NGOs) and social movements to fight these practices have struggled to emerge, with civil society organisations and political activists failing to mobilise resources in a large and effective scale (Scafuto and La Barbera, 2016; Lucchini and Membretti, 2016). Between the Neapolitan Mafia and the environmentalist activists, both the state and private businesses assumed a rather ambiguous role, contributing to the emergence of both the legal and illegal waste economies, on one hand, and the silencing and marginalisation of the environmentalist movement, on the other hand (Berruti and Palestino, 2020).

In our view, the emergence of the waste economy in the socio-ecological crisis of the Land of Fires offers an opportunity to reflect on what Karl Polanyi (1944) defined as the 'double movement' and the processes of embeddedness and dis-embeddedness of an economy. The double movement is often described as a two-stage mechanism (Goodwin, 2018): first, a process towards the creation of a market economy and the 'fictitious' commodification of key resources, such as land and labour, leading to the disruption of the social and political life of involved actors. Then, the emergence of a spontaneous 'counter-movement' which Polanyi indicates as stemming from the need of the involved actors to oppose the commodification process and to (re)establish socio-political relations and re-embed the economy in the social and political life (Polanyi, 1944). However, in the case of the waste economy of the Land of Fires we also observe another dimension in which 'the oscillation' between commodification and de-commodification takes place, because this is an economy in which the *embeddedness* process unfolds in diffused illegal and violent social relations, affecting various groups and organizations, and of which we still know very little. So, we suggest, the double movement does not only take place in the economic, social and political (environmental) spectrum of our life, but also in the legal and illegal dimension, as well as the violent and non-violent dimension, adding an interesting and so far, unexplored dimensions to the analysis of processes of embeddedness. Based on this intellectual premise and given the rich empirical context of the LoF crisis, our work tackles the broader question of whether we can better understand the emergence of an intertwined legal and illegal (waste) economy by mobilising both Polanyi's notions of anthropological and economic embeddedness (Vančura, 2011). In so doing, our work aims at contributing to the nascent literature on the role of institutions, and economic organisations, in the production and reproduction of socio-ecological crises, extending the rich Polanyian tradition (see Goodwin, 2018; 2022), and the different notions of anthropological and economic embeddedness, to contexts in which organised violence dominates social, political and economic life.

The chapter is organised as follows: section two presents a brief conceptual background to define our approach to embeddedness in context of diffused violence and socio-ecological crises. We then present the methodology adopted in our study. In section four, we present the key findings of our analysis. Section 5 is dedicated to the discussion of our findings and further conceptualisation of the notion of embeddedness.

EMBEDDING AN ECONOMY IN VIOLENT RELATIONS AND THE PRODUCTION AND REPRODUCTION OF *SOCIO-ECOLOGICAL CRISES*

Extant literature has started to recognise socio-ecological crises emerging in geographies of violence, where economic and social life have been exploited and violated through extended and prolonged relations of dispossession, victimization, abuse, corruption, and intimidation, amongst others (Kilby, 2013; Costas and Grey, 2019). In parliamentary democracies, contexts of crises due to organized crime are expected to be ruled and controlled by the state, producing, and reproducing the Weberian notion of 'state monopoly of violence' (Acemoglu et al., 2013; Bohm and Pascucci, 2020). However, the state can fail to establish or maintain such a 'monopoly' due to various conditions, for example historical, cultural, ethnical, and geographical reasons (Bohm and Pascucci, 2020). Moreover, the state can fail to establish or maintain its monopoly of violence as part of a wider process in which economic organisations, for example corporates, support the logic of d*is-embedding the economy from a system of legal and social relations*, by disrupting traditional forms of institutions, regulatory frameworks, and norms of social protection. In the Great Transformation, Karl Polanyi (1944) has addressed the process of embedding and dis-embedding economies through the lenses of commodification and de-commodification, and what he defines as double movement (Goodwin, 2018; 2022). Central to his argument there is the idea that an economy relying only on self-regulating markets, and anonymised relations, should be regarded as an utopic assumption, leading to provoke a 'counter-movement' and the re-establishment of some form of social structures and institutions (Block, 2003). The notion of embeddedness, in a wider Polanyian sense (Vančura, 2011; Wood 2019), is of relevance here. The key idea of Polanyi's analysis to embeddedness focuses on the relationship between the individual and society, of the place of the individual in society, and in the economy at various times in social history (Vančura, 2011). From this perspective, human nature requires that individual actions be "embedded" in social relationships, constituting the 'normal condition' of social existence throughout human history (Wood et al., 2019). However, Polnayi also mobilised an idea of 'economic embeddedness' in relation to the level (or degree) of social and political control over means of production and distribution, in a given economic organisation or economy (Vančura, 2011). He distinguished in this way, between different forms of production and distribution that are completely unaffected by forms of socio-political control, as such dis-embedded, like market economies, or more socially or politically controlled, as in the case of socialist economies (Vančura, 2011).

We argue that this Polanyian approach to the notions of embeddedness is crucial to understand the complex relation between state and organised crime in context of diffused violence. This approach offers a conceptual and analytical alternative to the Weberian notion of state monopoly of violence, to navigate the intertwined nature of an illegal and legal economy, where Mafia-like organizations, organised crime more in general, operate at the intersection of social, political and economic life. This intersectionality is a distinct factor in our view. It creates processes of commodification and de-commodification, for example of land and labour, influenced primarily by violence and subjugation, extreme alienation, and oppression where the expropriation of land and destruction of nature is coupled with diffused dispossession, public health disruption, and the erosion of the role of the state (Ağar and Böhm, 2018; Bohm and Pascucci, 2020). This dynamic is of relevance when considering how Mafia-like organizations have managed to create *markets in contexts of extreme violence, expulsion, displacement and dispossession.* Mimicking practices of necro-capitalism, these organizations thrive by dispossession and the subjugation of life to the power of death (Banerjee, 2008). Organized crime manages or protects illegal businesses such as drugs (Sandberg, 2012) or arms trafficking (Raab and Milward, 2003), but also infiltrates legal economies, creating partnerships and alliances with state representatives and private businesses (Vaccaro and Palazzo, 2015; Cavotta et al., 2021). Organized crime operates in markets such as toxic-waste processing, construction, renewable energies, banking, agriculture and sometimes control significant portions of these markets (Cavotta et al., 2021). These are (illegal) market economies that develop in parallel to legal ones. These economies tend to produce and reproduce an erosion of a collective 'sense of place' and belonging, leading to the disruption of social relations and the legitimization of dispossession and displacement for the victimised actors, with profound institutional and political implications (Scafuto and La Barbera, 2016; D'Alisa et al., 2017). In fact, when illegal and criminal practices are tolerated, or even encouraged by the absence or failure of the state to maintain a monopoly of violence, this is giving to organised crime the opportunity to 'socialise' markets based on dispossession and displacement (Armiero and D'Alisa, 2013). This process also creates conditions for a permanent socio-ecological crisis due to the positioning of the organised crime at the intersection of economic, social and political life. For example, while burning or dumping waste challenges the state's rules and norms and contradicts the very meaning of what is legal and socially acceptable, simultaneously it works as a process of legitimizing illegal practices by establishing norms emerging in the void of recognition of the state as a meaningful institution. In other words, burning and dumping waste in someone's property is violating the idea of a state monopoly of violence, while legitimizing organizations, like the Neapolitan Camorra, as an institutional and economic actor (D'Amato and Zoli, 2012; D'Alisa et al., 2017). The presence of competing legal and illegal market economies create continuous tensions not only between the state and violent organizations, but also among and between other social and economic actors, enacting processes of place dispossession, and displacement (Harvey, 2002). Looking at these tensions is of particular interest to theorize about how forms of social embeddedness emerge in the production and reproduction of socio-ecological crises (Ekers and Prudham, 2017; Ağar and Böhm, 2018; Bohm and Pascucci, 2020).

Starting from this initial conceptualisation, we engaged in the investigation of a rich empirical case based on data collected in the waste economy and socio-ecological crisis of the Land Fires in Naples (Italy). In so doing, we attempted to understand the emergence of an intertwined legal and illegal (waste) economy by mobilising both Polanyi's notions of embeddedness (Goodwin, 2018; Wood et al., 2019), and particularly the distinction between anthropological and economic embeddedness (Vančura, 2011). Based on our findings, in the discussion session we get back to this point and present our conceptualisation of embeddedness in context of violent relations and socio-ecological crises and reflect on the Polanyian notions of anthropological and economic embeddedness in contexts of organised violence, where relations of dispossession and displacement dominates social, political and economic life (Goodwin, 2018; 2022).

METHODOLOGY

Research Context

This paper is part of a broader research project aiming at understanding the complexity of the Land of Fires crisis, investigating its socio-ecological effects and particularly for providing evidence on the contamination of the environment, with the specific purpose of informing evidence-based public policies. In line with an inductive focus, this chapter reports the qualitative case study approach used to design the data collection and analysis and then to conceptualise embeddedness in context of violent relations and socio-ecological crises. Our case study focuses on how different actors, such as environmentalist activists and NGOs, the state, private businesses, and the Neapolitan Mafia (also called camorra) mobilised in the emergence of the waste economy in the unfolding of the socio-ecological crisis of the Land of Fires. This research context provided rich empirical evidence and data for our analysis and ambition to theorise processes of embeddedness of nascent market economies, in context of intense violent relations and a weak national state.

Data Collection and Analysis

We followed an inductive and interpretative approach to theorizing (Gehman et al., 2018), with an initial goal to understand, broadly speaking, processes of collective forms of protest in the Land of Fires, as well as state intervention, for example through legislative and policing acts, the Neapolitan Mafia and private businesses. In so doing, we used a chronological and process methodological approach (Langley 2009; Langley et al. 2013). When we started our data collection in 2013, the research team wanted to develop a case study and to map out the dynamics of the crisis through a longitudinal perspective. Two of the authors grew up in the metropolitan area of Naples, providing rich experience of and access to different actors involved in the crisis, local political activists, journalists and bloggers, as well as NGOs and social collectives. Hence, the research team collected data using multiple sources, starting from a wealth of secondary data, particularly archival data from researchers, journalists, bloggers and documentaries. Then the authors integrated these sources by interviewing activists and farmers. Table 1 below summarizes the types of data collected.

Table 1. Overview of data sources

Category	Data Sources	# Entries
Secondary data		
Press articles *Documentaries*	*Newspapers, blogs* *Web, TV*	25 12
Archival documents	*EU, Italian National parliament, regional council*	45
Academic publications	*Journal articles, chapters and monographs (books)*	34
Primary data		
Interviews	*Interviews with activists*	3
	Interviews with farmers representatives	2
	Interviews with farmers	11

In our analysis, we relied principally on retrospective accounts to reconstruct responses to the crisis, and any form of protest in the area or in relation to Land of Fires, starting from to the origin up to the date of the interview. First, we interviewed actors about their first-hand knowledge of the crisis and asked the same questions to all our key informants. Second, we asked informants to recall specific events rather than generalized information or opinions. Last, to reduce hindsight bias, we asked informants to remember a time when they thought that the Land of Fires crisis started, any episode that had affected the actors, events related to social unrests in the specific neighbourhood or area, and any other critical events. Ultimately, these interviews provided rich data on how interviewees experienced the crisis and how they positioned themselves with regard to contestation waves. Besides, to triangulate the data and to prevent the inaccuracy addressed above, we gathered a consequent data set based on multiple types of archival documents. Data encompasses a large variety of formats, amongst which newspapers articles, activist blog posts and public authorities archival documents including regulations, national and public laws, public reports, documentary videos, press releases, radio and television shows and press articles. This data helped not only to better comprehend the context in which the Land of Fires crisis arose but also to observe the different actors involved and their public positioning.

FINDINGS

Our findings inform our research focus on understand and theorize processes of embeddedness in a geography of socio-ecological crisis located in the heart of the metropolitan area of Naples. In this geography, an intertwined legal and illegal market economy has been established to manage waste, and at the same time defines an example of *contexts of extreme violence, expulsion, displacement and dispossession*. This analysis has helped the research team to identify the key turning points of the crisis and the key thematic dimensions in terms of embeddedness processes. In this section, we first present the chronological narratives of the crisis, using temporal bracketing. Then, we present how key events informing the crisis relate to forms of social, political and economic resistance and mobilization, particularly looking at the role of social movements, the state, private businesses, and Mafia-like organizations.

Temporal Analysis: Emergence of an Intertwined Legal and Illegal Waste Economy

In this section, key events characterizing the socio-ecological crisis of the Land of Fires have been reconstructed, documented and succinctly narrated. Figure 1 presents a timeline and overview of the key stages of the crisis in the Land of Fires, from its origin into the recent years.

Period I (80s – 1994): Emergence of the Illegal Waste Economy and Commodification of Land

The first stage of the crisis unfolded for roughly two decades, from the early 80s until the mid-90s, through illegal practices involving the Neapolitan Mafia organizations operating in the area of Naples and Caserta and connected to the increased demand for managing industrial waste streams, both nationally and internationally (Iacuelli, 2007; Armiero and D'Alisa, 2012). This first stage of the crisis can be considered as 'silent', unfolding 'under-cover', and without significant evidence of 'state interventions' to contrast the illegal activities, while the protest and opposition from civil society organizations is confined to the activism of a few environmental NGOs (Armiero and D'Alisa, 2012). This is the stage where an illegal market economy is established, at the intersection of the state inability to control violence and legality in this region, the interest of private businesses to dispose toxic and costly waste, and the limited capacity of environmentalists to contrast this process. The key process here is the commodification of land as 'space' for disposing the illegal waste streams, from creation of non-authorised/illegal landfills in farmlands, to the use of former mining sites and industrial estates, to the diffusion of micro-dumping and burning in peri-urban areas and neighbourhoods.

Figure 1. Timeline and key events of the socioecological crisis

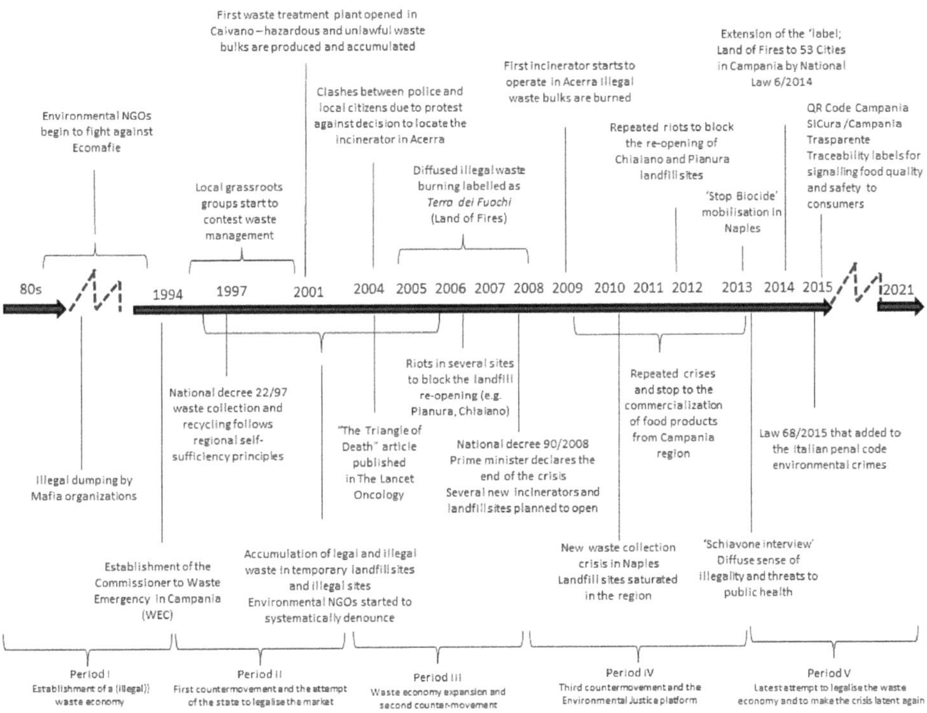

Period II (1994 – 2001): First Countermovement and the Attempt of the State to Legalise the Market

In 1994, the central government declared a regional waste emergency and delegated full power for waste management in Campania to a special authority: the Committee for the Waste Emergency (CWE) in Campania. A stage of formalised and politicized crisis began (Armiero, 2008; Armiero and D'Alisa, 2012). The Italian national parliament and government formally had to recognise the inadequacy of the regional council to address the waste management problems, amid increasing concerns for public health, and evidence of the connection between illegal waste management and dumping in peripheral urban areas and farmlands, and the activities of the

Neapolitan Mafia (D'Alisa et al., 2010). The reason behind the formalization of the crisis was the evident inability of the Campania's Regional Council to comply with rules and norms set in the Regional Law 10/1993, in particular the lack of the planned Regional Waste Disposal Plan, while the disposal capacity of the region was decreasing drastically (D'Alisa et al., 2010). In 1997 the crisis spread out dramatically also as a consequence of the national government decree 22/97 "Implementation of Directive 91/156 / EEC on waste, Directive 91/689 / EEC on hazardous waste and Directive 94/62 / EC on packaging and packaging waste". This act of national legislation introduced the obligation to implement a recycling plan at regional level through the management of 'separate waste collection streams' and within the administrative boundaries of the region. While this top-down approach had the purpose of mitigate the waste management crisis in Campania, it created the opposite effects, and in fact it exacerbated the crisis due to the absence of a system of collection and treatment plants, making the efforts of the population to differentiate waste steams useless, and imposing to continue to use landfill sites. In 2000 FIBE, a consortium of Italian and German enterprises, won a public tender for the construction of two incinerators and seven plants for transforming waste into refuse derived fuel, i.e. combustible waste blocks known popularly in Italy as "ecoballe", with the state outsourcing the control of the management of the entire waste cycle to private corporations (Armiero and D'Alisa, 2012). The system of public bids and tendering, such as the one awarded to FIBE had the purpose of legalise the waste market, also in light of emerging concerns form environmentalist NGOs and a nascent platform of grassroots movements opposing the waste management approach of the state and the CWE. However, this process failed to tackle the crisis by seeking long-term and participatory solutions, creating an ineffective, opaque and equally lucrative waste economy. The procedures for assigning the bids were particularly bureaucratises and lacking forms of basic transparency, and most importantly of social and environmental justice. For instance, the CWE awarded the tender to FIBE, based on the 'lowest cost of the project' principle, instead of seeking the 'most effective and efficient technology and equipment' rule. The tender also indicated a ''delivery or pay'' provisioning scheme for the regional municipalities, thus requiring each municipality to send a certain amount of garbage to the incinerator or pay a penalty, has contributed to the low rate of recycling in Naples and Campania (D'Alisa et al., 2010; Armero and D'Alisa, 2012). In parallel, waste bulks ('eco-balle') were produced without meeting the legal standards to be burned in the incinerators. Without incinerators, an ineffective waste collection, all existing landfill sites in the region reached their full capacity, and the ill-designed and treated waste bulks started to be accumulated in new sites. Moreover, without new sites and incinerators operating in the region the waste stopped to be collected in the metropolitan area of Naples and Caserta, with episodes of illegal burning and dumping spreading in many areas of the region. The scale of the crisis increased, reaching national and international attention, deeply affecting the political and social dynamics. The crisis unfolded in a vicious cycle of top-down and authoritarian decisions by the CWE and the regional council (Armiero and D'Alisa, 2012), with protests from local grassroots organizations being labelled as 'Not-In-My-Backyard' type of mobilization (D'Alisa et al., 2010). Several scholars have also pointed out at the hidden racism by which the crisis was narrated, with local citizens being depicted as lazy, violent, uncivil and acting as criminals.

Period III (2001 – 2008): Waste Economy Expansion and Second Counter-movement

In 2001 a new stage of the crisis started when, amid unclear public procurement rules and procedures, the first facility for waste treatment was officially opened in Caivano. As said, by tendering to FIBE waste treatment plants, CWE wanted to quickly fix the crisis by creating a cycle of differentiated waste streams, and the creation of two incinerators for energy recovery from the unrecyclable fraction of those streams. The continued emergency of the late 90s had pushed the CWE to increase the capacity of existing landfill sites in the region, and similarly the identification of new sites (Falcone et al., 2020). It is at the intersection of this continued emergency and increasing needs to identify 'quick fixes' under the pressure of a mounting tension with the local population, that the Neapolitan Mafia repositioned their business interests, profiting from both legal and illegal waste management practices (Armier and D'Alisa, 2012). Moreover, the more the pressure was mounting from below, the more urgent public interventions needed to be actualized, facilitating a rather scattered and ineffective public decision-making process (D'Alisa et al., 2010). The announcement of the opening of the first waste treatment plant, and the start of the construction of the first incinerator in the municipality of Acerra, a dozen kilometres away from Naples, fuelled the protests from local citizens and collectives (Falcone et al., 2020). Furthermore, the production of waste bulks not compliant with national and European environmental standards, created de facto a chain of illegal waste treatment practices within the boundaries of the state activities. The absence of any functioning incinerator also meant the rapid accumulation of waste bulks that were known to be toxic and dangerous for public health. In 2004 a prominent group of scientists published a paper in Lancet Oncology journal, indicated a disproportioned distribution of health risks, and cancer particularly, in the area of the crises, now labelled by the scientists as the 'Triangle of Death' (D'Alisa et al., 2010; Falcone et al., 2020). The report brought to light the detrimental socio-ecological conditions affecting public health as determined by several years of illegal waste disposal and landfill, coupled with diffused ecological problems. The need to identify areas to store the waste bulks led to the creation of 'temporary' open-air warehouses in former landfill sites or newly identify sites, mostly in using farmland in the metropolitan areas of Naples. In parallel, mounting evidence of the wrongdoing of the Neapolitan Mafia was becoming accessible to the wider public. The idea of considering the metropolitan area of Naples and Caserta, a wide contaminated area was making ground in the public opinion as well as in the political debate.

An intertwined illegal and legal waste economy is established and cemented at the intersection of the state intervention, private businesses and Neapolitan Mafia interests in this period. This 'movement' to further expand the waste economy, perpetrated by both 'legal' and 'illegal' actors, defines the emergence of the second 'counter-movement', this time originated and enacted by grassroots movements and environmental activists. During the period between 2004 to 2008 several clashes between local activists and the police took place, including riots at landfill sites in the region. Quite dramatic is the episode of significant police violence that took place on August 29, 2004, in Acerra at a demonstration against the building of the incinerator (Armiero and D'Alisa, 2013). Violent repression of citizens' protests took place in various sites through this period, and again in 2008 violent clashes were witnessed in Chiaiano and Pianura, again against citizens who were protesting the re-opening of landfill sites. In between 2002 and 2008, several grassroots organizations were established in this period, such as the Campania Network for Environment and Health (RCSA) and Waste Regional Coordination (CO.RE.RI), against the mounting evidence of the environmental and public health risks (see next section for a more detailed analysis of these organizations). However, and against any evidence, at the end of 2008 the Prime Minister, representing the national government, declared that the waste management crisis was over, and issued the Decree 90/2008. This legislative act authorised the establishment of ten new landfills, the building of four new incinerators in Campania, and the ordering of the national military to monitor waste facilities now defined as areas of national strategic interest and creating limitations to forms of protest and oppositions from activists (D'Alisa et al., 2010).

Period IV (2009 – 2013): Third Countermovement and the Environmental Justice Platform

Despite the numerous attempts to keep the emergency under control, and the opening of the first incinerator in Acerra in 2009, a new state of emergency was again declared in 2010, when waste collection was interrupted in the city of Naples due to the saturation of landfill sites. The need to identify new sites re-emerged in the public debate fuelling new forms of protests in the municipalities listed as suitable places. Both landfill sites and areas to store the waste bulks for the incinerators start to be placed in farming areas, while previously dismissed sites were re-opened in attempt to increase the regional capacity to stock waste. The decree 90/2008 and the violent riots in Chiaino and Pianura of the same year had accelerated the 'militarization' of the crisis by the state and particularly the CWE. Several organizations formed wider alliance to contrast the oppressive dynamics with the state. Collective forms of protests were embedded in diverse networks of activists and socio-political platforms due to the activism of local grassroots organizations in several municipalities in Campania, as well as Naples (Falcone et al, 2020). From these platforms, the 'Stop the Biocide' movement emerged to claim Environmental Justice to all citizens in Campania, and against the authoritative approach of the CWE and the state. In 2013, a huge mobilisation was organised in the city of Naples, probably representing the peak of street mobilization of the movement (Falcone et al., 2020). The crisis also affected groups that were not so active in previous periods, and particularly farmers and their representatives. During 2011 and 2012 the crisis had spread out into the 'countryside', and in 2013 a new stage of the crisis emerged, this time impacting the farming communities more directly. In an interview to a national media, the former head of one of Neapolitan Mafia organizations, Carmine Schiavone, declared that the practice of illegally landfill toxic wastes in farmlands around the urban fringe and countryside had started in the 80s and had been more extensive than the public authorities had thought, or NGOs has denounced. Despite the protests and contestations, and the attempt of farmers' organizations to enact food quality control and safety measures, as well as the support of national and regional authorities, many farmers were confronted with the prospect of economic bankruptcy, being unable to commercialise their products. This time, professional organizations and farmers representatives guided a parallel form of protest and lobbied both national and regional authorities for fixing the crisis and deploy economic compensations. In 2013-2014 a series of actions take place to put in place a traceability and food quality system ('QR Code Campania Sicura – QR Code Safe Campania'). After much lobbying and protesting, the crisis is contained into a problem of waste management and apparently decoupled from safety and quality issues related to agri-food production.

Period V (2014 - Present): The Latest Attempt to Legalise the Waste Economy and to Make the Crisis Latent Again

From the end of 2013 the crisis changed again, involving a series of legislative acts to re-organise the approach to environmental crimes in Italy and its regional administrations. In November 2013, for example, the massive mobilization in Naples forced the national legislator to declare the burning of waste a crime (Law Decree 136/2013), while before it was considered only a misdemeanour (Falcone et al., 2020). It also had indirectly contributed to introduce a new title in the Italian penal code dedicated to environmental crime (D'Alisa et al., 2017). After decades of political struggles and postponement, the movement for Environmental Justice in Campania forced an acceleration of the approval process, and the related legislative act of the Law 68/2015 (Falcone et al., 2020). In parallel, the regional council issued a resolution to update the Urban Solid Waste Management Plan, and to build new and more efficient biological treatment plants and enhance the recycling system at regional level. Although forms of collective protest are still present in various events, particularly in relation to the decision to build a biological treatment plant for the organic fraction in the industrial zone of Pomigliano d'Arco, near Acerra, they become dispersed, fragmented and sporadic. With the beginning of the Covid-19 emergency, in 2020, and a series of lockdowns and restrictions on mobility, forms of collective protest have practically disappeared.

An Intertwined Illegal and Legal Waste Economy Emerging From a Geography of Diffused Violence

Our chronological analysis maps out the key periods in which we observe the production and reproduction of a geography of socio-ecological crisis, affecting the territory of the Land of Fires over the past 40 years. Our data indicate a first stage of latent socio-ecological crisis, with the state, private businesses and Mafia organizations actively articulating their 'waste economies' amid an accumulation of social and political unrest. Then, we observe a stage of further expansion of an illegal waste economy, embedded in diffused relations of violence and dispossession, with the state attempting to legitimise a legal market economy for waste, amid social protest and opposition to the deterioration of public and environmental health. Then, a final stage of the crisis, where the legal and illegal markets are socially and economically intertwined neglecting forms of social participatory mechanisms or democratic processes. This quote summarises the overarching process:

The direct involvement of citizens in the development of the waste management plan is completely absent in Campania. Indeed, the 1994 declaration of the state of emergency regarding waste management has imposed an authoritarian system. Therefore, the environmental struggles in the region should be analyzed as a crisis of democracy rather than a case of waste emergency (Armiero and D'Alisa, 2013: 58)

All these stages have been emerging through what we have identified as three critical movements and counter-movements, shaped by the relations between the state, private businesses, the Neapolitan Camorra and grassroots organisations and the Environmental Justice movement. Figure 2 visualizes these key dynamics, and how they relate to processes of embeddedness, either anthropological or economic, at the intersection of legal and illegal practices. The first movement and countermovement is characterised by the state *attempting at establishing legal 'market's for waste collection and management*, by minimizing the relevance and urgency of the crisis, focusing solely on urban waste, and delegitimizing social unrest and protest through soft repression. The Neapolitan Mafia, instead, was focused on disrupting legal markets and facilitating continued crises for establishing illegal practices to manage waste, profiting from the illegal practices of burning and dumping waste. This is the stage where the waste commodification is coupled with the commodification of the land needed for the establishment of the illegal market economy. We identify this stage as *the emergent articulation of State – Mafia embeddedness of the waste economy (Theme 1)*, in which social unrest and contestation was accumulated amid illegal practices from both the state, private businesses and the organized crime:

The case of the struggles over garbage disposal and incinerators in Campania [...] is the by-product of the combination between the inefficiency and corruption of local institutions and the criminal activities of the Neapolitan mafia, the camorra. (Armiero, 2008: 6).

Our findings indicate that a process of production and reproduction of a geography of crisis was shaped by the state increased authoritarianism to establish a market economy of waste, based on state-support of corporate investments, and amid evidence of its inefficiency and lack of democratic procedures. Hence, while the State is 'dis-embedding' the waste economy from its social context, away from the citizens who are embodying the crisis, with the deteriorating of their health and living conditions, the Mafia organizations are deploying all their strengths to socially and economically embed an illegal market economy, and create fixes to the crisis. What is emerging in this stage are the conditions for the establishment of an economy of violence and dispossession, enacted in parallel by the state, private businesses and the Mafia organizations:

[...] the authoritarian regime had the social effect of fuelling the resentment of the local communities by excluding them from decisional processes and undermining the participation of the uncorrupted segment of the population. People from the Land of Fires found themselves trapped between the militarization of their area by the national government and the spread of criminal organizations engaged in the illegal quarrying of building materials, producing quarries extremely well suited to recycling as unauthorized waste dumps (Berrutti and Palestino, 2019: 279)

In 2008, despite the evidence of an unresolved crisis, the garbage accumulating in the streets of Naples, and the need to provide quick fixes, the State escalated the level of intervention and *control of the waste economy through a coercive and observable repression* (Earl, 2003). In parallel, and to react to the prospect of an ever increasing number of landfill sites and incinerators, as established by the authoritarian act of the Decree 30/2008, grassroots organizations and social collectives formed a wider and more visible platform, an articulated social movement for Environmental Justice, *to re-affirming the need of a legalised waste economy*, reclaiming the right to use the territory and the farmland to enhance both public and environmental health, thus emphasizing the relevance of webs of relations between humans and the environment (Armiero and D'Alisa, 2013). In parallel, Mafia organizations continued their *institutional and social manoeuvring to keep exploiting the waste economy and the commodification of its resources, particularly land,* and navigating through legal and illegal practices to take advantage of the expansion of the waste crisis:

The architects of this plan appeal to modernization, scientific knowledge, and promise a win-win scenario in the form of monetary compensation and/or jobs for the communities sacrificed to host the waste infrastructures. They characterize the Environmental Justice activists in the opposite way technophobic, unscientific, and NIMBY-oriented. (Armiero and D'Alisa, 2013: 61)

This is a stage of *emerging of social embedded illegal markets and the establishment of a geography of dispossession and violence* (Theme 2). While citizens organized in groups of protesters were accused to support or even being mobilised by the organized crime, creating a false sense of blurriness between activists and the Neapolitan Mafia's practices, the state and private businesses were illegally producing waste bulks, bringing illegal practices within the boundaries of 'legalized procedures', and Mafia representatives increasingly investing in side activities to profit from public tenders and procurement schemes.

When the dumps were managed by the Camorra, no one has ever opposed them . . . Our right to be cowards includes the possibility to protest only if on the other side there is the law, which does not scare us too much (original citation from Durante 2008 reported in Armiero and D'Alisa, 2012: 61).

The final stage of the crisis, after the great mobilization of 'Stop the Biocide' movement in 2013, is characterized by a profound *re-organization of the waste economy* enacted by the state, private businesses, and the Neapolitan Mafia, contributing to the *emergence and establishment of an intertwined (mixed) economy of legal and illegal waste management* (Theme 3).

Figure 2. Chronological themes around the emergent of an intertwined legal and illegal waste economy

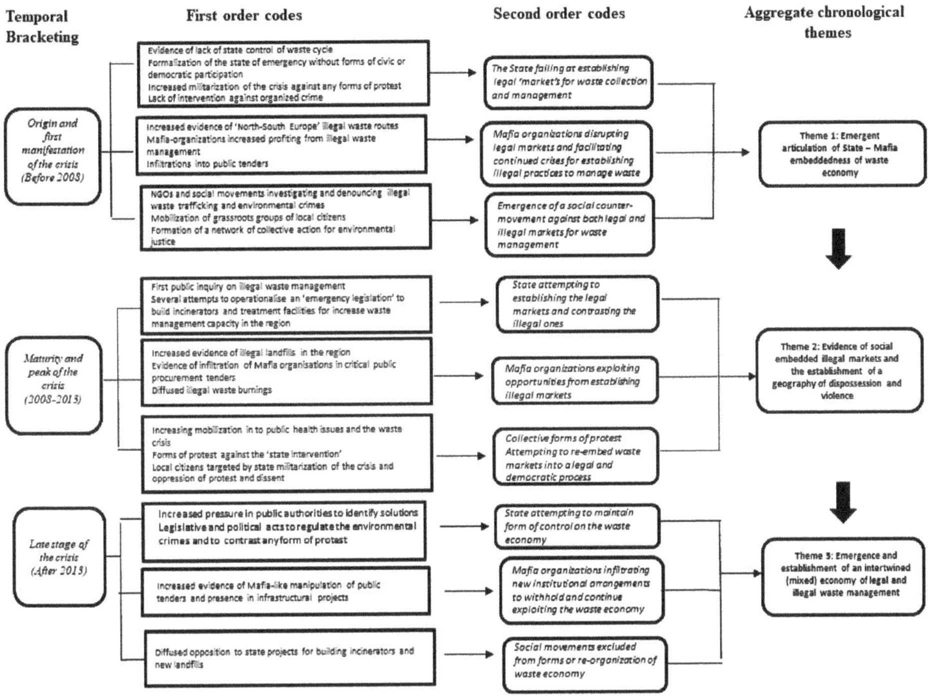

DISCUSSION AND CONCLUDING REMARKS

Our findings narrate the emergence of a waste economy in the socio-ecological crisis of the Land of Fires. Our interpretative approach has led the research team to identify key dynamics between the involved actors and to anchor their interpretation and conceptualisation with the Polanyian notion of 'double movement': a processes of embeddedness and dis-embeddedness, commodification and de-commodification, in the making of an economy in a given historical and social context (Goodwin, 2022). Particularly, our findings indicate the presence of multiple and recursive 'oscillations' – e.g. commodification/de-commodification processes - which we believe are key to understand, and thus conceptualise, why an illegal and legal economy may emerge.

In the analysed case of the emergence, establishment and expansion of a waste economy in the Land of Fires, we observe that these 'oscillations' are taking place in a geography of diffused (pre-existing) illegal and violent relations, affecting various groups and organizations. We believe this is a key point to begin the conceptualisation of the socio-ecological crisis and the establishment of the waste economy. Particularly our inductive work supports the further conceptualisation of the Polanyian idea of (dis-)*embeddedness* of a market economy, however particularly concerning contexts of diffused illegal and violent social and economic relations. We believe this adds to the nascent literature in this specific field of inquiry, for instance looking at dynamics of commodification of land and natural resources in the Global South, as well as the exploitation and marginalisation of indigenous communities, minorities and various social groups in market economies (Goodwin, 2018; 2022).

Contribution to the Notion of Double Movement and Embeddedness

Our first attempt to extend the notion of 'embedded economy' builds on the initial work of Polanyi (1944), presented in the Great Transformation, and extensively debated in the economic sociology literature (Goodwin, 2018). Particularly we focus on the idea, mobilised by some scholars in recent years (Vancura, 2011), of the distinction present in Polanyi's work between an 'anthropological' and 'economic' embeddedness. If we look at on our findings, and the temporality of events and 'oscillations', this distinction can become useful to understand the role of the different actors in the crisis, and the overarching process of emergence and establishment, and further expansion of a waste economy. In fact, the first tension between commodification and de-commodification manifest at the intersection of the economic activities of the organised crime (e.g. Neapolitan mafia), on one hand, and the state/private businesses, on the other hand. In this stage there is still very limited mobilisation of social actors, mostly confined to environmentalist NGOs. In our view, the establishment of the waste economy, as an economic mechanism to cope with the socio-ecological crisis of the waste disposal and management can be largely explained by the idea of commodification of waste and land, which takes place in the accumulation of the crisis and its first manifestation. Using a Polanyian metaphor, the waste becomes a lucrative commodity because creates the economic need of being disposed at lower possible costs, thus leading to the commodification of land, as place for disposal and incineration. This creates the condition for transforming the territory of Naples and Campania region into a 'satanic mill' of oppression, exploitation, and violence in order to produce and reproduce waste disposal of any sort. From this standpoint, the Neapolitan Mafia, with the complicity of the state and the collusion of interested businesses accelerate a process of commodification of land through dispossession, subjugation, and marginalisation of other actors, particularly farmers and local citizens, particularly by dumping and burning waste illegally. Equally, from looking at the notion of 'economic embeddedness', these criminal organisations manage an illegal waste market through social relations of diffused violence and forms of abuse and exploitation. In the initial stage of the crisis, it is the state to attempt to enact a form of countermovement, not because challenging the idea to resolve the waste management problem through a market economy approach but trying to dis-embed this economy from criminal and illegal social and economic practices. Like the idea of creating a 'duopoly' in the waste economy, the outcome of this attempt by the state is the *establishment of the waste economy, both legal and illegal, through the articulation of state-Mafia social, political, and economic relations.*

The second double movement, instead, assumes the more 'standard' Polanyian connotation, with social groups spontaneously reacting to the persistence of the socio-ecological crisis, unresolved by the newly established waste market, and exacerbated by the initial effect of the 'satanic mill': diffused pollution, land degradation, victimisation and exploitation, deterioration of public and environmental health. The increased evidence of the commodified land, coupled with the effect of deterioration of the quality of life, health, and ecology of the place, is the trigger for this reaction, which takes places prevailing in the dimension of the legal waste market. However, the economic embeddedness perpetrated by the Neapolitan Mafia to manage the illegal waste market, through violent practices of dispossession, through the expropriation of land and destruction of nature, is not directly address by the countermovement. Instead, it is the more evident overarching 'dis-embeddedness' of the overall waste economy to mobilise social unrest, making the state the more obvious target for the protest and forms of contestation. It seems to emerge an impossibility by these social groups to identify and challenge the embeddedness of practices of violence and dispossession in the social fabric of this geography. This is what we have defined as *emergence of social embedded illegal markets and the establishment of a geography of dispossession and violence.*

Finally, during the last part of the analysis crisis, the process of commodification accelerates. The state and the mafia are practically hardly distinguishable in their practices of land expropriation, dispossession, and exploitation. There is a further disarticulation or erosion of the role of the state by criminal organizations such as the Neapolitan mafia, while an increased separation and hostility manifests between social groups and movements of local citizens, the state and its representatives. Again, a new process of commodification and de-commodification takes place, at a larger scale, involving more communities and places, and creating an even larger 'satanic mill' of waste production and reproduction. This is a stage where the entire region is the 'satanic mill' where dispose, burn, dump, manage waste as economically needed. The line between what is legal and what is now is blur and practically undistinguishable to the eyes of citizens, social movements and various forms of protest that constitute the 'Stop the Biocide' platform. From their point of view, the state, private business and the Mafia organizations all key economic actors managing a profitable and lucrative waste economy. They have little or no interest to preserve public health and the environment. They have little or no interest to challenge the diffused violence and exploitation which takes place in the 'satanic mill' of the Land Fires. They can only try to oppose to the *emergence and establishment of an intertwined (mixed) economy of legal and illegal waste management.*

Looking at our study, we suggest considering to further theorise the notion of double movement. The Polanyian idea of alternating processes of commodification and de-commodification does not only affects the economic, social and political (environmental), but should also consider a legal and illegal dimension (e.g. the rules and norms in place, and more in general regulatory regimes), as well as a violent and non-violent dimension. Adding these dimensions makes the notion of double movement even more powerful and insightful, allowing scholars to navigate an interesting and so far, unexplored dimension to the analysis of processes of embeddedness. Particularly, mobilising the debate around the distinction between 'anthropological' and 'economic' embeddedness is promising (Vančura, 2011).

Contribution to Understanding Socio-ecological Crisis in Diffused Violent Relations

Based on the considerations presented so far, in this concluding section we reflect on the role of institutions and economic organisations in the production and reproduction of socio-ecological crises, extending the rich Polanyian tradition to contexts in which organised violence dominates social, political, and economic life (Goodwin, 2018). This section develops presents our considerations in two ways. First, we acknowledge the role of organised crime, namely Mafia-like organizations, as relevant actors in processes of social and economic embeddedness. The establishment of an illegal market of waste is based on the opportunity created by the state in dis-embedding the legal economy from its social context, thus creating a window of opportunity for social and economic actors, like Mafia organizations, and simultaneously using social mechanisms of violence and dispossession to embed, instead, the illegal economy. This 'movement' and 'counter-movement' assumes some conceptual relevance from a Polanyian perspective: recognizing the role of organised crime is particularly important as the state and private companies did enact limited (direct) violence themselves in the attempt to establish a legal waste economy. However, the entanglement of illegal and legal activities of our case (D'Alisa et al, 2010; Armiero and D'Alisa, 2012) indicate they contributed to (and perhaps profited from) the establishment of a geography of socio-ecological crisis.

Second and as a consequence of this first point, our studies provide a more fine-grained analysis of two distinct forms of embeddedness, often referred to as 'anthropological' and 'economic' embeddedness (see Vančura, 2011) both relevant to understand the violent access to natural resources to manage waste by different actors in the economic geography of the Land of Fires. On one hand we suggest that the state has failed to facilitate the embedding of the waste economy in a legal process of negotiation and democratic participation with social and political actors in this geography, and simultaneously identifying 'quick fixes' to the crisis even outside legally sounding procedures. On the other hand, we point at how, in the shadow of state's failures, the mafia organizations have been able to legitimise the establishment of an illegal waste economy, and to continue enhancing profit accumulation in the region. This process of dis-embeddedness and (re-)embeddedness have led to the emergence of an intertwined legal and illegal waste economy.

This result also contributes to existing knowledge that aims at unpacking the geography of socio-ecological crises, by exploring how social and economic dynamics may hinder collective responses to the crisis. Our research provides an illustration of a geography of violence and dispossession for which social and economic practices, and policies, led by co-existing legal and illegal institutionalized agents, here the Mafia and the state. This resulted in the emergence and sustaining of a major crisis while overall hampering the emergence of effective and creative responses led by civil society to the environmental issues. Our analysis suggests more specifically that the increasing clashes in the interactions between the state and the environmental justice movement elided any forms of the mafia organization regarding the crisis. Indeed, after a long period of neglect of the Neapolitan territory, the state exercised power to repress civil society collective action rather than channelled or promoted new social or economic relations to address the crisis. In that sense, the solutions led by the state remained predominantly dis-embedded from the local social context, while initiatives proposed by local communities stayed at the local level and never scaled into effective economic mechanism to tackle the crisis at regional or national level. The mafia, on the other hand, engaged in strategic ambiguity, using its positioning at the intersection of legal and illegal, mobilising form of diffused violence and oppression, to spur the crisis while remaining out of public (state and social movements) scrutiny.

ACKNOWLEDGMENT

This research was funded by LIFE11/ENV/IT/275 - ECOREMED "IMPLEMENTATION OF ECOCOMPATIBLE PROTOCOLS FOR AGRICULTURAL SOIL REMEDIATION IN LITORALE DOMIZIO-AGRO AVERSANO NIPS".

The authors would like to thank the anonymous interviewees and the dr. Luigi Zagaria for his kind and fruitful cooperation provided to carry out the survey required for the implementation of this research.

REFERENCES

Acemoglu, D., Robinson, J. A., & Santos, R. J. (2013). The monopoly of violence: Evidence from Colombia. *Journal of the European Economic Association, 11*(suppl_1), 5–44. doi:10.1111/j.1542-4774.2012.01099.x

Ağar, C. C., & Böhm, S. (2018). Towards a pluralist labor geography: Constrained grassroots agency and the socio-spatial fix in Dêrsim, Turkey. *Environment and Planning A. Economy and Space, 50*(6), 1228–1249.

Armiero, M. (2008). Seeing like a protester: Nature, power, and environmental struggles. *Left History, 13*(1). Advance online publication. doi:10.25071/1913-9632.24610

Armiero, M., & D'Alisa, G. (2012). Rights of resistance: The garbage struggles for environmental justice in Campania, Italy. *Capitalism, Nature, Socialism, 23*(4), 52–68. doi:10.1080/10455752.2012.724200

Armiero, M., & D'Alisa, G. (2013). Voices, clues, numbers: Roaming among waste in Campania. *Capitalism, Nature, Socialism, 24*(4), 7–16. doi:10.1080/10455752.2013.851262

Böhm, S., & Pascucci, S. (2020). It's Not Just About the Mafia! Conceptualizing Business–Society Relations of Organized Violence. *The Academy of Management Perspectives, 34*(4), 546–565. doi:10.5465/amp.2019.0029

Berruti, G., & Palestino, M. F. (2020). Contested land and blurred rights in the Land of Fires (Italy). *International Planning Studies, 25*(3), 277–288. doi:10.1080/13563475.2019.1584551

Berrutti, G., & Palestino, M. (2019). Contested land and blurred rights in the Land of Fires (Italy). In International Planning Studies. Routledge.

Block, F. (2003). Karl Polanyi and the writing of the Great Transformation. *Theory and Society, 32*(3), 275–306. doi:10.1023/A:1024420102334

Bobby Banerjee, S. (2008). Necrocapitalism. *Organization Studies, 29*(12), 1541–1563. doi:10.1177/0170840607096386

Cavotta, V., Palazzo, G., & Vaccaro, A. (2021). Mobilizing After Corporate Environmental Irresponsibility in a Community of Place: A Framing Microprocess Perspective. *Journal of Business Ethics*, 1–15. doi:10.100710551-021-04983-1

Costas, J., & Grey, C. (2019). Violence and organization studies. *Organization Studies, 40*(10), 1573–1586. doi:10.1177/0170840618782282

D'Alisa, G., Burgalassi, D., Healy, H., & Walter, M. (2010). Conflict in Campania: Waste emergency or crisis of democracy. *Ecological Economics*, *70*(2), 239–249. doi:10.1016/j.ecolecon.2010.06.021

D'Alisa, G., Germani, A. R., Falcone, P. M., & Morone, P. (2017). Political ecology of health in the Land of Fires: A hotspot of environmental crimes in the south of Italy. *Journal of Political Ecology*, *24*(1), 59–86.

D'Amato, A., Mazzanti, M., & Nicolli, F. (2015). Waste and organized crime in regional environments. *Resource and Energy Economics*, *41*, 185–201. doi:10.1016/j.reseneeco.2015.04.003

D'Amato, A., & Zoli, M. (2012). Illegal waste disposal in the time of the mafia: A tale of enforcement and social wellbeing. *Journal of Environmental Planning and Management*, *55*(5), 637–655. doi:10.1080/09640568.2011.620324

Earl, J. (2003). Tanks, Tear Gas, and Taxes: Toward a Theory of Movement Repression. *Sociological Theory*, *21*(1), 44–68. doi:10.1111/1467-9558.00175

Eisenhardt, K. M., & Graebner, M. E. (2007). Theory building form cases: Opportunities and challenges. *Academy of Management Journal*, *50*(1), 25–32. doi:10.5465/amj.2007.24160888

Ekers, M., & Prudham, S. (2017). The metabolism of socioecological fixes: Capital switching, spatial fixes, and the production of nature. *Annals of the Association of American Geographers*, *107*(6), 1370–1388. doi:10.1080/24694452.2017.1309962

Falcone, P. M., D'Alisa, G., Germani, A. R., & Morone, P. (2020). When all seemed lost. A social network analysis of the waste-related environmental movement in Campania, Italy. *Political Geography*, *77*, 102114. doi:10.1016/j.polgeo.2019.102114

Gehman, J., Glaser, V. L., Eisenhardt, K. M., Gioia, D., Langley, A., & Corley, K. G. (2018). Finding theory–method fit: A comparison of three qualitative approaches to theory building. *Journal of Management Inquiry*, *27*(3), 284–300. doi:10.1177/1056492617706029

Goodwin, G. (2018). Rethinking the double movement: Expanding the frontiers of Polanyian analysis in the Global South. *Development and Change*, *49*(5), 1268–1290. doi:10.1111/dech.12419

Goodwin, G. (2022). Double movements and disembedded economies: A response to Richard Sandbrook. *Development and Change*, *53*(3), 676–702. doi:10.1111/dech.12698

Harvey, D. (2002). *Spaces of capital: Towards a critical geography*. Routledge. doi:10.4324/9780203821695

Iengo, I., & Armiero, M. (2017). The politicization of ill bodies in Campania, Italy. *Journal of Political Ecology*, *24*(1), 44–58. doi:10.2458/v24i1.20781

Kilby, J. (2013). Introduction to special issue: Theorizing violence. *European Journal of Social Theory*, *16*(3), 261–272. doi:10.1177/1368431013476579

Langley, A. (1999). Strategies for theorizing from process data. *Academy of Management Review*, *24*(4), 691–710. doi:10.5465/amr.1999.2553248

Langley, A. N. N., Smallman, C., Tsoukas, H., & Van de Ven, A. H. (2013). Process studies of change in organization and management: Unveiling temporality, activity, and flow. *Academy of Management Journal*, *56*(1), 1–13. doi:10.5465/amj.2013.4001

Lucchini, F., & Membretti, A. (2016). The land of fires. Evaluating a state law to restore the narrative power of local communities. *Partecipazione e conflitto, 9*(2), 640-665.

Misangyi, V. F., Weaver, G. R., & Elms, H. (2008). Ending corruption: The interplay among institutional logics, resources, and institutional entrepreneurs. *Academy of Management Review*, *33*(3), 750–770. doi:10.5465/amr.2008.32465769

Raab, J., & Milward, H. B. (2003). Dark networks as problems. *Journal of Public Administration: Research and Theory*, *13*(4), 413–439. doi:10.1093/jopart/mug029

Scafuto, F., & La Barbera, F. (2016). Protest against waste contamination in the 'Land of Fires': Psychological antecedents for activists and non-activists. *Journal of Community & Applied Social Psychology*, *26*(6), 481–495. doi:10.1002/casp.2275

Vaccaro, A., & Palazzo, G. (2015). Values against violence: Institutional change in societies dominated by organized crime. *Academy of Management Journal*, *58*(4), 1075–1101. doi:10.5465/amj.2012.0865

Vančura, M. (2011). *Polanyi's Great Transformation and the concept of the embedded economy*. IES Occasional Paper, No. 2/2011. Charles University in Prague, Institute of Economic Studies (IES).

Wood, A. J., Graham, M., Lehdonvirta, V., & Hjorth, I. (2019). Networked but commodified: The (dis)embeddedness of digital labour in the gig economy. *Sociology*, *53*(5), 931–950. doi:10.1177/0038038519828906

Chapter 6
We Know More Than We Can Zoom:
Challenges for Young Professionals During the COVID-19 Pandemic

Anouk Mols
https://orcid.org/0000-0003-0355-9849
Erasmus University, Rotterdam, The Netherlands

Yosha Wijngaarden
Erasmus University, Rotterdam, The Netherlands

Imke Greven
Erasmus University, Rotterdam, The Netherlands

Marloes van Wijnen
Erasmus University, Rotterdam, The Netherlands

ABSTRACT

Measures to curb the COVID-19 pandemic forced many young professionals to work from (often small and sometimes shared) homes. On the basis of in-depth interviews in the Netherlands, this chapter aims to unpack how working from home in times of COVID-19 affects the whole personhood of young knowledge workers. Three important insights are provided. First, when it comes to around boundary sculpting practices, many respondents' boundary negotiations between personal and professional spheres entail personal, collective, temporal, and spatial borders. Second, interpersonal connections prove to be of vital importance because a lack of face-to-face interactions not only causes a lack of interpersonal contact and emotional connection to colleagues, but also a lack of tacit knowledge. Third, additional spheres like the public sphere are crucial for providing motivation and inspiration. This research shows that working from home can be detrimental to the whole personhood of young professionals.

DOI: 10.4018/978-1-6684-2364-6.ch006

INTRODUCTION

In the early 2020s, the global COVID-19 pandemic changed the work practices for large groups of workers within the Western world and beyond. Where millions of people set their alarms in the early mornings, ran their errands, and commuted to work almost synchronously, the measures to halt the pandemic also halted their collective behaviour in offices, classrooms, and workplaces. Instead, they mutually attuned to each other using digital means, working from their home offices, kitchens or even bedrooms, switching from cacophonous Zoom meetings to stifled solitude in seconds. The measures to stop the COVID-19 virus from spreading have harmed mental well-being and increased feelings of loneliness globally (Hu & Qian, 2021). Forced working from home affects workers' personhood and household dynamics. For instance, people can experience stress from the collapsing of boundaries between private and professional contexts, or, in other words, their home and work (Schieman et al., 2021). Moreover, enforced working from home can reduce productivity and cause feelings of isolation (Waizenegger et al., 2020). And how do people find the essential inspiration and motivation for their work when there is little to see beyond their houses' walls?

While researchers have studied the implications of working from home in times of COVID-19 for mothers or caregivers (Hjálmsdóttir & Bjarnadóttir, 2021), couples (Qian & Hu, 2021), students (Elmer et al., 2020), and precarious workers (Han & Hart, 2021), other groups have received less academic interest. One of these groups is young professionals. Young professionals are usually not burdened by demanding family responsibilities, child rearing or assisting in their childrens' online education. Yet, considering their budding careers and often relatively small-scale way of living (in solitary apartments or shared environments), they face challenges of their own. Their position in the labour market transformed from being a starting professional as part of a physical workplace to being an individual in a makeshift work environment as part of a digital team.

This transformation brings insecurity, alienation from the organisation, a dependence on digital communication platforms, a lack of inspiration and motivation to build a career, and halts interpersonal connections and opportunities. Moreover, the alienation from collective spheres caused by social distancing accelerates a trend of individualisation which is characterised by a decreasing sense of community (Faludi & Crosby, 2021). To study the precarious and challenging situation for young professionals who are forced to work remotely, this chapter poses the question: How does working from home in times of COVID-19 affect the whole personhood of young knowledge workers? Looking at the whole personhood means taking not only work and private contexts into account, but all spheres of life, and how these interact and intertwine. Specifically, this chapter poses three sub questions: 1) how do young professionals sculpt the boundaries between their private and professional spheres, 2) how do they seek to connect with their professional contacts from their – lockdown induced – private spheres, and 3) how do they cope with the lack of other spheres (e.g. the public realm) when working from home?

This chapter focuses specifically on the tensions that emerge out of the enforced working from home in times of COVID-19 which blurs the boundary between personal and professional contexts (Clark, 2000; Mols & Pridmore, 2021; Nippert-Eng, 1996), impedes the exchange of (tacit) knowledge (M. Polanyi, 2009 [1966]), and requires young professionals to retain the energy and inspiration to build and sustain a career without being able to draw upon connections to others (cf. Bhansing et al., 2018; Collins, 2020). This research takes the socio-economic context of working from home into account and follows Wood et al.'s (2019) integrated approach to K. Polanyi's notion of embeddedness by zooming in on interpersonal relations and experiences while considering how platform economies thrive on the commodification of labour and data (Grabher & König, 2020).

Building upon 22 interviews with young knowledge workers from The Netherlands. the analysis highlights how systematic changes affect the everyday work life and whole personhood of young knowledge workers. Specifically, it zooms in on three major developments: the convergence of the professional and personal spheres while having to work from (often small and limited workspaces at) home, the difficulties of establishing personal ties with co-workers for starting employees and freelancers, and the challenge of finding motivation and inspiration when working in monotonous and sedentary work settings.

BACKGROUND

Working from home is highly dependent on communication technologies. During the COVID-19 lockdown, platformed solutions for work communication, connections and collaboration became the context of almost all work practices. Regular opportunities for communication and collaboration, and sources of inspiration and motivation in a dedicated work environment were suddenly replaced by a solitary home office. This theoretical framework reflects on the implications on knowledge workers' whole personhood, the collapse of boundaries between work and professional life, work practices during the COVID-19 pandemic, and challenges regarding a sudden lack of tacit knowledge and sources of inspiration and motivation.

Digital Communication in the Context of Platform Economies

Knowledge workers were able to continue their work during lockdown situations because they can conduct their work via digital communication. For many, work communication in pre-Covid times already partly took place via the infrastructures of big tech companies like Alphabet-Google, Apple, Facebook, Amazon, and Microsoft. They shifted all communication to digital spheres when they started to do all work from home. In other words, their work is embedded in a platform society, wherein societal, social, and economic traffic primarily moves via online platforms (Van Dijck et al., 2018). Platforms (the aforementioned big five as well as many other companies) are programmable digital architectures "designed to organise interactions between users – not just end users but also corporate entities and public bodies." (Van Dijck et al., 2018, p. 4) In the platform society, private and public interest as well as commercial and public interests are almost always intertwined, while they are difficult to separate (Van Dijck et al., 2018). The business models of most platforms rely on automatically collecting and processing user data, in order to target and profile individual users as well as user groups (Van Dijck et al., 2018).

In line with K. Polanyian viewpoints, platforms can be seen as part of a global political-economic system wherein labour and data in particular are commodified (Grabher & König, 2020). The proliferation of platforms is seen as a global political-economic system and described as *platform capitalism* (Srnicek, 2017). Furthermore, Zuboff (2019) elaborates on the role of commercial data collection within this system in her account of *surveillance capitalism*. Surveillance capitalism entails a society dominated by internet companies (platforms) for whom consumer (behavioural) data form surveillance revenue which offers profits as well as informs markets in future behaviour (Zuboff, 2019). According to Zuboff (2019), this system threatens human autonomy and freedom by subjecting people to maximised extraction of personal data and using this to influence their actual behaviour. What matters here is that while shifts to platform societies and surveillance capitalism are a long-term process, the fast shift towards fully depending on platforms to conduct work changes the nature of work by adding a commercial surveillance layer to the everyday practices of (young) knowledge workers. Moreover, as indicated, the move towards working from home causes alienation from the workplace, which becomes a fictitious space rooted in a commodified system. The aim is to understand how these changes transform the whole personhood of young knowledge workers and how they are personally affected by their forced way of working on a (social) distance alienated from their work environment and sources of inspiration.

Whole Personhood and Spheres

This chapter's point of departure follows the idea of Weber (1978a) that societies are organised around several spheres, including the economic sphere, political sphere, and the intellectual sphere. In this section, particular spheres are highlighted that influence young knowledge workers. Following K. Polanyi, the economic sphere can be characterised as a market that governs through material production and reproduction of society. In other words, the economic organisation of capitalist societies entails a commodification of labour, land and money (Lacher, 1999).

Another crucial sphere is the public sphere which, as Habermas (1971) developed, is the place where public debate happens. Originally, it concerned coffee houses and salons in 17th and 18th century Europe, though many of such exchanges now occur also via mass or social media (see also Habermas, 2016, who raises some doubts on the effectiveness of especially mass communication). What is important, nonetheless, is that in the public sphere, people are exposed to new ideas and developments. Moreover, others have also included the sphere of the family, such as Gorski (2013) and Scaff (1992). Current distinctions often describe the private sphere, referring to this family sphere as well as the household.

Each of these spheres, Weber argues, have their own internal way of working, which potentially leads to clashes with other spheres. Historically, Weber's spheres functioned as a macro-level ideal-type, a means to serve as a point of orientation in research endeavours – particularly to understand and argue the increasing rationalisation of each of these spheres (Terpe, 2020). However, Terpe (2020) underscores how such spheres can also function as a means to conceptualise the life of individual actors. Collective entities, in the work of Weber, are meaningful on the individual level, and often have a decisive influence on the actions of individual people (Weber, 1978b). On a micro-level these spheres translate to individual experiences of public, professional, and personal spheres. Individuals navigate between these spheres, with some spheres taking a big chunk out of their personal life (think about a full-time workweek or care for children and the household) and others being of importance, but less prevalent in day-to-day planning and practices. This goes well-beyond the idea of increasing rationalisation of all life-spheres, but rather takes an actor-centred perspective looking at the ideas and experiences 'in the minds' of individuals (Terpe, 2020).

What is here described as whole personhood is the full human experience, in which all of these spheres have their place, but also compete for time and attention. A whole person has the agency to balance these spheres and to reach their own personal human potential. In practice, this means that individuals have the capacity to decide how to distribute their time but are also impacted by the more structural arrangement of these spheres in society. Meta as well as micro level spheres are interdependent and often interact. For instance, the economic sphere causes a commodification of time which, on a micro level, can make salaried time more pressing in the balancing of different personal spheres. While different spheres often interact or even collapse, this became more prevalent with the use of digital technologies. Digital communication allows for the collapsing of time and space and of different contexts (Pagh, 2020). More specifically, when working from home, people exist and act simultaneously in their personal and their professional sphere. The COVID-19 measures enforced social distances between different spheres while simultaneously collapsing the essence of different spheres. This is especially the case for professional and personal spheres which affects the whole personhood of young professionals. On the other hand, this collapse also hampers a full emergence in the work sphere, as face-to-face interactions, *seeing* people work and taking part in the informal practices have suddenly been carved out of day-to-day work life. In order to understand the consequences of this convergence *and* divergence of spheres and interactions, this chapter includes existing research about boundary work, tacit knowledge, inspiration and motivation, and other challenges for young knowledge workers.

Convergence: Boundary Work

The collapsing of professional and personal spheres entails a dissolving of boundaries between these spheres. For young professionals who are forced to work from home, this creates challenges and pressure. More specifically, when their home suddenly becomes the location where their personal and professional spheres collapse, they need to renegotiate the boundaries between those contexts. Boundary theory provides helpful tools to understand how workers deal with blurring boundaries. Nippert-Eng (1996) describes the concept of boundary work as “strategies, principles and practices that we use to create, maintain and modify cultural categories” (p. 564). Boundaries can be seen as sociocognitive boundaries which are permeable; elements from one sphere (category) can enter other spheres (Clark, 2000). Boundaries can be thick (strong) when they form a high and strong distinction between personal and professional life or thin (weak) when the borders between different spheres are blurred (Jahn et al., 2016). In other words, boundary work happens in an “integration-segmentation continuum” (Nippert-Eng, 1996). When home and work are fully integrated, their existence is practically the same and there are no boundaries that separate content or practices. In contrast, when one’s home and work are completely segmented, particular people, things, and tasks belong exclusively to home or work contexts. Objects, activities, and tasks are tangible markers of different spheres and of how people segment or integrate those, for instance, the use of keys can differ across employees—employees who separate work from private life might use two sets of keys, while people who integrate the two contexts might have a mixed set of keys (Nippert-Eng, 1996). Digital functionalities and tools can also be used to create tangible segmentations between work and personal spheres or to maintain integration between the two (Mols & Pridmore, 2021).

For young professionals, boundary work and engagement in boundary negotiations are challenged when they manage their work roles (e.g. as an employee), their personal roles (e.g. as a roommate or friend), and the transition between the two (Jahn et al., 2016). The greater the dissimilarity between the identities of different roles, the harder the transition between these roles (Duxbury et al., 2014). This can also be described as 'territories of the self' to classify certain aspects or context-specific versions of one's identity (Nippert-Eng, 1996). Often there are distinctions between who someone is in the home sphere and their work sphere. These distinctions are based on mentality as well as influenced by certain triggers. For example, conversations can be a trigger that blurs the boundaries between work and home territories of the self and therefore someone could choose to avoid work talk in their home (Nippert-Eng, 1996).

When people work from home, the boundaries between personal and professional spheres are automatically blurred. This brings additional challenges when it comes to boundary work and managing different spheres in life. Many people working from home find it hard to ensure that their hours and work intensity are visible to their team and management and their urge to prove themselves often creates a pressure to overwork themselves (Ciolfi et al., 2020; Wheatley, 2012). The rise of remote work over the past decades already changed ways of working for many. The COVID-19 pandemic accelerated these changes when working from home was enforced for the multitude of knowledge workers. Kerman et al. (2021) indicate that people working from home during the COVID-19 pandemic struggled to manage both home and work demands. Violations of work-home boundaries caused unfinished tasks in both spheres and decreased satisfaction about the investment across the board (Kerman et al., 2021). For working student mothers, decreased satisfaction in work, school, and home spheres had to do with the lack of dedicated and sufficient amounts of time for the demands in each sphere and the spill over between their three roles as students, mothers, and workers (Andrade & Lobo Fernandes, 2021). Especially in families with children, the spatial and temporal boundaries between home and work blurred to such an extent that they partly disappeared whereby mothers most often carried the largest load in arranging and coordinating work shifts and childcare (Otonkorpi-Lehtoranta et al., 2021). This indicates that the exceptional circumstance in the pandemic increases the pressure and demands put on home-based knowledge workers.

Divergence: Challenges of Online Communication in Working From Home

Another - yet totally different - issue with enforced digital communication is the difficulties of conveying anything beyond codified knowledge. Codified knowledge refers to explicit forms of knowledge that are formal and systematic - and that can be conveyed over large distances and stored in various types of media. Think for instance about the product specifications of a software package or formal work procedures (Nonaka, 2007). Obviously, such knowledge is relatively easily transferred in online settings. Walkthroughs or procedures for certain situations are well captured in for example word processing files and can be shared via email or digital collaboration platforms. For the exchange of codified knowledge, online work is less of a serious barrier.

Nevertheless, there are also different forms of knowledge that do not thrive as well in online settings. Everyone who ever learned to ride a bicycle or bake a sourdough bread knows: only reading the guidelines makes at best a challenging, and at worst an impossible learning experience. In the words of chemist turned philosopher M. Polanyi (2009 [1966], p. 4): "*[w]e can know more than we can tell*" [italics in original text]. This more intangible form of knowledge is often called tacit knowledge. Nonaka (2007) discerns two aspects of tacit knowledge. First, it consists of technical skills and technical *know-how* - not the science behind the technologies, but rather the experience one has 'at the fingertips'. Second, and this is even more important for the research topic at hand, tacit knowledge has a cognitive dimension, consisting of "mental models, beliefs, and perspectives so ingrained that we take them for granted and therefore cannot easily articulate them" (p. 165). Organisational cultures are very much shaped by such mental models and being able to understand and participate in them requires the acquisition of a fair amount of this tacit knowledge. What are acceptable ways of addressing senior or junior staff? How often and how long do people meet? How much discretion does one have? What is considered 'common sense', and what is not? What are the organisation's best practices? Only by being part of an organisation for some time, through observation, imitation and practicing, can these more nuanced, cognitive forms of knowledge be transferred.

Learning this tacit knowledge is dependent upon relational conditions, including face-to-face interactions, trust, and cultural proximity. Such relational conditions are primarily facilitated and promoted by spatial proximity (see among others Banks et al., 2000; Bathelt et al., 2004; Ettlinger, 2003; Gertler, 2008) which is something that has been strikingly absent during the pandemic. Wijngaarden et al. (2020) show that frequent face-to-face interactions lead to informal and serendipitous learning. Even for people that do not necessarily collaborate (such as freelancers), sharing ideas, gossip and news at the water cooler or coffee corner provides fertile sources of individual or organisational knowledge exchange. Especially for relatively new entrants to the labour markets, a lack of access to an organisation's cumulative stock of tacit knowledge could be detrimental. They, obviously, have had much less time to be socialised into the mores and practices of their colleagues. Because the acquisition of tacit knowledge takes time, this group includes very recent graduates, but also those that have been working for a short period of time. Thus, young professionals might know the *know-what,* but might feel less confident or experienced in the *know-how.*

Besides a lack of *know-how,* the impossibility to fully immerse in the sphere of work might also lead to a decrease of inspiration and motivation - which both are important aspects of individual professional development. Straume and Vittersø (2012), for example, show that motivation is key for personal growth and for functioning optimally in the workplace. Motivation is often seen as being energised or activated to do a certain activity (Bhansing et al., 2018). Deci and Ryan's (2008b, 2008a) assumption is that motivation is related to cultural and social environments, and that processes of motivation are influenced by contextual factors, such as social climates such as peers (see e.g. Taylor & Lobel, 1989). Especially when working from home, this obviously becomes more pressing, as pushing yourself to get things done is, for many people at least, more difficult in living rooms, kitchens, or bedrooms than in designated office environments. Straume and Vittersø (2012) show that it is key for personal growth and for functioning optimally in the workplace.

Inspiration is often thought of as being "evoked in response to getting a creative idea and that compels the individual to transform the creative idea into a creative product" (Thrash et al., 2010, p. 470). While this refers to creative products, for all knowledge workers, developing and implementing ideas is part of their work practices. Inspiration - seen from the field of psychology - contains three aspects (Thrash and Elliot, 2004): it is evoked by a stimulus object, it implies transcendence beyond ordinary routine behaviour, and it entails motivation to complete the ideas. Economic geography adds the importance of specific, geographical locations to this, such as the look and feel of a place (Heebels & Van Aalst, 2010) or the vicinity of other workers (Bhansing et al., 2018; Drake, 2003; Wijngaarden et al., 2021). Without real access to either, inspiration will presumably wither away. Based on this, the presumption rises that the COVID-19 pandemic did not only affect the personal and professional spheres of young workers, but also hamper them in their creative and inspirational development.

Challenges of Young Knowledge Workers During COVID-19

As outlined throughout the chapter so far, the COVID-19 pandemic has tremendous effects on entire societies. The sudden move towards home-based work affected almost half of Dutch workers – who were working from home by the end of 2020

(TNO, 2021). This is in line with the European average of 50% (Ahrendt et al., 2020). Many of those were knowledge workers. Knowledge workers are usually conceived as people whose work is based on "information processing, problem solving and the production of knowledge" (Benson & Brown, 2007, p. 122). Even prior to the pandemic, knowledge work often took place at home (Ipsen et al., 2021). Existing research shows that workers voice various positive aspects of working from home, including an improved work-life balance (due to reduced commute time and being closer to family), increased work efficiency (due to e.g. reduced interruptions and lengthy meetings), and having a higher sense of work control (autonomy over planning and breaks) (Eddleston & Mulki, 2017; Wheatley, 2012). Negative aspects include home office constraints (lack of social interaction and exercise), work uncertainties (unclarity about expectations and continuation of work, having to do less interesting work) and inadequate tools (lacking physical equipment or access to data or documents) (Byrnes et al., 2020; Marlow et al., 2017).

Research comparing the effects of working from home on different groups frequently highlight the profound effects on families, especially women, with children (Ipsen et al., 2021; Galanti et al., 2021). This includes not only child rearing, but also home schooling, preparing meals for the entire family and solving technical issues with online teaching (Galanti et al., 2021). Very few studies, however, specifically look at age and career stage in assessing the effects of the lockdowns on workers. This is a lacuna, as Ipsen et al. (2021) highlight that young workers (18-30 years old) significantly experience more work uncertainties and – to a lesser extent – also home office constraints.

What makes these young professionals stand out? Compared to professionals that are further in their careers and have been able to invest in larger residences, young workers often lack the space and financial means to transform one part of their home into a workplace. This indicates that they are more likely to struggle with the breakdown of clear distinctions between work/home and professional/private lives. As a result, compared to other age groups, they tend to be more hindered in their opportunity to sculpt boundaries between personal and professional contexts (Clark, 2000; Nippert-Eng, 1996). Moreover, enforced working from home puts young adults in precarious positions because they started their careers not too long ago. Recent graduates lacked the opportunity to 'settle' in a physical workplace in the first place and had to start their career without being able to attune to the workplace's mores, demeanour, and the discrete and less discrete gossip at the water cooler. As such, these young professionals are currently in a precarious position of starting and building a career in an uncertain work situation with limited guidance and social support.

DATA AND METHODS

In order to explore the challenges faced by early career knowledge workers, this research is based on semi-structured interviews with 22 higher educated young professionals. Purposive and snowball sampling were used (Luborsky & Rubinstein, 1995; Robinson, 2014) to recruit young knowledge workers (age 23-31, see Table 1 in Appendix 1); on the one hand salaried young professionals with a dedicated work environment (office) and, on the other hand, freelancers with a more nomadic work life. Fourteen respondents identified as women, eight as men. The interviews were conducted between Spring 2020 and Summer 2021, and most interviews were conducted digitally (e.g., via Zoom), as during the lockdowns, working from home and decreased social interactions were the norm. All respondents consented to the recordings and transcriptions, and to protect their privacy, pseudonyms are used. The analysis is based on a three-stage inductive constructivist grounded theory coding procedure (Charmaz, 2006) including open, axial, and selective coding. In the first round of open coding a collection of verbatim descriptive codes was created (such as 'constantly in workplace'), which were organised in mutually exclusive more conceptual categories (such as 'hindrance for creativity/productivity') via axial coding. In the results section, the three resulting selective codes are presented.

RESULTS

The analysis of the interviews indicates that young knowledge workers are facing three particular challenges in their enforced working from home in line with the literature discussed above: sculpting boundaries between work and personal spheres, maintaining social connections with a lack of tacit knowledge in professional spheres, and acquiring motivation and inspiration from public spheres. What follows is a description of these themes to provide an in-depth account of how enforced working from home affects the whole personhood and household dynamics of young professionals.

From Professional to Personal Spheres: Boundary Sculpting

Young professionals often have a small living space that is sometimes shared with others (but rarely their families). Working from home forces them to live and work in the same space and collapses the contexts between these spheres (Pagh, 2020). Therefore, the first sub question inquires how young professionals sculpt the boundaries between private and professional spheres. This proves to be challenging for most respondents, as Nadine explains:

It is quite hard to work from home there, with your laptop on your bed or I don't know. We have more girls in the house that are studying or working. So, everyone kind of needs their space, so you cannot really move to the living room. Especially with meetings, yeah, if I were to have calls all day in the living room, that would be very annoying also for my flat mates, so it was quite a challenge. (Nadine, marketing employee)

Working from home means that Nadine needs to negotiate space with her housemates and multiple respondents are in a similar situation. Their boundary sculpting processes taking place in shared homes not only have to do with creating distinctions between the individual personal and professional sphere (Nippert-Eng, 1996) but also with those of their housemates. Living together with other young professionals requires interpersonal boundary negotiations between the personal and professional spheres of all household members. Moreover, all people involved constantly have to switch between their roles as professionals and as housemates even more than they would have to do if they are living alone (Jahn et al., 2016).

While living in a shared and small environment, young professionals constantly have to manage 'territories of the self' (Nippert-Eng 1996) as well as spatial territories. For Nadine, her bedroom is also her workspace which complicates efforts to separate between personal space and professional space. Markedly, this is not something that only applies to young professionals in shared homes. Respondents with a solitary living environment also struggle with combining work and personal spheres in their homes. Joris (consultancy employee) draws a clear picture:

My laptop is on my dining table, so when I am not working, I take it off and it turns into a dining table. What is annoying is that I don't really have a comfortable chair or something like that, it is something that I can still arrange…But then it is: where am I going to put this thing? I live in a tiny apartment, where would I put a giant chair? (Joris, consultancy employee)

Joris' example shows that the presence and absence of his laptop transforms his table into a working and a dining area. The boundaries between his personal and professional sphere are born out of the necessity to work and to eat. Moreover, when working from home means working from your bed or dining table, there is no room for a second screen, or an ergonomic chair. Across the interviews, work comfort proved to be an important factor for being productive, the respondents mention proper chairs, decent tables, enough electric sockets, high-functioning internet connections, a toilet nearby, proper daylight, good coffee, and good food as key ingredients for a comfortable working environment. When young professionals lack the space and facilities to create a comfortable workspace, working from home can also harm them physically.

Furthermore, while for students engaging in lectures from their dorm is acceptable, young knowledge workers have to navigate more professional work environments which sometimes conflict with their ways of living. Environments like Joris' studio and Nadine's bedroom show personal items because these are not dedicated workspaces. Their living environments can work against the professional roles that young professionals want to uphold (Jahn et al., 2016). And even though self-employed professionals are used to working from home, the freedom to work in other places proved crucial for the respondents. COVID-19 induced lockdowns took away their freedom to vary workspaces, in other words they no longer have the autonomy to switch between different spatial territories of work. This which can reduce productivity, as Marlie indicates:

Variety is one of the main reasons I am working as a freelancer. I would go mad... Well, maybe now I am overreacting, but I would not like working five days at an office. Although I do like to go there now and then. [...] To me, it is important that there is some sort of balance. I know that I'll get stuck when I constantly work from home, so that's why I prefer to work at extended workplaces some days of the week. (Marlie, freelance journalist and copywriter)

The challenge to manage boundaries between personal and professional spheres in shared, ill-equipped, and monotonous spaces amplifies the increased demands and pressure COVID-19 places on workers (Kerman et al., 2021).

From Personal to Professional Spheres: Social Connections and Tacit Knowledge

Despite the issues of retaining the boundary between work and private life, social interactions between colleagues or between freelancer, peer and client appear to be crucial elements in having an enjoyable work life. The second sub question aims to examine how young professionals connect with their professional contacts from their – lockdown induced – private spheres. The interviews show that relationships with direct colleagues or professional connections are perceived as crucial for their professional success. Michelle indicates why this is the case:

You know, what you see, there are a lot of positions that are extremely dependent on the colleagues with whom they work. And if you do not know anyone and you are also not inclined to make the first step, you will most likely not feel connected with the company. You might be working for the company, but you would have no idea with whom, merely by name. (Michelle, HR employee)

It is therefore no surprise that especially the salaried workers expressed that they found it challenging to build relationships with their colleagues now that direct interactions - besides occasional Zoom meetings - have become rare. This is especially the case for more informal interactions - those that go beyond the mere sharing of facts or codified knowledge (M. Polanyi, 2009 [1966]). Bart, for example, described how emotional connections are not easy to establish via online connections. For him, a face-to-face meeting proved to be critical to build a relationship of trust with his colleague:

I also notice that people behave differently in video calls, I have that less, but one of my colleagues always had a very defensive attitude. I once went on a walk with him in a park and we talked about our private lives for an hour, and I really see that it made our work relationship better. There is a lot less suspicion and a lot more trust. This really made it a lot better. (Bart, consulting)

This lack of connection also trickles down to how young professionals felt connected to the organisational culture and knowledge. That is, they felt that they found it difficult to obtain the tacit knowledge required to fully integrate in the company. Two interviewees explicitly mentioned that they missed informally hearing about updates from different departments, as they felt like currently, they have no idea what is going on. For example, on certain days Paulina (marketing employee) would physically overhear her colleagues talking about their work and engage in with them. Now, when people update her on their work activities, she finds it harder to understand what they mean and as a result feels more distanced from them and the projects they work on.

An interesting point that three of the respondents pointed out is the possibility of a virtual office. Paulina (marketing employee) also mentioned that the energy from an office influenced her to get into a better workflow. She, and other respondents, engaged in 'open hangouts', in which workers, informally, could interact while working. Employees in these hangouts are quietly working with their microphones off but can just turn them on if they want to ask a question or make a comment. The general consensus of these calls was also that this type of interaction was allowed and therefore a certain type of office simulation was accomplished. This idea of creating a virtual office on demand seems to be something which could combat the lack of social facilitation. Though, respondents emphasised, it could never replace the office in other respects, such as providing visual cues and inspiration - which will be explained in the next section.

Including Public Spheres: Acquiring Motivation and Inspiration

The third sub question explores the impact of a lack of other spheres like the public realm in working from home in times of COVID-19. A lack of face-to-face social connections can not only harm well-being (Waizenegger et al., 2020) or the vulnerability on the labour market (Ipsen et al., 2021), but also influences the motivation and inspiration of young professionals. Therefore, besides the importance of boundaries between work life and private life, and access to knowledge, there is a third important aspect of work that is often overlooked in existing literature on teleworking (Baruch, 2000; Mann & Holdsworth, 2003): how 'buzzing' environments lead to the crucial motivation and inspiration to get work done. This is something the freelance respondents - who often have ample experience working from home - already observed prior to the pandemic. From the interviews with freelancers, it has become clear that multiple participants prefer to work amongst others because being your own boss can make you feel alone. Martin, for example, explains how working from home constantly or too often makes him feel sad. He longs for social belongingness (Blagoev et al., 2019; Liegl, 2014) and working from home takes away the aspects of work that make him enjoy it:

Working from home can be pretty lonely. That I go to bed and think: tomorrow, new day, same workplace: my home, yay. That makes you feel less motivated and less happy. No, you'd rather go to a café with Henk and Ingrid, talk some bullshit, make some jokes, and do some work. (Martin, freelance digital graphic designer)

In order to reap the full benefits of working in more social settings, it is important that people surround themselves with others who are also working independently. One reason for that is that in 'normal' cafés, people seem to pay more attention to them, which makes the respondents feel uncomfortable. However, most importantly, they work in social work-oriented settings because it provides a work ethic that they feel is not available working alone, from their homes. Kirsten and Pim make this very implicit when talking about their ideal work situations:

Yes, I prefer to work amongst others who are working too. Well, it is not the case that I would not go to a specific place where others are just having coffee, but when others are working too, it creates this kind of ambience, like: we are all working, we are all in the same boat. That creates some sort of work ethic, while it takes away the feeling of: oh, I am working amongst people who are just having lunch and coffee. That creates a whole other ambience. (Kirsten, 26, freelance journalist and copywriter)

When I see other people working, or calling, or whatever, that motivates and inspires me to work hard too, and to push my creativity a little bit further. I do not think that is peer pressure, but well, you can compare it, because it makes me feel, like: well, I cannot shop online when I see other people around me working very hard. (Pim, 24, freelance journalist)

Romy, in turn, feels the complete opposite of the ideal situation described above now that she is working from home. This indicates that not only self-employed professionals, but also salaried workers thrive on connections with others to make their work enjoyable. A lack of interaction with her co-workers deprived Romy of nearly all motivation. These findings fit the existing research indicating that when people work around others, their motivation increases. This is dubbed a 'social facilitation' effect: people work harder when they are not alone (Morrison-Smith & Ruiz, 2020).

I remember thinking, for what and for who am I even doing this? Because I wasn't hearing anything. I thought: "If I hand in poop, you won't look at it anyway." So, my motivation really decreased due to that, those [engagement from co-workers] are things that I really appreciate. (Romy, accounting employee)

Nevertheless, besides a lack of work ethic and motivation to continue working (and not indulging in online shopping), a lack of social interaction also reduced the inspiration of young professionals. Stijn (freelance journalist), for example, explains how he relies upon the vicinity of other people for his creative endeavours.

I prefer to have other people around me because they inspire me. When I for example am thinking about how to arrange a photoshoot, and I see a girl in a pink sweater, I think: oh, well, maybe I can work with something pink. Other people thrive my creativity in that sense. (Stijn, freelance journalist)

Though obviously inspiration is connected to arts and creative production, many of the young professionals often feel that they need inspiration to come up with new ideas and projects to work on, as well as developing new ways to tackle problems they are encountering. Verena, for example, explains that she is dependent upon social interactions not only to gain the relevant knowledge for her work, but also to gain the inspiration to do her work:

When I work from home too much, my creativity level goes down. I think that happens because... Well, inspiration comes from other people. For example, that you see other people, with different clothes, in a different environment, where you see different things on the wall. Or you talk to others, who have different ideas than you. That is what thrives your creativity. (Verena, freelance journalist)

However, it is not only the people that drive inspiration and motivation. Also, just the plain idea of going *somewhere else* with different visual stimuli already strongly affects self-perceived work satisfaction. Kirsten (freelance journalist and copywriter) for example explains that grey, boring spaces do nothing to spark her enthusiasm for work, while Lieve emphasises that she misses such inspiration and colours (besides the social aspects) now that she has to work from home: "I miss that energy, the inspiration that a workplace can give me when a lot is happening. Colours, people, employees, and the inspiration they give me." (Lieve, freelance marketing and communication professional).

SOLUTIONS AND RECOMMENDATIONS

While some of the abovementioned issues might also be applicable for knowledge workers in more advanced career stages, they are detrimental to the development of young professionals. Because for them, their twenties are formative years in the sense that especially when they do not yet have family obligations, they have the time and opportunity to fully engage in other spheres of life; social, professional, and public spheres. At this moment the full cohort is affected equally, however, the longer the measures will take, the more especially women will endure the negative effects of the pandemic (Otonkorpi-Lehtoranta et al., 2021). Whereas labour participation is relatively equal for men and women in the Netherlands in their early 20s (*StatLine - Arbeidsdeelname; kerncijfers*, 2021), this changes once they hit the childrearing age (which averages around 30 in the Netherlands for higher educated women). This, in general, makes career continuation difficult, but without the networks, tacit knowledge, and social capital acquired in the preceding years, it is expected that labour participation differences in ten to fifteen years for women will be much more pronounced in this cohort.

These findings are especially relevant because (partially) working from home will most likely be a norm rather than an exception in future post-COVID societies. While most young professionals managed to do a good job while working from home, this does not mean that employers can enforce working from home in the future. Instead, young workers should be rewarded with the autonomy to sculpt their working lives and to have a say in their own working times and locations. For young professionals, it is important that employers or clients facilitate them in working in inspiring and healthy environments.

FUTURE RESEARCH DIRECTIONS

This study is exploratory in nature and therefore limited in scope. Obviously, interviews with 22 Dutch young knowledge workers provide some insights in the experiences of this generation, but do not account for the intersectionality of all young workers' experiences. For example, though gender differences might not be as profound before potentially children are born, women of all ages endure setbacks on the labour market (see e.g. Bradley, 1989) and higher expectations in terms of household chores (Cerrato & Cifre, 2018). There are many cultural differences too, affecting the family responsibilities, autonomy, and cultural capital of young workers. Finally, social class differences of course have a major impact on the ability to deal with labour market vulnerability and a lack of access to professional, ergonomic workspaces at home. Future research could further unpack socio-cultural differences within this generation, or systematically assess the differences between young knowledge workers vis-à-vis other generational groups.

Moreover, for knowledge workers, communication and collaboration platforms are indispensable when working from home. However, they simultaneously alienate people from their workspaces because of the aforementioned lack of face-to-face interactions, tacit knowledge, and inspiring buzz. None of the respondents brought the role of commercial platforms up in the interviews, which shows how digital platforms are taken for granted and fully embedded in everyday work spheres. Their embeddedness in commercial ecosystems thriving on the commodification of personal data (Grabher & König, 2020) is rarely considered by workers. This, however, should not be overlooked. Not only does the use of commercial platforms sustain, from a K. Polanyian viewpoint, a capitalist platform economy (Grabher & König, 2020) and surveillance capitalism (Zuboff, 2019), it also affects the daily life of workers. Knowledge workers are exposed to far-reaching commercial surveillance via company-supported channels and hence become lucrative subjects for third parties while they are just doing their jobs. Future research could further unpack the increasing effect of such platform economics on the whole personhood of workers – both freelance and employed. Companies should reconsider the use of commercial platform providers and take responsibility in protecting their employees against enforced monitoring practices.

CONCLUSION

This research aims to answer the question how working from home in times of COVID-19 affects young knowledge workers and adds three important insights. First, when it comes to around boundary sculpting practices (the focus of sub question

1), many respondents' boundary negotiations between personal and professional spheres entail personal, collective, temporal, and spatial borders. In other words, young professionals often have to negotiate not only their personal time and space but also those of their housemates. And together with switching between territories of the self (the changing of roles in particular spheres), respondents have to transform their spatial territories continuously to make sure that their workspace corresponds with their professional role.

Second, interpersonal connections prove to be of vital importance (in answer to sub question 2). A lack of face-to-face interactions not only causes a lack of interpersonal contact and emotional connection to colleagues, but also a lack of crucial knowledge. The research findings indicate that if tacit knowledge is not being transferred, this seemingly affects everything. Especially at the start of their career, people learn a lot through face-to-face interactions and seeing others working. Working from home prevents the transmission of crucial information.

Third, apart from whole personhood depending on a healthy balance between the personal and professional sphere, this study shows that additional spheres are crucial (as inquired by sub question 3). What this chapter includes as the public sphere refers to external sources that prove to be essential sources of motivation and inspiration. The opportunity to work in a vibrant environment contributes to a productive and comfortable working life. Vibrant spheres contribute to young professionals' whole personhood because they can prevent loneliness and feelings of unproductivity.

To conclude, the interview findings show that working from home can be detrimental to the whole personhood of young professionals. Whole personhood is dependent on a healthy balance between different life spheres. This became impossible when the COVID measures put a halt to the social lives of young professionals and collapsed personal and professional spheres. Moreover, the lack of a physical work sphere made the transition from being a student to being a professional more difficult than ever. Many respondents perceived themselves to be in a liminal career phase, and struggled to feel at home at work, and to work at home. And the longer this takes, the more pressing the concerns that come to light in this chapter will be. At the time of writing, enforced working from home has been advised/enforced for two years in the Netherlands, and is expected to (partially) remain the norm for many knowledge workers.

REFERENCES

Ahrendt, D., Cabrita, J., Clerici, E., Hurley, J., Leončikas, T., Mascherini, M., Riso, S., & Sándor, E. (2020). *Living, working and COVID-19* (report COVID-19 series). Publications Office of the European Union. https://www.eurofound.europa.eu/publications/report/2020/living-working-and-covid-19

Andrade, C., & Lobo Fernandes, J. (2021). Role boundary management during COVID-19 pandemic: A qualitative analysis of focus group data with working-student mothers. *Psicologia, 35*(1), 175–162. doi:10.17575/psicologia.v35i1.1694

Banks, M., Lovatt, A., O'Connor, J., & Raffo, C. (2000). Risk and trust in the cultural industries. *Geoforum, 31*(4), 453–464. doi:10.1016/S0016-7185(00)00008-7

Baruch, Y. (2000). Teleworking: Benefits and pitfalls as perceived by professionals and managers. *New Technology, Work and Employment, 15*(1), 34–49. doi:10.1111/1468-005X.00063

Bathelt, H., Malmberg, A., & Maskell, P. (2004). Clusters and knowledge: Local buzz, global pipelines and the process of knowledge creation. *Progress in Human Geography, 28*(1), 31–56. doi:10.1191/0309132504ph469oa

Benson, J., & Brown, M. (2007). Knowledge workers: What keeps them committed; what turns them away. *Work, Employment and Society, 21*(1), 121–141. doi:10.1177/0950017007073623

Bhansing, P. V., Hitters, E., & Wijngaarden, Y. (2018). Passion inspires: Motivations of creative entrepreneurs in creative business centres in the Netherlands. *The Journal of Entrepreneurship, 27*(1), 1–24. doi:10.1177/0971355717738589

Blagoev, B., Costas, J., & Kärreman, D. (2019). 'We are all herd animals': Community and organizationality in coworking spaces. *Organization, 26*(6), 894–916. doi:10.1177/1350508418821008

Bradley, H. (1989). *Men's work, women's work: A sociological history of the sexual division of labour in employment.* University of Minnesota Press.

Byrnes, K. G., Kiely, P. A., Dunne, C. P., McDermott, K. W., & Coffey, J. C. (2021). Communication, collaboration and contagion: "Virtualisation" of anatomy during COVID-19. *Clinical Anatomy (New York, N.Y.), 34*(1), 82–89. doi:10.1002/ca.23649 PMID:32648289

Cerrato, J., & Cifre, E. (2018). Gender inequality in household chores and work-family conflict. *Frontiers in Psychology, 9*(1330), 1–11. doi:10.3389/fpsyg.2018.01330 PMID:30123153

Ciolfi, L., Gray, B., & Pinatti de Carvalho, A. F. (2020). Making home work places. *Proceedings of 18th European Conference on Computer-Supported Cooperative Work*. 10.18420/ecscw2020_ep10

Clark, S. C. (2000). Work/Family Border Theory: A New Theory of Work/Family Balance. *Human Relations*, *53*(6), 747–770. doi:10.1177/0018726700536001

Collins, R. (2020). Social distancing as a critical test of the micro-sociology of solidarity. *American Journal of Cultural Sociology*, *8*(3), 477–497. doi:10.105741290-020-00120-z PMID:33101676

Deci, E. L., & Ryan, R. M. (2008a). Facilitating optimal motivation and psychological well-being across life's domains. *Canadian Psychology*, *49*(1), 14–23. doi:10.1037/0708-5591.49.1.14

Deci, E. L., & Ryan, R. M. (2008b). Self-determination theory: A macrotheory of human motivation, development, and health. *Canadian Psychology*, *49*(3), 182–185. doi:10.1037/a0012801

Drake, G. (2003). 'This place gives me space': Place and creativity in the creative industries. *Geoforum*, *34*(4), 511–524. doi:10.1016/S0016-7185(03)00029-0

Duxbury, L., Higgins, C., Smart, R., & Stevenson, M. (2014). Mobile Technology and Boundary Permeability. *British Journal of Management*, *25*(3), 570–588. doi:10.1111/1467-8551.12027

Eddleston, K. A., & Mulki, J. (2017). Toward understanding remote workers' management of work–family boundaries: The complexity of workplace embeddedness. *Group & Organization Management*, *42*(3), 346–387. doi:10.1177/1059601115619548

Elmer, T., Mepham, K., & Stadtfeld, C. (2020). Students under lockdown: Comparisons of students' social networks and mental health before and during the COVID-19 crisis in Switzerland. *PLoS One*, *15*(7), e0236337. doi:10.1371/journal.pone.0236337 PMID:32702065

Ettlinger, N. (2003). Cultural economic geography and a relational and microspace approach to trusts, rationalities, networks, and change in collaborative workplaces. *Journal of Economic Geography*, *3*(2), 145–171. doi:10.1093/jeg/3.2.145

Faludi, J., & Crosby, M. (2021). The Digital Economy of the Sourdough. Housewifisation in the Time of COVID-19. *TripleC*, *19*(1), 113–124. doi:10.31269/triplec.v19i1.1222

Galanti, T., Guidetti, G., Mazzei, E., Zappalà, S., & Toscano, F. (2021). Work From Home During the COVID-19 Outbreak: The Impact on Employees' Remote Work Productivity, Engagement, and Stress. *Journal of Occupational and Environmental Medicine, 63*(7), e426–e432. doi:10.1097/JOM.0000000000002236 PMID:33883531

Gertler, M. S. (2008). Buzz Without Being There? Communities of Practice in Context 1. In *Community, Economic Creativity, and Organization*. Oxford University Press. doi:10.1093/acprof:oso/9780199545490.003.0009

Gorski, P. S. (2013). Beyond the fact/value distinction: *Ethical naturalism and the social sciences. Society, 50*(6), 543–553. doi:10.100712115-013-9709-2

Grabher, G., & König, J. (2020). Disruption, Embedded. A Polanyian Framing of the Platform Economy. *Sociologica, 14*(1), 95–118. doi:10.6092/issn.1971-8853/10443

Habermas, J. (1971). *Toward a rational society: Student protest, science, and politics*. Beacon Press.

Habermas, J. (2016). *Time of transitions*. John Wiley & Sons.

Han, W.-J., & Hart, J. (2021). Job precarity and economic prospects during the COVID-19 public health crisis. *Social Science Quarterly, 102*(5), 1–18. Advance online publication. doi:10.1111squ.13031 PMID:34908614

Hjálmsdóttir, A., & Bjarnadóttir, V. S. (2021). "I have turned into a foreman here at home": Families and work–life balance in times of COVID-19 in a gender equality paradise. *Gender, Work and Organization, 28*(1), 268–283. doi:10.1111/gwao.12552 PMID:33041540

Hu, Y., & Qian, Y. (2021). COVID-19, Inter-household Contact and Mental Well-Being Among Older Adults in the US and the UK. *Frontiers in Sociology, 6*, 143. doi:10.3389/fsoc.2021.714626 PMID:34381838

Ipsen, C., van Veldhoven, M., Kirchner, K., & Hansen, J. P. (2021). Six Key Advantages and Disadvantages of Working from Home in Europe during COVID-19. *International Journal of Environmental Research and Public Health, 18*(4), 1826. doi:10.3390/ijerph18041826 PMID:33668505

Jahn, K., Klesel, M., Lemmer, K., Weigel, A., & Niehaves, B. (2016). Individual Boundary Management: An Empirical Investigation on Technology-related Tactics. *PACIS 2016 Proceedings*, 268–271.

Kerman, K., Korunka, C., & Tement, S. (2021). Work and home boundary violations during the COVID-19 pandemic: The role of segmentation preferences and unfinished tasks. *Applied Psychology*, 1–23. Advance online publication. doi:10.1111/apps.12335 PMID:34548734

Lacher, H. (1999). The politics of the market: Re-reading Karl Polanyi. *Global Society*, *13*(3), 313–326. doi:10.1080/13600829908443193

Liegl, M. (2014). Nomadicity and the Care of Place—On the Aesthetic and Affective Organization of Space in Freelance Creative Work. *Computer Supported Cooperative Work*, *23*(2), 163–183. doi:10.100710606-014-9198-x

Mann, S., & Holdsworth, L. (2003). The psychological impact of teleworking: Stress, emotions and health. *New Technology, Work and Employment*, *18*(3), 196–211. doi:10.1111/1468-005X.00121

Marlow, S. L., Lacerenza, C. N., & Salas, E. (2017). Communication in virtual teams: A conceptual framework and research agenda. *Human Resource Management Review*, *27*(4), 575–589. doi:10.1016/j.hrmr.2016.12.005

Mols, A., & Pridmore, J. (2021). Always available via WhatsApp: Mapping everyday boundary work practices and privacy negotiations. *Mobile Media & Communication*, *9*(3), 1–19. doi:10.1177/2050157920970582

Morrison-Smith, S., & Ruiz, J. (2020). Challenges and barriers in virtual teams: A literature review. *SN Applied Sciences*, *2*(6), 1096. doi:10.100742452-020-2801-5

Nippert-Eng, C. E. (1996). *Home and Work: Negotiating Boundaries Through Everyday Life*. University of Chicago Press. doi:10.7208/chicago/9780226581477.001.0001

Nonaka, I. (2007). The Knowledge-Creating Company. *Harvard Business Review*. https://hbr.org/2007/07/the-knowledge-creating-company

Nooteboom, B. (2000). Learning by Interaction: Absorptive Capacity, Cognitive Distance and Governance. *The Journal of Management and Governance*, *4*(1), 69–92. doi:10.1023/A:1009941416749

Otonkorpi-Lehtoranta, K., Salin, M., Hakovirta, M., & Kaittila, A. (2021). Gendering boundary work: Experiences of work–family practices among Finnish working parents during COVID-19 lockdown. *Gender, Work and Organization*, gwao.12773. Advance online publication. doi:10.1111/gwao.12773 PMID:34898870

Pagh, J. (2020). Managing Context Collapses: The Internet as a Conditioning Technology in the Organization of Practices. *International Journal of Communication*, *12*, 2810–2827. https://ijoc.org/index.php/ijoc/article/view/11872

Polanyi, M. (2009). *The Tacit Dimension.* The University of Chicago Press. https://press.uchicago.edu/ucp/books/book/chicago/T/bo6035368.html

Qian, Y., & Hu, Y. (2021). Couples' changing work patterns in the United Kingdom and the United States during the COVID-19 pandemic. *Gender, Work and Organization, 28*(S2), 535–553. doi:10.1111/gwao.12661 PMID:34230781

Scaff, L. A. (1992). *Fleeing the Iron Cage: Culture, Politics, and Modernity in the Thought of Max Weber.* University of California Press.

Schieman, S., Badawy, P. J. A., Milkie, M., & Bierman, A. (2021). Work-Life Conflict During the Covid-19 Pandemic. *Socius: Sociological Research for a Dynamic World, 7*, 1–19. doi:10.1177/2378023120982856

Srnicek, N. (2017). *Platform Capitalism.* John Wiley & Sons.

StatLine—Arbeidsdeelname; kerncijfers. (2021, November 16). *CBS.* https://opendata.cbs.nl/statline/#/CBS/nl/dataset/82309NED/table?dl=56E36

Straume, L. V., & Vittersø, J. (2012). Happiness, inspiration and the fully functioning person: Separating hedonic and eudaimonic well-being in the workplace. *The Journal of Positive Psychology, 7*(5), 387–398. doi:10.1080/17439760.2012.711348

Taylor, S. E., & Lobel, M. (1989). Social comparison activity under threat: Downward evaluation and upward contacts. *Psychological Review, 96*(4), 569–575. doi:10.1037/0033-295X.96.4.569 PMID:2678204

Terpe, S. (2020). Working with Max Weber's 'spheres of life': An actor-centred approach. *Journal of Classical Sociology, 20*(1), 22–42. doi:10.1177/1468795X18789328

Thrash, T. M., Maruskin, L. A., Cassidy, S. E., Fryer, J. W., & Ryan, R. M. (2010). Mediating between the muse and the masses: Inspiration and the actualization of creative ideas. *Journal of Personality and Social Psychology, 98*(3), 469–487. doi:10.1037/a0017907 PMID:20175625

TNO. (2021). Bijna een kwart van de thuiswerkers wil ook na corona grotendeels thuis blijven werken [Almost a quarter of the homeworkers wants to work mostly from home even after corona]. *TNO.* Retrieved 22 September 2021, from https://www.tno.nl/nl/over-tno/nieuws/2021/2/kwart-thuiswerkers-na-corona-deels-thuis-blijven-werken/

Van Dijck, J., Poell, T., & De Waal, T. (2018). *The Platform Society: Public Values in a Connective World.* Oxford University Press. doi:10.1093/oso/9780190889760.001.0001

Waizenegger, L., McKenna, B., Cai, W., & Bendz, T. (2020). An affordance perspective of team collaboration and enforced working from home during COVID-19. *European Journal of Information Systems*, *29*(4), 429–442. doi:10.1080/0960085X.2020.1800417

Weber, M. (1978). *Gesammelte Aufsätze zur Religionssoziologie* (Vol. 1). Mohr.

Weber, M. (1978). *Economy and society: An outline of interpretive sociology* (Vol. 2). University of California Press.

Wheatley, D. (2012). Good to be home? Time-use and satisfaction levels among home-based teleworkers. *New Technology, Work and Employment*, *27*(3), 224–241. doi:10.1111/j.1468-005X.2012.00289.x

Wijngaarden, Y., Bhansing, P. V., & Hitters, E. (2021). Character trait, context or… create! Innovative practices among creative entrepreneurs. *Industry and Innovation*, *28*(8), 1077–1097. doi:10.1080/13662716.2021.1949964

Wijngaarden, Y., Hitters, E., & Bhansing, P. V. (2020). Cultivating fertile learning grounds: Collegiality, tacit knowledge and innovation in creative co-working spaces. *Geoforum*, *109*, 86–94. doi:10.1016/j.geoforum.2020.01.005

Wood, A. J., Graham, M., Lehdonvirta, V., & Hjorth, I. (2019). Networked but Commodified: The (Dis)Embeddedness of Digital Labour in the Gig Economy. *Sociology*, *53*(5), 931–950. doi:10.1177/0038038519828906

Zuboff, S. (2019). *The Age of Surveillance Capitalism: The Fight for a Human Future at the New Frontier of Power*. Public Affairs.

KEY TERMS AND DEFINITIONS

Boundary Work: Building on the work of Nippert-Eng, boundary work refers to practices to create, manage, and adjust the boundaries between different life spheres, like work and personal contexts.

Codified Knowledge: Codified knowledge refers to explicit forms of knowledge that are formal and systematic – and that can be conveyed over large distances and stored in various types of media.

Knowledge Workers: Knowledge workers can be seen as people whose work is based on the production of knowledge, information processing, and problem solving. Knowledge workers are sometimes also referred to as white collar workers.

Motivation: Motivation refers to being energised or activated to do a certain activity. It is influenced by contextual factors, such as cultural and social environments.

Public Sphere: Described by Habermas in 1971, the public sphere is the place where public debate happens and where people are exposed to new ideas and developments.

Tacit Knowledge: A more intangible form of knowledge that consists of technical skills and know-how, and of beliefs and knowledge that people take for granted.

Whole Personhood: Whole personhood is the full human experience, in which all (societal, personal, micro, and macro level) spheres have their place, but also compete for time and attention. A whole person has the agency to balance these spheres and to reach their own personal human potential.

APPENDIX

Table 1. Respondent overview

Pseudonym	Identify as	Age	Work Field / Occupation
Salaried Workers			
Henk	Male	26	Accounting
Romy	Female	27	Accounting
Anita	Female	24	Marketing
Nadine	Female	25	Marketing
Paulina	Female	26	Marketing
Joyce	Female	28	HR
Michelle	Female	28	HR
Joris	Male	26	Consulting/HR
Gerrit	Male	26	Consulting
Bart	Male	23	Consulting
Anne	Female	23	Sales
Roberto	Male	29	Sales
Self-employed Professionals			
Verena	Female	27	Journalist
Marlie	Female	29	Journalist & copywriter
Anneloes	Female	26	Journalist & social media professional
Kirsten	Female	26	Journalist & copywriter
Pim	Male	24	Journalist
Britt	Female	23	Social media & marketing professional
Stijn	Male	21	Journalist & photographer
Martin	Male	31	Digital graphic designer
Lieve	Female	23	Marketing and communication professional
Vivian	Female	27	Copywriter & marketing professional & photographer

Chapter 7
Can Music Save Lives?
The Experience of COVID-19 and the Impacts of Music-Making on Young People in Their Home Environment

Paula Guerra
Faculty of Arts and Humanities, University of Porto, Portugal

ABSTRACT

Against the background of the global COVID-19 pandemic, this chapter presents an in-depth vision of the relationship between music-making and the domestic life of Portuguese artists. The chapter presents and discusses data from an international project related to the Portuguese reality. Then, on the basis of some 40 semi-structured interviews with Portuguese musicians, the author reflects on the impacts of the pandemic on their musical careers and potential impacts on music-making processes more generally, as well as on family and domestic life. Finally, the chapter highlights the scarcity of this kind of research in the Portuguese reality, making it imperative that other dimensions of music-making and artists' lives are explored and made perceptible, not just the economic losses suffered.

INTRODUCTION

Several discourses have stated that COVID-19 has introduced a "new normality" (Guerra et al., 2021). This materializes in the establishment of unprecedented social, economic, political, family, and mental conditions. Employment, mental health, wellbeing, and daily and domestic experiences were all impacted by the pandemic, including for young musicians[1] (Howard et al., 2021). Simultaneously,

DOI: 10.4018/978-1-6684-2364-6.ch007

culture – including music – has been an important escape route because, while not vital for the preservation of life, it is vital for the preservation of a sense of life (Banks, 2020) when there is a return to the domestic space. In that sense, we intend to show that the COVID-19 pandemic exacerbate the social and economic conditions of inequality, insecurity, and risk experienced in the public and private spheres by social actors, mainly young musicians/music-makers. This chapter reports on the experiences of young musicians during their period of isolation and social estrangement, focusing on topics such as mental health, wellbeing, and experiences in the domestic space, in other words, we intend to show that the market failed, but that online as an alternative was not viable for most musicians, thus accentuating their precariousness and the uncertainty of their lives. In the following section, I'll explore how the restrictions faced by young musicians have impacted not only their ability to perform live, but also to rehearse, collaborate and create. In exploring the short- and long-term consequences of COVID-19 for young musicians, the following sections demonstrate that the long-term impacts represent more economic instability and unemployment for the coming years, an aspect that accentuates the precariousness inherent in a music career (Beatfreeks, 2020) and consequently affect domestic and family experiences.

Our results were obtained by conducting 40 semi-structured interviews in Portugal, which we'll present in more detail later[2]. These interviews were conducted in a period of isolation and post-isolation, that is, between the second and third waves of the pandemic in Portugal. This study adopted a qualitative design with the data extracted from semi-structured interviews with young people between 18 and 35 years of age in Portugal. This age group was chosen as it conforms to the current parameters of emerging adulthood and late youth (Arnett, 2014). The research sites (different Portuguese cities) were chosen to examine if and how differing national rates of COVID-19 infection and steps to curb its spread have impacted the daily experiences of youth and how they have used music as a means of coping with measures including lockdown and social distancing. This research project also intended to understand the inequalities between different cities and between different types of musicians. Given the advice concerning health and safety at the time of data collection, all interviews were conducted online using Zoom and Skype taking about 40 minutes on average. The interview protocol included questions on basic demographics (e.g. age, gender), music involvement (e.g. type, level, frequency of live performance), the impacts of COVID-19 crisis on music-making activity together with questions surrounding the role of music-making in shaping wellbeing and precarity during the pandemic (e.g. "Have there been ways in which music-making has helped you cope more positively with the COVID-19 crisis?"). The interviews were audio recorded and transcribed verbatim for data analysis. Deep content analysis was used (Bardin, 1977), and platforms of analysis such as NVivo.

Authors such as Mas-Herrero et al. (2020) state that the COVID-19 pandemic has been responsible for an increase in uncertainty, anxiety and depression, resulting from the long months of isolation, but also from a return to the domestic family space. For the young musicians who found themselves without constant and systematic income, and with no state support, music and music-making processes became a way to resist the uncertainty of daily life, and to cope with these feelings, although they do not provide financial capacity/stability as one would expect. On this point, it is important to introduce Polanyi's (1957) contributions, mainly at the level of the concept of embeddedness, so that we can understand how the system failed these musicians. In fact, based on Polanyi's definition of embeddedness, the economy is only embedded in the economic system, whereas it should be based on social relations. This concept is very important for us to frame the discourses of our interviewees at the level of the difficulties they experienced during the pandemic, not least because embeddedness is not only an analytical term, but also an attitude that alludes to a political task and to stabilise the organisation of a given society, through the social regulation of markets, something that in our case study failed (Beckert, 2007).

Young artists focused on a routine of shows, tours, performances, recordings, and productions found themselves confined to improvised studios inside their homes, confronted with constant contact with their children or spouses, creating obstacles to the music-making process. Others took on responsibilities as caregivers for children and/or the elderly. In the process, music and music-making for these young artists acquired an ambivalence (Frith, 2003). For some it became a creative outlet, for others a torment, as the intense domestic life hindered creativity, and even participating in fund-raising campaigns or livestreams. Music-making became an individual rather than collective endeavour devoid of audiences, prompting a change in relationship with their instruments. The individualisation of the music-making process can also be attributed to an acceleration of the nature and pace of work in the cultural and creative sector, since production logics were intensified to respond to the needs gradually being imposed (Dillon, 2007). However, this individualisation and the closer, more introspective relationship of musicians with their instruments also stemmed from an intensification in inequalities of resources: with no physical workplace, there are few mechanisms and little time to promote collective engagement. Undoubtedly, the pandemic has emphasized our dependence on others and the role of home environments in individual, experiential, emotional, and experiential terms in the performance of our professional lives. Through the interviews, we account for these dimensions, to offer a complex and reticular view of the impacts of the pandemic, focusing on a micro dimension of domestic family sociabilities – the social actors – rather than the meso or macro dimension – the collective or society.

KEEP IT REAL IN THE PANDEMIC: THE STRUCTURAL WEAKNESSES OF THE CREATIVE SECTOR AND MUSIC INDUSTRY

In early 2020, the music industry began to feel the first impacts of the pandemic, which quickly spread globally, however, our premise is that not everyone has experienced it in the same way. Over time, several control measures were implemented, including social isolation and the closure of non-essential services; consequently, several workers found themselves without work for long periods. In Portugal, hotel services, tourism, and the cultural sector were deeply affected by these restrictions. As Strong (2021) states, the impacts of the pandemic on musical ecosystems remain unknown.

Strong and Cannizzo (2020) document in their Australian research a similar reality to the Portuguese one. These authors assess that the cultural sector was one of the most affected by the pandemic, and one of the least supported/subsidised by the state. According to Guerra et al. (2021), many cultural workers received no government support. Many indie rock musicians were left with no job prospects or stable incomes, and their careers were thrown into limbo, with no idea when it would be possible to return to normality. The social inequality and exclusion accentuated by the pandemic is even more evident in the independent and alternative music universe, marked by do-it-yourself (DIY) and amateur practices (Guerra, 2015, 2017, 2018, 2021). To some extent, Polanyi's definition of social order (Streeck, 2006) is precarious, as it is assumed to be an unstable outcome of social and political struggles, something that is visible by the lack of support offered to artists in Portugal, especially independent artists. Online emerged as an alternative; an alternative that almost seemed to exempt the role of the state in regulating and providing social and economic support to individuals and households affected by the pandemic. During the pandemic, the online was seen as a market replacement mechanism, however, as we will see later, it also failed because there was no regulation. The very notion of "double movement" fits into this analysis, as it corresponds to political intervention in the markets in the light of their social consequences. Moreover, Sound Diplomacy (2020) warns about the impacts on the music industry, listing several reasons why cities should support music professionals and create strategic action. The artistic-cultural sector is at a turning point, needing effective policies for a possible victory in the face of a (post-)pandemic scenario. As Cirillo and Tullio (2021) affirm, workers in the cultural and artistic sector face countless difficulties in staying active, leaving them to rely on the support of family and friends. There is a need to rethink the status of workers in the artistic and cultural sector; to raise awareness about the importance of culture and the arts in life; to definitively assume the weight of music and the arts in urban planning, urban regeneration and development policies; and to demonstrate the importance of creative activities and music in the economy.

NOT ONLY HOME SWEET HOME: IMPACTS OF COVID-19 ON MUSIC-MAKING AND FAMILY-DOMESTIC LIFE

The impacts of the pandemic on the incomes of the young musicians are indisputable, and in most cases both our interviewees and their partners worked in the cultural sector. This threatened sustainability of the professional future of the interviewees. Given that our focus is to show that the market failed, but that online as an alternative was not viable for most musicians, thus accentuating their precariousness and the uncertainty of their lives, I introduce here the contributions of Gielen (2018), because they show that cultural work is only sustainable when there is a balance between the intimate spaces of production, the market, and the social and civil dimensions of the arts. In other words, we are before a level of abstraction that marks these three poles, and the final product - music - can be seen as a component of personhood (Louth, 2012). Here the concept of personhood comes from the informal knowledge that is obtained and mobilized for the creation of personal epistemologies of individuals as musicians The novelty of this model is its view of the importance of life as a whole: giving prominence to the intimate, personal, domestic, and family sphere of artists and musicians. Since the 2008 economic and financial crisis, working in Portugal in the cultural and creative sector has become synonymous of great precariousness, so many artists and musicians have had to work in other areas to earn a stable income and continue to pursue their music as a hobby. One example is Rui, a 34-year-old musician with two young daughters, whose only professional activity was music. His wife also works in the cultural sector. Due to a lack of support from the Portuguese state, Rui and his wife saved money on fuel, as they could not leave home, and on food, as they did not go out to rehearse or attend concerts. They only received extraordinary support due to the reduction of professional activity as self-employed workers[3].

I continue to work only on music. This year has not been easy at all. When the pandemic broke out, just from what I had already booked, I lost 14,000 Euros. That's a whole year! I have two daughters. You always must have income coming in ...And my wife does the same ... We are surviving with the extraordinary support for the reduction of the activity of independent workers, from social security, but it's very little money. We've been holding on, but we haven't managed to save any money. (Rui, 34 years old, musician)

Although in reports and works such as Strong and Cannizzo (2020) only the negative impacts of the containment measures of COVID-19 are reported, in individual spheres, positive aspects emerge. This shows the isolation and the pandemic were not experienced by everyone in the same way, demonstrating that social impacts do not follow a linear path. Indeed, the measures to combat the pandemic can be seen from two perspectives. With reference to what we mentioned earlier about the regulation of markets, we can already see that even before the pandemic, the market was already failing to regulate the careers and economic remuneration of these artisans (Polanyi, 1957). The first concerns musicians who only survived from live performance of music and who suddenly found themselves with nothing, which is the case of António; the second concerns musicians who had artistic and musical activity as a second job and, with the cancellation of concerts and the imposition of isolation, ended up dedicating themselves more to the creative processes of music-making, like Rafael. The first group of musicians battled the most against depression and anxiety, while those in the second group have a positive view of the impacts of the pandemic. It all depends on the proportion that live music occupies in their careers.

It all happened at the same time. The last concert I gave was on March 6, 2020. I had a concert on March 11, which didn't happen, then I didn't have anything else ... The normal concerts were all cancelled. Some were postponed. (António, 35 years old, musician)

I wrote a lot more than I played. Mainly that was it. I focused much more on writing and as I haven't played as much, the idea part of the songs merged more with the drawings, the films, the paintings and so there is a big idea floating around that can branch out into all areas and the music I start making will certainly be affected by that and will be in an ambience that is perhaps a bit denser, with more words and a greater focus on the idea of music than something quicker and more fleeting. (Rafael, 22 years old, musician, and visual artist)

The pandemic put many families' lives on pause, causing plans to be postponed. In Pedro's case, as his wife also works in the cultural sector, they have had to postpone their dream of buying a house. Others have found themselves in even more precarious situations – for example, musicians who have been fired from their bands, and to survive have had to look for jobs in areas such as construction. Several academic studies (e.g. Guerra, 2010) have documented the precariousness of musicians' careers in Portugal, in the sense that most are forced to have another professional activity for economic stability and to be able to maintain their musical activity, because work in the cultural sector is seasonal, and between November and April there are few job opportunities.

If, for some interviewees, isolation and online working were seen as a springboard for fostering creativity (Howard et al., 2021); for others they had a profoundly negative impact on creativity, due to financial difficulties and being apart from the outside world. At the same time, motivation is also complementary to the direct impacts of the pandemic. Some musicians were motivated by the possibility of producing more, so in the future they would have more opportunities to do concerts and shows, while other artists were completely unmotivated, asking "What am I going to create and produce for?" and "There are no concerts, so what's the point?" Conflict between the music-making process and family life also emerged, with demands intensifying and posing new challenges (Blum, 2020; Guerra et al., 2021; Rocco, 2020). Working at home - especially for those with children - became a challenge, as there was no separation between individual and collective spaces. Family life and work life ended up being a continuum, as we can see from the excerpts presented below,

In the beginning, it was very difficult to work with the children at home ... The first few days I could still work, but then I couldn't. It's an intensity! Even more so in a tiny flat, with a screaming baby, always knocking at the door. (João, 33 years old, musician)

We were in a phase where we were rehearsing and composing every week, making new songs. And when this came up, it was at the time when I was a father, Afonso was a father, then João was a father, which means half the band was a father. So, reconciling the pandemic with fatherhood, we stopped completely and now we're seeing if we'll start up again and if we'll resume composing. But there's been an almost complete stop. We kept in touch every day. But the composition part was completely stopped. In terms of the solo project, I took advantage of the paternity and the two months to compose. I made some songs. Now I don't know if I can continue or not. For now, I'm in a more precarious situation in professional terms, so I can't give priority to something that's not going to make me any money. (Salvador, 33 years old, musician)

THE FIGHT FOR LIFE: WELLBEING AND RESISTANCE

Picking up on the end of the previous section, which refers to the difficulties experienced by the interviewees who had children, in this section, we look for to demonstrate alternative courses of action and which modes of resistance and overcoming were used by the interviewees to face these difficulties, as well as others. For most of the interviewees, the difficulty of reconciling various social roles within one single space has been overwhelming. Wellbeing and mental health were affected (Li & Wang, 2020, Salari et al., 2020), although some young musicians have been able to fight back. According to Terasawa et al. (2021), these changes through had a deep impact on daily routines and behaviors – visible mainly in the domestic sphere, where loneliness and sadness tended to be highlighted given that concerts disappeared, music lessons ended, and live rehearsals were suspended. This is demonstrated in the speech of Pedro,

In terms of mental health I would say that it affected me – the fact of not being able to leave home and not being on the road because it's something I have been doing for seven years ... suddenly I lose that right of being able to be outside my own city and that of knowing new spaces and new people ... being locked at home affected me pretty much and not having the freedom – music was one of my first escapes ... yes, I had my guitar at home and to distract myself ... I played and that would eventually calm me down a bit. (Pedro, 28 years old, musician and sound technician)

Authors like Sloboda (2010) describe music as something to be experienced in communal settings, generating a series of emotional experiences (DeNora, 2000); the pandemic suspended this. Terasawa et al. (2021) argue that a change in the location of music impacts the musical experience and causes changes in musical behaviors. The pandemic showed the act of listening to music is accessible to most people through new technologies and digital platforms; however, the act of making music is only available to those with the economic power to acquire suitable equipment and technologies to record at home. For some, isolation served as an opportunity to deepen the creative process. In this section, we consider how the practice of music creation is a kind of moderator of dispositions and emotions and, as such, a combat tool against depression, isolation, loneliness and sadness (Thoma et al., 2012).

For now, from a personal level, it is funny because it suddenly made me listen again to the CDs at home. I bought a bunch of vinyls in this period, and re-listened to vinyls. I had time to listen to music and have also a session and all this is very personal, we had a session of listening to our childhood music in the car, Pearl Jam, Red Hot Chili Peppers, Nirvana, Radiohead ... Me and my partner did this thing, both screaming in the car and it was very good for surviving COVID. (André, 33 years old, musician and researcher)

This excerpt from Andre's interview reveals Swarbrick et al.'s (2018) view of music as a universal phenomenon. Although music has a physical component, including live events, it acquired new significance during isolation. The interviewees described music during COVID-19 as an alternative to the stress of the family context. Many articles have been published by musicians portraying their losses and their fight to maintain mental health (Neller, 2021). It is relevant to highlight the work of Brunt and Nelligan (2021), who discuss pandemic media narratives of cultural workers. The first narrative articulated musicians' personal accounts of grief and loss, and the direct impact on mental health. The use of first-person language helped to capture the feelings of despair. Although this study was carried out in Australia, the situation in Portugal was similar, with interviewees stating that they felt swamped by the quantity of news about COVID-19's impact on the music industry.

The second narrative identified by Brunt and Nelligan (2021) was the creation of web pages supporting creativity and the wellbeing of the artists, something that was completely neglected in Portugal. While non-musicians enjoyed free online or streamed musical productions during isolation, in professional musicians were running out of opportunities to maintain their activities (Terasawa et al., 2011), which led many musicians to the digital universe. Among the interviewees, men generally tried to obtain revenue digitally, while female artists were more discouraged – perhaps due to more family pressure (Strong & Cannizo, 2020). When questioned about their online usage, men tended to refer to problems such as a lack of instruments or specialized equipment, or a lack of public exposure, while women referred to aesthetic worries, clothes, or the number of visualizations they had, for example Ana refers that,

Afterwards I was able to make a live stream concert for a gig at Antenna3 but I thought it was horrible, it's very strange to give a concert for people you are not seeing via mobile phone, through their Instagram, and they are far away ... you can't even capture anyone's reaction ... you can just see yourself on the screen and it is a 1x1 very strange conversation ... it is super different and a completely different mindset because I am not thinking in the future or if I am looking hot. (Ana, 25 years old, musician and singer)

Lindsey et al. (2021) demonstrate that art served as an escape during the pandemic, offering opportunities for the individuals to express their emotions, something evident in the discourses of our younger women interviewees, who saw themselves distanced from their parents and friends,

Music is what saves my mental health, the truth is, pre-pandemic, during the pandemic, post-pandemic... it was the way I figured to be able to express everything ... for me it was always music and it is basically my psychologist. (Inês, 28 years old, singer)

For our interviewees, music was essential for mental health and wellbeing. Those who continued to produce artistic content during the pandemic saw themselves affected by isolation in a positive way, whereas others saw themselves unable to produce and create, and as affected negatively by isolation. Artistic production and creativity became popular topics during isolation, with Braus and Morton (2020) identifying artistic practice as beneficial during the crisis, leading to self-awareness and a perception of control of the situation. Gupta (2020) says such artistic creation allowed an invisible virus to be given tangibility.

CAN WE WORK IT OUT? CAREERS, PRECARITY AND DOMESTIC LIFE

Arriving at this section, we resume the idea that the online universe emerged as an alternative to traditional markets and the economic sector that underlies the music industry. Thus, we intend here to demonstrate the ways in which the digital universe can be seen as a continuation of the failures of the economic market and the music industry sector, as the precariousness of careers continued or became even more accentuated, as well as causing numerous constraints on home life (space, schedules, equipment, etc.).

Many musicians turned to the digital universe during COVID-19, livestreaming (Vandenberg et al., 2021), and releasing albums and songs to sell merchandise. For artists with families, the digital was seen as a possible path to earn revenue, though for many it failed. But for the majority of our interviewees, the digital was seen more as a way to battle depression and isolation because it enabled contact with other artists, to share ideas and perfect other competencies, such as voice training, marketing, and mastering.

Why is it that musicians must be obliged to offer a concert when concerts are a way for them to gain a living? Why is it that the artist has the social responsibility to entertain people that are confined? I think that people relied too much on livestreams. It is much easier to say "make a video of a concert" when there is no infrastructure to support that. And even small artists, as well as big ones had big losses. And nobody thinks about the technicians. A band is not just the musicians. (Catarina, 26 years old, manager and student)

Even within a group affected profoundly by the pandemic and that is disadvantaged compared with other workers, deep inequalities exist. While some artists were able to engage in upskilling, for others a lack of quality recording equipment or finances impeded their ability to record. The ambivalence and duality of the interviews materialized the inequality in and of the artistic careers evidenced by the pandemic. Those musicians who were able to improve their musical and production capabilities during the pandemic as a possible 'window of opportunity' for a better future (Strothers, 2021) tended to be those without family or financial commitments, or intense domestic activities, like it happened with Diogo,

When the quarantine began, the first thing that I thought was: I'll record a new album. The second thought was: I'll be investing in myself, in the time I never had, to be a better singer, to speak better English. I applied that … I trained my singing

and started to have good results ... Today I feel I am a much more prepared artist than before the pandemic. Nevertheless, if I had kids and a house to support ... I wouldn't have done all this. (Diogo, 35 years old, musician, actor)

If some saw in the pandemic an incentive for artistic and creative production, many interviewees also mentioned that the digital complicated things because they were not familiar with it and were unable to take advantage of it. Others also said their personal lives impeded an effective digital presence. The excerpt below demonstrates the idea of precarious careers that we talked about at the beginning of the section, i.e. it emphasises the idea that the digital universe is presented as a democratic tool available for everyone to take advantage of, however, it is not very often that we hear reports of this kind that, to a certain extent, highlight the ways in which digital media also deregulate the market and accentuate inequalities. This assumption is clear in the case of Tiago.

During the pandemic I just made two streaming transmissions because when you have another job and other responsibilities, sometimes it is difficult to remember that I am a musician. I also discovered I should have learned much more about what playing with an acoustic guitar in my room and with just my computer microphone implied. (Tiago, 35 years old, musician and office clerk)

Thinking about the inequalities and about the digital universe, Levstek et al. (2021) refer to the amplified impacts of music's collective dimension (Collins, 2004). The creation of group and collective identities during the pandemic was another point raised. Through the digital universe, artists found support and identification with other artists; nevertheless, this deeply affected family life, since many artists focused on this conviviality and sharing and relegated family life to a second place. Indeed, artists started seeing in the digital, alternative scenarios new realities similar to those pre-pandemic. Turino (2008) describes this as sonic bonding, something that can be seen in the Manuel's speech,

We have discussed among ourselves the need to produce at home and we started exchanging music through the internet. One would compose, leave a folder in Dropbox and the others would listen and began adding their parts. I went first, then the bassist, then the guitarist solo and finally the drummer. We tried to put together a scheme so as not to stand still and to continue to have production. In that period, we were able to make three songs we play at rehearsals. (Manuel, 32 years old, musician and researcher)

The sharing of music with other artists via the internet was considered positive by some interviewees, as leading to the release of more work, more concerts and more stable careers post-pandemic. Moreover, this sonic bonding would ultimately imply a process of reinvention of the industry by artists, in the sense that the platforms such as Facebook, Instagram or Bandcamp would end up being the new stages, the new rehearsal rooms and the platforms of discussion and content sharing. New ways of making music, but also of communicating, were generated – aspects that in the medium and long term would affect the careers of the musicians.

Even being at home, we weren't very active. We are part of the Pandemonium Platform[4] which integrates many artists and came to be to give opportunities for these artists to remain active, to produce and compose and even, perhaps, to join their art and make some interesting work together, that is what happened eventually. So I ended up remaining active in this aspect and ended up giving myself those distraction moments at the end of the day, where I left work and husband aside and only concentrated on myself. (Ana, 30 years old, musician and music teacher)

It is clear that music was used as a way for individuals to remain socially connected (MacDonald et al., 2021) and the digital was seen by some as an alternative to economic precarity (Strong & Cannizzo, 2021). The truth is that the pandemic came to accentuate the need for Portuguese musicians to reinvent their careers and ways of life, generating new processes of resistance and resilience (Anacin, 2021; Guerra, 2021). As Hunt and Gedgaudas (2020) advocate, there will never be a uniform model to confront the crisis by the musicians and their families, partly because each departs from a different experiential context. However, it was clear that the digital was seen negatively by most of our interviewees. From the outset, this was due to the precarity of their careers, which in the interviewees' understanding was materialized in low wages and poor working conditions – in other words, the absence of employment ties and a lack of recognition of the importance of music and those who work in music. In periods of crisis, the artistic field suffers the most, due to a lack of support and the absence of an entity that represents the interests of cultural workers. COVID-19 has led to major concern with the survival of the music sector and those who are part of it. There is, on the one side, a critical and attentive view of the possible impacts of the proliferation of livestreams (Frenneaux & Bennett, 2011), particularly regarding the devaluation of live concerts. In this sense, a question emerges: has digital led to the devaluation of live concerts? How will the careers and the lives of these artist be sustained? And what will the impact of these changes be on their families and their domestic life? These issues need to be studied in the future. At the level of economic sustainability, a small glimpse of the Portuguese reality is already available in the excerpt below,

I participated at a friend's live and afterwards we split the earnings between the two. I won't tell you that it was an awful quantity, but it also wasn't enough to fulfil the basic needs of my family in a month. It is also understood that people were passing through difficulties, but I think the problem was having made this in a voluntary logic, kind of like who wanted gave and whatever he wanted to give ... we should have made something closed, kind of like them paying a fix sum to attend. (Luís, 30 years old, musician, graffiti, and tattoo artist)

On the other side, some interviewees presented a more optimistic view of the role of technologies in the long term, for both individuals and music careers, as well as in the domestic space. Many interviewees recognized that the digital will be the path to follow, primarily because of economic factors; they indicated a view that the family life conditions would improve, leaving uncertainty and precarity less obvious. This group of interviewees argued that the online would not substitute for the live, but rather complement it, as it provides other types of stimuli, interactions, creations and ways of sharing. From the beginning of the pandemic, technology evolved in an abysmal and unpredictable way, to respond to the lived experiences of artists. The online is still the main means to promote concerts or sell merchandising, but it also took on the role of alerting artists to other emergent public needs. For our interviewees, the exponential increase in the number of series and movies available on platforms such as Netflix changed music and musicians' careers.

It is not streaming that will replace live shows, for example. Now the digital will help the exponential growth of series; I think there are many more ways and many more ramifications through which music can go and through which people who want to make art can eventually go. I think that this partly individual and partly communitarian. More and more people [are affected] ... and perhaps this confinement could even bring us lots of alterations in in this aspect, because we already perceive that the digital world will not be the same, or will not substitute for the real life. We already perceive that we don't have the same stimuli, we don't have the same relationship with the world digitally as we have with the real world. Technology also evolved in an unpredictable manner and very quickly to do justice to this need of the digital life that people suddenly were obliged to have. But I think we can take good things from here. (Miguel, 35 years, musician, songwriter, and producer)

PERHAPS EVERYTHING WILL NOT BE ALRIGHT: CONCLUSIONS

This chapter was based on the question of whether music can save lives. Although we cannot definitively answer this, it did become possible to infer that it can have an effect: music and music-making (Howard et al., 2021) produce deep impacts in the sense that they can soften social, economic, political, family, living, and mental conditions. Our interviewees enabled us to verify that the cultural and creative sector was deeply impacted by the pandemic, and consequently musicians were among the groups who suffered most – especially given the lack of economic support by the state. Even though this research provides a glimpse of the pandemic's impact on the musical ecosystem (Strong, 2021), there are still many unknowns in relation to living experiences and the domestic space. What is certain is that within the literature review undertaken when writing this chapter, we came across many studies in other countries that provided accounts – in a wider and deeper way – of the impacts of the pandemic on the lives of musicians, their creative processes and their family lives. Our interviewees were left without work prospects and without stable wages, and saw their careers being thrown into the kind of limbo associated with not knowing when it will be possible to go back to some kind of normality. In addition, the pandemic also came to accentuate many other kinds of social inequalities that had not previously been considered.

The double precarity was accentuated in the case of our interviewees – that is, it existed frequently as a discourse about partners also working in the cultural sector, which made them see their professional and personal futures as unfeasible. This chapter has demonstrated that isolation and the pandemic were not lived in the same way by everyone, with some musicians who usually survive only through their musical activities suddenly seeing themselves with nothing, while others who had artistic and musical activity as a second job found that, with concerts cancelled and with the imposition of isolation, they had the opportunity to dedicate more to their own creative processes and music-making. If some do see a future online, it is generally as a complement to live shows – when these come back; others understand that the digital has just worked to devalue concerts. There were musicians who took advantage of the digital switchover to dedicate themselves to learning music and study; others were unable to reconcile their domestic life with their presence on social networks. At the level of mental health there were also many differences that – due to page limitations – could not be addressed in depth: some artists used artistic practice and creativity to remain active and to alleviate social isolation, while others saw their mental health deeply affected by having no future work prospects. For those without children, immersion in creative processes occurred in a natural way, while parents who were in charge of their children 24/7 often felt defeated by the accumulation of social roles within a small physical space. Moreover, not all musicians had the physical conditions or the necessary means to continue producing and making music. Yet, despite all these differences, and with so many uncertainties and precarious futures in play, music was always in a highlighted spot and was appointed as a point of salvation.

REFERENCES

Anacin, C. (2021). I lost a gig "pero ok lang": Filipino migrant musicians in Australia during the COVID-19 pandemic. *Perfect Beat*, *21*(1), 33–39. doi:10.1558/prbt.19260

Arnett, J. J. (2014). *Emerging Adulthood: The Winding Road from the Late Teens Through the Twenties*. Oxford. doi:10.1093/acprof:oso/9780199929382.001.0001

Banks, M. (2020). The work of culture and C-19. *European Journal of Cultural Studies*, *23*(4), 648–654. doi:10.1177/1367549420924687

Bardin, L. (1977). *Análise de conteúdo* [Content analysis]. Edições 70.

Beatfreeks. (2020). *Take the temperature: A national youth trends report understanding the impact of coronavirus on young people in the UK*. Retrieved from: https://www.beatfreeksyouthtrends.com/take-the-temperature

Beckert, J. (2007). The great transformation of embeddedness. Karl Polanyi and the New Economic Sociology. *Max Planck Institute for the Study of Societies*, *7*(1), 1–25. doi:10.2139srn.2465810

Blum, D. (2020). Burnt-out parents brace for a cruel summer. *New York Times*. Retrieved from: https://www.nytimes.com/2020/06/23/parenting/kidssummer-burnout-coronavirus.html

Braus, M., & Morton, B. (2020). Art therapy in the time of COVID-19. *Psychological Trauma: Theory, Research, Practice, and Policy*, *12*(1), 267–268. doi:10.1037/tra0000746 PMID:32478544

Brunt, S., & Nelligan, K. (2021). The Australian music industry's mental health crisis: Media narratives during the coronavirus pandemic. *Media International Australia*, *178*(1), 42–46. doi:10.1177/1329878X20948957

Cirillo, R., & Tullio, M. F. (Eds.). (2021). *Healing culture, reclaiming commons, fostering care: A proposal for EU cultural policies*. Italian Institute for the Future Press.

Collins, R. (2004). *Interaction rituals*. Princeton University Press. doi:10.1515/9781400851744

DeNora, T. (2000). *Music in everyday life*. Cambridge University Press. doi:10.1017/CBO9780511489433

Dillon, S. (2007). *Music, meaning and transformation*. Cambridge Scholars Publishing.

Frenneaux, R., & Bennett, A. (2021). A new paradigm of engagement for the socially distanced artist. *Rock Music Studies*, *8*(1), 65–75. doi:10.1080/19401159.2020.1852770

Frith, S. (2003). Music and everyday life. *Critical Quarterly*, *44*(1), 35–48. doi:10.1111/1467-8705.00399

Gielen, P. (2018). Safeguarding creativity: An artistic biotope and its institutional insecurities in a global market orientated Europe. In Y. Watanabe (Ed.), *Handbook of Cultural Security* (pp. 398–416). Edward Elgar. doi:10.4337/9781786437747.00028

Guerra, P. (2010). *A instável leveza do rock: génese, dinâmica e consolidação do rock alternativo em Portugal* [The unstable lightness of rock: genesis, dynamics and consolidation of alternative rock in Portugal] [Unpublished doctoral dissertation]. University of Porto.

Guerra, P. (2015). Keep it rocking: The social space of Portuguese alternative rock (1980–2010). *Journal of Sociology (Melbourne, Vic.)*, *52*(4), 615–630. doi:10.1177/1440783315569557

Guerra, P. (2017). 'Just can't go to sleep': DIY cultures and alternative economies from the perspective of social theory. *Portuguese Journal of Social Science*, *16*(3), 277–282. doi:10.1386/pjss.16.3.277_2

Guerra, P. (2018). Raw power: Punk, DIY and underground cultures as spaces of resistance in contemporary Portugal. *Cultural Sociology*, *12*(2), 241–259. doi:10.1177/1749975518770353

Guerra, P. (2021). So close yet so far: DIY cultures in Portugal and Brazil. *Cultural Trends*, *30*(2), 122–138. doi:10.1080/09548963.2021.1877085

Guerra, P., Oliveira, A., & Sousa, S. (2021). Um Requiem pelas músicas que perdemos: Percursos com paragens pelos impactos da pandemia na produção musical independente em Portugal [A Requiem for the songs we lost: journeys with stops by the impacts of the pandemic on independente music production in Portugal]. *O Público e o Privado: Caderno dos Nucleos e Grupos de Pesquisa Vinculados ao Mestrado Academico em Politicas Publicas e Sociedade da Universidade Estadual do Ceara*, *38*, 171–198.

Gupta, N. (2020). Singing away the social distancing blues: Art therapy in a time of coronavirus. *Journal of Humanistic Psychology*, *60*(5), 593–603. doi:10.1177/0022167820927807

Howard, F., Bennett, A., Green, B., Guerra, P., Sousa, S., & Sofija, E. (2021). "It's turned me from a professional to a 'bedroom DJ' once again": COVID-19 and new forms of inequality for young music-makers. *Young*, *29*(4), 417–432. doi:10.1177/1103308821998542

Hunt, M., & Gedgaudas, L. (2020). *Initial impacts of the COVID-19 crisis on the music industry in Colorado and the Denver metropolitan region*. Colorado State University.

Levstek, M., Bamby, R. M., Pocock, K. L., & Banerjee, R. (2021). "It all makes us feel together": Young people's experiences of virtual group music-making during the COVID-19 pandemic. *Frontiers in Psychology*, *12*, 1–18. doi:10.3389/fpsyg.2021.703892 PMID:34421756

Li, L. Z., & Wang, S. (2020). Prevalence and predictors of general psychiatric disorders and loneliness during COVID-19 in the United Kingdom. *Psychiatry Research*, *291*, 113267. doi:10.1016/j.psychres.2020.113267 PMID:32623266

Louth, P. (2012). Personal knowledge, personal epistemology, and informal music learning. In S. O'Neill (Ed.), *Personhood and Music Learning. Connecting Perspectives and Narratives* (pp. 17–32). Canadian Music Educators' Association.

Lindsey, I., Mahammadie-Sabet, S., & Rademacher, N. (2021). *Art-making and wellbeing with professional artists during a pandemic* [Unpublished doctoral dissertation]. Loyola Marymount University.

MacDonald, R., Burke, R., DeNora, T., Donohue, M. S., & Birrell, R. (2021). Our virtual tribe: Sustaining and enhancing community via online music improvisation. *Frontiers in Psychology*, *11*, 1–19. doi:10.3389/fpsyg.2020.623640 PMID:33708151

Mas-Herrero, E., Singer, N., Ferreri, L., McPhee, M., Zatorre, R. J., & Ripollés, P. (2020). *Rock'n'roll but not sex or drugs: Music is negatively correlated to depressive symptoms during the COVID-19 pandemic via reward-related mechanisms*. Retrieved from: https://psyarxiv.com/x5upn

Neller, M. A. (2021). Life on pause: Coping with loss as a musician in a pandemic. *Rock Music Studies*, *8*(1), 3–6. doi:10.1080/19401159.2020.1852775

Polanyi, K. (1957). *The great transformation*. Beacon Press.

Rocco, P. (2020). Let me go to the office! An investigation into the side effects of working from home on work–life balance. *International Journal of Public Sector Management*, *33*(6/7), 771–790. doi:10.1108/IJPSM-06-2020-0150

Salari, N., Hosseinian-Far, A., Jalali, R., Vaisi-Raygani, A., Rasoulpoor, S., Mohammadi, M., Rasoulpoor, S., & Khaledi-Paveh, B. (2020). Prevalence of stress, anxiety, depression among the general population during the COVID-19 pandemic: A systematic review and meta-analysis. *Globalization and Health*, *16*(1), 57. doi:10.118612992-020-00589-w PMID:32631403

Sarkar, P. (2021). Being a DJ in a time of zero social huddling: Tales from a locked-down India. *Perfect Beat*, *21*(1), 47–55. doi:10.1558/prbt.19347

Sloboda, J. A. (2010). Music in everyday life: The role of emotions. In P. N. Juslin & J. A. Sloboda (Eds.), *Handbook of music and emotion: Theory, research, applications* (pp. 493–514). Oxford University Press.

Sound Diplomacy. (2020). *Music cities – resilience handbook*. Retrieved from: https://www.sounddiplomacy.com/better-music-cities

Strong, C. (2021). Introduction: Music history and the COVID-19 pandemic. *Popular Music History*, *14*, 5–8.

Strong, C., & Cannizzo, F. (2020). *Understanding Challenges to the Victorian Music Industry During COVID-19*. RMIT University.

Strong, C., & Cannizzo, F. (2021). Pre-existing conditions: Precarity, creative justice and the impact of the COVID-19 pandemic on the Victorian music industries. *Perfect Beat*, *21*(1), 10–24. doi:10.1558/prbt.19379

Strothers, S. R. (2021). Virtual shakuhachi with dai-shihan Michael Chikuzen Gould: Shakuhachi learning before and during the pandemic. *Perfect Beat*, *21*(1), 81–86. doi:10.1558/prbt.19346

Swarbrick, D., Bosnyak, D., Livingstone, S. R., Bansal, J., Marsh-Rollo, S., Woolhouse, M. H., & Trainor, L. J. (2018). How live music moves us: Head movement differences in audiences to live versus recorded music. *Frontiers in Psychology, 9*. https://www.frontiersin.org/articles/10.3389/fpsyg.2018.02682/full PMID:30687158

Teixeira, N., Vianna, G. M., Lima, R., Jáuregui, C., Furtado, L., Alberto, T. P., & Medeiros, R. (2021). COVID-19 impact on the music sector in Belo Horizonte (Minas Gerais, Brazil). *Frontiers in Sociology*, *6*, 1–21. doi:10.3389/fsoc.2021.643344 PMID:34268350

Terasawa, H., Matsubara, M., Goudarzi, V., & Sadakata, M. (2021). Music in quarantine: Connections between changes in lifestyle, psychological states, and musical behaviors during the COVID-19 pandemic. *Frontiers in Psychology*, *12*, 1–18. doi:10.3389/fpsyg.2021.689505 PMID:34707530

Thoma, M. V., Ryf, S., Mohiyeddini, C., Ehlert, U., & Nater, U. M. (2012). Emotion regulation through listening to music in everyday situations. *Cognition and Emotion*, *26*(3), 550–560. doi:10.1080/02699931.2011.595390 PMID:21902567

Turino, T. (2008). *Music as social life: The politics of participation*. Chicago University Press.

Vandenberg, F., Berghman, M., & Schaap, J. (2021). The “lonely raver”: Music livestreams during COVID-19 as a hotline to collective consciousness? *European Societies*, *23*(sup1), 141–153. doi:10.1080/14616696.2020.1818271

ENDNOTES

1. This chapter is part of the Transnational Research Project entitled “Until COVID-19 do us apart: Music Scenes in Lockdown”, the result of a partnership between Portugal, Australia, and the United Kingdom. This transnational project aims to understand how the creative and working lives of people in the music industry have been impacted by the pandemic. For further information, see https://www.kismifcommunity.com. This chapter was supported by FCT – Foundation for Science and Technology within the scope of UIDB/00727/2020.
2. This article complies fully with the guidelines included in the Charter of Fundamental Rights of the European Union (2000/C364/01), including any information, private or professional, concerning an identified or identifiable natural person (Article 2(a) of EU Directive 95/46/EC). We also comply with the guidelines contained in the General Data Protection Regulation No. 2016/679. The collection, processing, management, and exploitation of data

will similarly be based on the guidelines provided by the Codes of Ethics of the International Sociological Association and the Oral History Association and International Council on Archives, in addition to the Code of Ethics of the International Sociological Association and the Statement of Ethics of the American Anthropological Association. All the interviewees' names are fictitious.

3 In fact, most of the musicians we interviewed were self-employed, making them the target of greater inequality and therefore one of the groups most affected by the pandemic, as they were excluded from most state support (Guerra et al., 2021; Sarkar, 2021).

4 An artistic creation collective that bets on the expansion of new artists and on a new creative approach that privileges multidisciplinarity. This platform appeared during the pandemic as a disengaged initiative, as a vehicle in the construction of an alternative through true communitarian and collaborative meaning, but also a strategy and real implementation. For more information, see https://plataformadopandemonio.com/quem-somos.

Chapter 8
Gender Violence in Mexico Before and During the COVID-19 Pandemic:
A Multidimensional Analysis

Ingrid N. Pinto-López
https://orcid.org/0000-0002-1580-1375
UPAEP Universidad, Mexico

Cynthia Maria Montaudon-Tomas
https://orcid.org/0000-0002-2595-6960
UPAEP Universidad, Mexico

Alicia L. Yáñez-Moneda
UPAEP Universidad, Mexico

ABSTRACT

This chapter analyzes gender-based violence in Mexico before and during the COVID-19 pandemic. Various indicators related to the 2030 Sustainable Development Goals, particularly Goal 5, "Achieve gender equality and empower all women and girls," are analyzed. The fuzzy ordering method of Subjective Preferences is used to perform two multidimensional analyses, a global analysis that identifies the position of Mexico with regards to other countries in the American continent and an analysis that identifies the position of each of the states of the Mexican Republic. The results allow the authors to identify the countries with the lowest and highest prevalence of gender-based violence as well as the states of the Mexican Republic with the lowest and highest prevalence of gender-based violence.

DOI: 10.4018/978-1-6684-2364-6.ch008

INTRODUCTION

Women and girls constitute half of the world's population, yet they continue to suffer discrimination and violence (UN, 2021). Gender-based violence is a generalized burden that women begin to suffer at a very young age and that has worsened with the confinement conditions derived from social distancing measures due to the COVID-19 pandemic. Approximately 736 million women (one out of three) suffer physical or sexual violence inflicted by an intimate partner or sexual assaults perpetrated by others, a figure that has remained stable over the last decade (WHO, 2021). According to data from the United Nations UN (2021), one in four young women between 15 and 24 years old that have had an intimate relationship has suffered gender violence from their partner.

A study conducted by UN Women (2021b), established that distancing conditions potentially locked women down with their abusers, creating conditions in which violence against women escalated, suggesting that 45% of women (or a woman they know) have experienced a form of gender-based violence and that one in four participants stated that household conflicts became more frequent during the pandemic making them feel insecure or unsafe in their own homes.

This phenomenon is generalized and complex. It is related to economic inequalities, socio-cultural patterns linked to norms, values, roles, and meanings surrounding being a woman and being a man. Violence against women manifests itself in different ways and different spheres and deprives the enjoyment of rights and freedoms under equal conditions between women and men (INMUJERES, 2021).

The 2030 Agenda for Sustainable Development and its 17 Sustainable Development Goals (SDGs), approved by world leaders in 2015, proposes a roadmap to achieve sustainable progress that leaves no one behind. In this sense, achieving gender equality and the empowerment of women is an integral part of the agenda, guaranteeing respect for the rights of women and girls through these objectives is a very important way to achieve inclusion and justice, as well as promote economies that benefit all people (UN Women, 2021).

Mexico has long been regarded as one of the world's most violent countries and one with the highest level of inequalities (Valencia-Londoño, Nateras-González, Bruno-Solera, Strom-Paz, 2021), and violence against women has been escalating every year. According to statistics, two-thirds of women in Mexico have experienced some form of violence (INEGI-b, 2020). Before the pandemic started, 2019 was declared the most violent year, with a 2.5% increase in violent crimes in 2018 (Fry, 2020).

In Mexico, violence against women is a public problem. According to the National Information System (INEGI, 2016), 66% of women aged 15 years or older have faced at least one act of violence in their lifetimes, and the majority of the violent acts had occurred in their community or public spaces. This information seems to be corroborated by international sources, which suggests that two thirds of women in Mexico have experienced violence and live in a climate of impunity and lack of response from the state (Murray, 2021). The National Information System (INEGI, 2016) also reported that 43% of violent acts against women in Mexico were carried out by their partners and 53% by other aggressors.

According to data from the National Survey on the Dynamics of Household Relationships ENDIREH (INEGI, 2016), the women with the highest propensity to experience violence by any aggressor throughout their lives are those who reside in urban areas (69.3%), in ages between 25 and 34 years (70.1%), those with a higher education level (72.6%) and those who do not belong to an indigenous household (66.8%).

Results of the National Survey of Urban Public Safety ENSU (INEGI, 2020) estimate that, between January and September 2020, 9% of Mexican households experienced some situation of family violence. On the other hand, the Government Censuses reveal that, of the alleged crimes registered, the main crimes committed against women are sexual abuse in relationships (42.6%) and rape (37.8%) (INEGI, 2021).

During the COVID-19 pandemic, the number of violent acts against women has escalated substantially in Mexico. Emergency calls related to violence against women in Mexico rose (Raygada & Mendoza, 2021) more than 30% in 2020, as COVID-19 lockdowns kept families at home (Murray, 2021). An increasing number of women were seeking help and refuge due to increased domestic violence during lockdown and quarantines (Yourke, 2021). The National Network of Shelters has received 80% more calls since the pandemic started, and the number of women and children admitted to shelters increased by 50% (Sánchez & Rodríguez, 2020).

Women faced numerous problems in Mexico while being in lockdown with their abusers because they could not make a call for help which led to underreporting of these crimes (Valencia, Martínez, Bruno & Storm, 2021). In Mexico, most domestic violence cases are not reported (Statista, 2021). Still, when comparing March 2020 versus March 2019, there was a 25% increase in domestic violence and abuse reports in Mexico based on police reports (Statista, 2021). Additionally, women have been overloaded with domestic tasks while under pressure from their aggressors (CIVICUS, 2020).

This chapter analyzes gender violence in Mexico, before and during the COVID-19 pandemic, based on studying the indicators proposed in Goal 5, "Gender Equality" of the Sustainable Development Goals. Mexico signed the 2030 Agenda in September 2015, and to monitor the progress of the Sustainable Development Goals, it developed the monitoring system " Sustainable Development Goals Information System" (SIODS, acronym in Spanish), which provides georeferenced information on the progress made in relation to the monitoring of the 2030 Agenda (INEGI, 2021). Secondary information available in the SIODS monitoring system is used for the analysis.

BACKGROUND

Theoretical Framework: Gender Violence

The World Health Organization (WHO) defines violence as:

The deliberate use of physical force or power, whether threatening or effective, against oneself, other people or a group or community, that causes or is likely to cause injury, death, psychological damage, developmental disorders or deprivation (WHO, 2002, p.5).

Gender, on the other hand, can be defined as a:

Category that analyzes how sexual differences are defined, represented and symbolized in a given society. It alludes to the historical and socio-cultural ways women and men construct their identity, interact and organize their functions. These forms vary from one culture to another and are transformed over time (INMUJERES, 2007).

Gender violence can be described as a type of aggression that women and girls face, that can be either physical, verbal, psychological, sexual, or patrimonial, among other types, which can end up in femicide (Alvarado & Guerra, 2012), and is characterized by the control of power from male to female (Bravo, 2004). According to the United Nations (1994), in its Declaration on the Elimination of Violence against Women, violence against women is:

Any act of gender-based violence that results in, or is likely to result in, physical, sexual or psychological harm or suffering to women, including threats of such acts, coercion or arbitrary deprivation of liberty, whether occurring in public or in private life (UN, 1994)

Violence against women, in any of its forms, is a violation of human rights, as recognized by the United Nations (Carreras, 2019). Violence against women has been considered a *shadow pandemic* (UN Women, 2021a) which has exacerbated the preexisting violence crisis in which women are no longer safe in their homes or public spaces. It has also been regarded as a *pandemic of violence* (Prusa, García-Nice

& Soledad, 2020), the *patriarchal pandemic* (Fernández, 2021), a *silent pandemic*, and a *pandemic within a pandemic* (Stephen, 2020).

The COVID-19 pandemic and gender violence have been connected in numerous ways, and together, they have been called the two global pandemics. The difference between them is that the first is sudden and unpredictable, while the second is constant and predictable (Weil, 2020). Gender violence has also been depicted as a *collateral issue* of COVID-19 (Guerra-Lund, Manica & Manica, 2020), and family violence, more specifically that directed towards women during confinement, has been called *the perfect storm* (Usher, Bradbury, Bhullar, Durkin, Gyamfi, Fatema, & Jackson, 2021).

Gender is an important inequality that offers valuable insights into social relationships exacerbated by globalization and also by the pandemic, in which it has become a visible category for analyzing violence. Women have traditionally been the most affected by health crises and pandemics (Fernández, 2021). The pandemic made preexisting forms of discrimination and inequalities for women more visible (CIVICUS, 2020).

Polanyi's (1944) great transformation can be associated with the COVID-19 pandemic since this is a crisis with a magnitude like the great depression. It is a time of massive change with multiple effects (Meier, 2008), especially based on gender differences, gender violence, the feminization of the workforce across the world and the emergence of the "economic woman" and female behavior as part of the engendered considerations in Polanyi's works (Beneria, 1999). Polanyi's concept of embeddedness based on changes in social relationships and social structures, including kinship, gender, age, organizations, the economy, education, and other issues (Barber, 1995), following the 'new economic sociology' and Granovetter's (1985) use of embeddedness, referred to as the 'soft' Polanyi, (Peck, 2013),which can be useful in understanding gender differences and violence against gender in the COVID-19 pandemic.

Domestic violence became more prevalent during the first year of lockdown of the pandemic because disagreements tend to become exacerbated when families spend more time together. Additionally, financial situations became destabilized, increasing stress and opportunities for abuse. Isolation weakened support networks, and being in close quarters sometimes prevented the possibility of reporting the abuse (Felbab-Brown, 2020).

Furthermore, previous study suggests that verbal and physical abuse by a partner became more common according to 70% of the participants. Women aged 19 to 49 were the group most affected by domestic violence, and 52% of those reporting domestic violence were unemployed, compared to 43% of employed women reporting the same problem. Furthermore, 41% of the participants suggested that lockdown conditions due to the pandemic negatively affected their mental health.

Gender Violence and 2030 SDGs

In all parts of the world, women and girls should have the same rights and opportunities and should lead a life free of violence and discrimination. In this sense, along with other areas that need attention, the UN established a set of goals to be achieved by member countries by 2030. Goal number five of the 17 Sustainable Development Goals (SDG) aims to achieve gender equality and empower all women and girls (UN Women, 2021). SDG 5 comprises 9 targets and 14 indicators (see Table 1) (UNSTATS, N/D) that help measure specific conditions related to this issue around the world.

Table 1. Goals and indicators of Sustainable Development Goal five

Goal	Description	Indicator
5.1	End all forms of discrimination against all women and girls around the world.	5.1.1 Determine whether or not there are legal frameworks to promote, enforce and monitor equality and non-discrimination based on sex.
5.2	Eliminate all forms of gender-based violence against all women and girls in the public and private spheres, including sex trafficking and other types of exploitation.	5.2.1 Proportion of women and girls aged 15 and over who have suffered physical, sexual, or psychological violence at the hands of their current or former partner in the last 12 months, broken down by the form of violence and age. 5.2.2 Proportion of women and girls aged 15 and over who have suffered sexual violence at the hands of people who were not their partners in the last 12 months, broken down by age and place of the act.
5.3	Eliminate all harmful practices, such as child, early and forced marriage, and female genital mutilation.	5.3.1 Proportion of women between the ages of 20 and 24 who were married or in a stable union before their 15th birthday and before their 18th birthday, respectively. 5.3.2 Proportion of girls and women aged 15-49 who have undergone female genital mutilation or cutting, disaggregated by age.
5.4	Recognize and value unpaid care and domestic work through public services, infrastructure, and social protection policies, promoting shared responsibility in the home and family, as appropriate in each country.	5.4.1 Proportion of time dedicated to unpaid domestic and care work, broken down by sex, age, and location. Women perform four times more unpaid work than men, and homes have become the sole functional economic unit filling the gap imposed by the state, including schooling (Faludi & Crosby, 2021).
5.5	Ensure the full and effective participation of women and equal leadership opportunities at all decision-making levels of political, economic, and public life.	5.5.1 Proportion of seats held by women in a) national parliaments and b) local governments. 5.5.2 Proportion of women in managerial positions.

Continued on following page

Table 1. Continued

Goal	Description	Indicator
5.6	Ensure universal access to sexual and reproductive health and reproductive rights as agreed in accordance with the International Conference on Population and Development's Action Program, the Beijing Platform for Action, and the outcome documents of its review conferences.	5.6.1 Proportion of women aged 15-49 who make their own informed decisions about sexual intercourse, contraceptive use, and reproductive health care. 5.6.2 Number of countries with laws and regulations that guarantee men and women from the age of 15 full and equal access to sexual and reproductive health services and to information and education in this regard.
5. a	Undertake reforms that give women equal rights to economic resources and access to ownership and control of land and other types of goods, financial services, inheritance, and natural resources, in accordance with national laws.	5.a.1 a) Proportion of the total agricultural population with secure property rights or rights over agricultural land, disaggregated by sex; and b) proportion of women among owners or holders of agricultural land rights, broken down by type of tenure. 5.a.2 Proportion of countries whose legal system (including customary law) guarantees equal rights for women to own or control land.
5. b	Improve the use of technology, particularly information and communications technology, to promote the empowerment of women.	5.b.1 Proportion of people who own a mobile phone, broken down by sex.
5. c	Pass and strengthen sound policies and applicable laws to promote gender equality and the empowerment of all women and girls at all levels.	5.c.1 Proportion of countries with systems for monitoring gender equality and women's empowerment and the allocation of public funds for this purpose.

SDG Measurement and Monitoring System

Since the development of the 2030 Agenda, the United Nations established a list of indicators that should complement the regional and national measurement systems. IAn agreement was reached with regards to the establishment of an Inter-institutional Group of Experts in charge of proposing the indicators that will measure progress in the achievement of the 17 Sustainable Development Goals. The High-Level Group for Collaboration, Coordination and Capacity Building was also established, made up of 22 representatives of national statistical offices and international regional organizations, in order to promote national ownership of the SDG progress indicators (CIDOB, 2022).

In January 2017, the Global Action Plan for the treatment of data on Sustainable Development Goals was launched, approved by the United Nations Statistical Commission. This plan establishes a framework for the planning and implementation of statistical capacities necessary to achieve the scope of the purposes of the 2030 agenda at the national level, so that regional and national statistical organizations can adjust to the Global Action Plan and monitor the SDGs (UN, 2019).

In 2018, the United Nations Statistical Commission launched the Open SDG Data Hub to promote the exploration, analysis, and use of authoritative SDG data sources for evidence and data-driven decision-making and review. The new tool allows the best presentation and dissemination of data and statistics of the SDGs (UN, 2020).

By mid-2018, the Global SDG Indicators Database was launched, presenting data at the country level, as well as global and regional aggregate data compiled through the United Nations System and other international organizations (UN, 2018). in addition to submitting global information to the Global SDG Indicators Database, Mexico built a platform called the Sustainable Development Goals Information System SIODS (INEGI, 2022) that allows to consult and download information on indicators broken down into different types: Indicator of the global framework, specific indicator for Mexico, breakdown by state, breakdown by state and municipality, breakdown by state and main cities, and breakdown by state and self-represented metropolitan areas.

To date, the SIODS platform has integrated the information of some indicators, those that are missing will be fed as the data is obtained.

Research in the Field of Gender Violence

In order to identify the behavior and impact of scientific research over time on gender violence, a bibliometric analysis was carried out considering the publications stored in the SCOPUS database (2021). The search was carried out with the keywords "gender violence" and "gender violence & Mexico" and all publications that contain any of the keywords in the title of the article, the abstract of the article, or the article keywords. Regarding the types of documents, articles, book chapters, reviews, books and conference papers were considered.

Considering the aforementioned variables for the period from 1984 to 2021, results show that 2037 documents have been published in the field of gender violence, of which 35.29% are found currently in open access. Some of these publications have over 500 citations. The documents are classified as follows: 74.71% articles, 9.13% reviews, 8.25% book chapters, 3.34% books, 2.16% conference papers.

The publications on the topic of gender violence are mainly related to Social Science (65.53%), Arts and Humanities (22.53%), Medicine (20.47%), Psychology (15.95%), and Nursing (3.44%). The countries with the most publications on the subject are Spain (25.38%), the United States (22.97%), Brazil (10.01%), the United Kingdom (8.05%), and Mexico (5.00%). A great number of organizations are involved in gender violence research, primarily universities. The most productive universities, in terms of the number of publications, are Universitat de Barcelona

(2.8%), Universidade de Sao Paulo (1.76%), Universidad de Granada (1.67%), Universidad Complutense de Madrid (1.57%), Universitat Autónoma de Barcelona (1.52%) and the National Autonomous University of Mexico (1.18%).

The annual distribution of the publications is shown in Figure 1.

Figure 1. Articles published in the field of gender violence
Source: Elaborated by the authors with data from the Scopus obtained on 25/11/2021

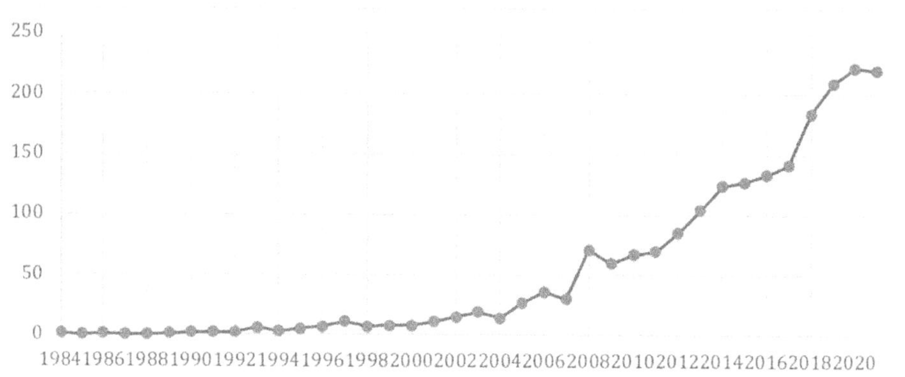

As can be seen in Figure 1, the number of publications has followed a growing trend. The increase has been more significant since the beginning of this century, a period in which approximately 96.86% of publications on this topic have been generated. In the period associated with the COVID-19 pandemic (2020-2021), 446 scientific documents related to gender violence have been published, which corresponds to 21.89% of the total publications.

When generating a search on Scopus using the keywords "gender violence" and "Mexico," 110 results are identified, of which 24.54% have been published between 2020 and 2021 (see Figure 2), and 39 publications are identified as open access.

Figure 2. Articles published containing the terms gender violence and Mexico
Source: Elaborated by the authors with data from Scopus obtained on 25/11/2021

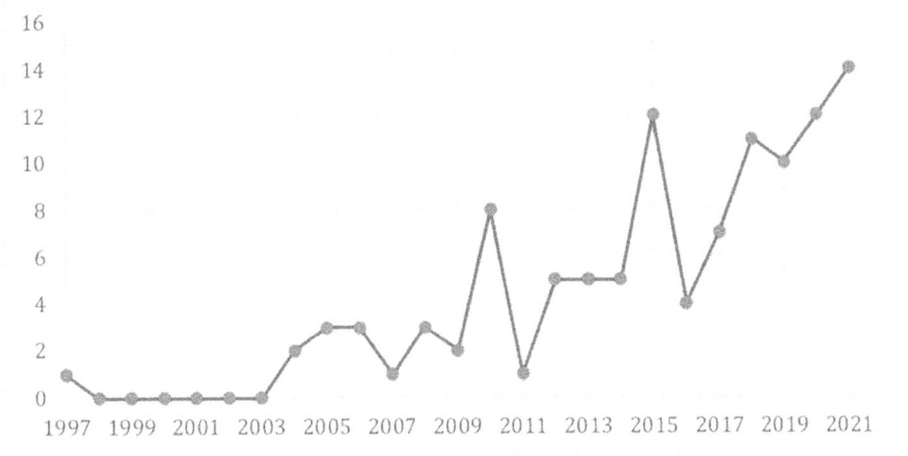

According to Scopus data, the distribution of publications refers mainly to areas of Social Sciences (70%), Medicine (22.72%), Arts and Humanities (18.18%), Psychology (11.81%), and Environmental Sciences (2.72%). The main organizations involved are the National Autonomous University of Mexico, with 14.54% of the total publications, and the National Institute of Public Health with 7.27%.

METHODOLOGY

The main focus of the chapter is to carry out a multidimensional descriptive analysis on gender violence in Mexico. The multidimensional analysis is carried out through the fuzzy ordering method of subjective preferences. Its purpose is to locate the position of each of the 32 states of the Mexican Republic in relation to gender violence, identifying those states that present lower and higher indexes of gender violence. In the same way, the subjective preferences method allows locating the position of Mexico with regard to other countries in the American continent in relation to gender violence.

The fuzzy ordering method of subjective preferences is used to carry out multi-dimensional analyses (Pinto-López et al., 2022; Gil-Lafuente et al., 2019; Gil-Aluja 1999; Kaufmann & Gil-Aluja, 1986; Gil-Lafuente & Alexander-López, 2015). The method used in the present study is an ordering method, its foundation lies in properties of the matrix calculation (Saaty, 1978; Dinh, 1984). The characteristics of the subjective preferences method allow to analyze, at first, the position of each of the states of the Mexican Republic from studying a set of indicators on gender violence. Finally, an ordered list is obtained from highest to lowest value with the position of each of the states of the Mexican Republic with regards to the best positioned state. Then, the position of Mexico is analyzed with respect to some other countries of the American continent and the countries with the lowest and highest prevalence of gender-based violence are analyzed. Both studies seek to answer questions such as which states of the Mexican Republic show the greatest progress in the fight to address gender violence? And, how is Mexico compared to countries in the American continent in relation to gender violence?

For the multidimensional study by state, secondary data provided by the Government of Mexico through the National Institute of Statistics and Geography (INEGI) published in the repository of the National Information System of Sustainable Development Goals (SIODS, 2021) is considered. The data was collected in the month of November 2021.

For the global multidimensional study, secondary data provided by the United Nations Department of Economics and Social Affairs published in the SDG Global Data Base repository (UN-b, 2021) is considered. The countries chosen were those that have information in the database and in all the indicators considered for the study, countries such as Argentina, Chile, and Colombia, were not considered because they did not have information available in the system for all the indicators used in the analysis, data was collected in the month of November 2021.

Global, national and regional indicators are analyzed with information from Goal 5, which is made up of 9 goals and 14 indicators. Descriptive studies, carried out with Excel 365 software, are also included in the analysis.

Subjective Preferences Ordering Method

The Subjective Preferences (SP) method proposes an algorithm that allows ordering physical or mental objects according to the importance of their characteristics, it consists of the following stages (Gil-Aluja, 1999; Gil-Lafuente et al., 2019):

It starts from two finite referential sets, representative of the objects to be ordered and of the characteristics:

$$\left[W_1\right]$$

$$E_1 = \left\{P_1, P_2, \ldots, P_m\right\}$$

For each characteristic C_j, j = 1, 2, ..., n a comparison is made between the selected objects, 2 by 2, C_i, C_k; i, k = 1, 2, ..., n by means of a quotient that determines the times that one object is preferred to the other.

$$E_2 = \{C_1, C_2, \ldots, C_n\}$$

Will represent the times that C_i is preferable to C_k. Evidently being:

$$\mu_{ik} = \frac{f_i}{f_k}; i, k = 1, 2, \ldots, n = \mu_{ki} = \frac{f_k}{f_i}$$

The gathering of all the $\frac{1}{\mu_{ik}}$, i, k = 1,2,…,n will lead to a matrix in R^+ for each characteristic C_j, j = 1,2,…,n, which, by construction, they will be reciprocal and coherent, and fulfill the following properties: a)

$$\mu_{ik}$$

b) All its rows (and also its columns) are proportional to the first row (and also to the first column); therefore, every row (and every column) is equal to another row (and another column) multiplied by a coefficient.

A reciprocal and coherent square matrix is of rank 1, since it has an "eigenvalue", unique and equal to n, since the remaining n-1 are equal to 0. On the other hand, if the eigenvalues of a matrix [M] are $\sum_{k=1}^{n} \mu_{ik} * f_k = \sum_{k=1}^{n} \left(\frac{f_i}{f_k}\right) * f_k = n * f_i$, we get:

$$\lambda_1, \lambda_2, \quad , \lambda_n$$

Where tr [M] is the trace of [M], that is, the sum of the elements of the main diagonal. As in the case of the reciprocal and coherent square matrices tr [M] = n, by construction, if a value is equal to n the remainder will be null.

Any positive square matrix has a positive eigenvalue, whose modulus is greater than all the others that can be real or complex. This dominant positive real eigenvalue, which will be denominated $\sum_{i=1}^{n} \lambda_i = tr\left[M\right]$ is unique, as proposed by the Perron_ Frobenius theorem. If n is the order of the matrix it will be λ_1 > = n.

The eigenvector corresponding to the dominant eigenvalue λ_1 is also made up of positive terms and when normalized, it is unique.

Therefore, if there is a positive and reciprocal square matrix of order n, its dominant eigenvalue will be λ_1. When λ_1 is very close to n it can be considered that the matrix is almost coherent. In this regard, it is customary to consider as a coherence index the relationship: λ_1

Thus, from the referential objects to be ordered E_1 and with characteristics E_2 there will be a reciprocal matric for each characteristic C_j, j=1,2,...,n, with an eigenvalue $I_c = \frac{(\lambda_1 - n)}{n}$ each and a coherence index:

λ_1^j

Such as:

$$I_c^{(j)} = \frac{\left(\lambda_1^{(j)} - m\right)}{m}, j = 1, 2, \ldots, n$$

Where:

	P_1	P_2	$\cdots$	P_m
P_1	1	μ_{12}	$\cdots$	μ_{1m}
P_2	μ_{21}	1	$\cdots$	μ_{2m}
$\cdots$	$\cdots$	$\cdots$	$\cdots$	$\cdots$
P_m	μ_{m1}	μ_{m2}	$\cdots$	1

If the coherence index $\mu_{ik} = \frac{1}{\mu_{ik}}, i, k = 1, 2, \ldots, n$ is sufficiently small, the corresponding eigenvector will be accepted as valid.

Being $I_c^{(j)}, j = 1, 2, \ldots, n$ the corresponding eigenvectors, with an acceptable coherence index:

$\left[V^{(j)}\right]$

Grouping the corresponding n eigenvectors provides a matrix such as the following:

$$\left[V^{(j)}\right] = \begin{array}{c|c} P_1 & V_{1j} \\ P_2 & V_{2j} \\ \cdots & \cdots \\ P_m & V_{mj} \end{array} ; j = 1,2,\ldots,n$$

Each column of the matrix (eigenvector relative to each characteristic $\left[V\right] = \begin{array}{c|cccc} & C_1 & C_2 & & C_n \\ \hline P_1 & V_{11} & V_{12} & \cdots & V_{1n} \\ P_2 & V_{21} & V_{22} & \cdots & V_{2n} \\ & \cdots & \cdots & \cdots & \cdots \\ P_m & V_{m1} & V_{m2} & \cdots & V_{mn} \end{array}$) highlights the relative preference of the objects C_j in relation, of course, to the respective characteristic. Then, if only a single characteristic was considered for the ordering, it would be enough to establish the order of the values of the cells of the chosen column (from highest to lowest or from lowest to highest, as appropriate) to make the appropriate decision. However, the most general assumption normally requires taking into account all the characteristics at a certain level, that is, considering the importance for the decision of each one of them in relation to the others.

To take this aspect into account, a reciprocal square matrix is constructed, in which the rows and columns will represent the $P_i, i = 1,2,\ldots,m$ characteristics. Thus, if a 3 is put in the cell $C_j, j = 1,2,\ldots,n$, for example, it will indicate that the characteristic i is 3 times more important or interesting to the decision than the characteristic k. Thus, there will be a matrix [C] such as the following:

$$\left(i,k\right)$$

This matrix will have a dominating eigenvalue $\left[C\right] = \begin{array}{c|cccc} & C_1 & C_2 & & C_n \\ \hline C_1 & 1 & c_{12} & \cdots & c_{1n} \\ C_2 & c_{21} & 1 & \cdots & c_{2n} \\ & \cdots & \cdots & \cdots & \cdots \\ C_n & c_{n1} & c_{n2} & \cdots & 1 \end{array}$ and a corresponding vector $\lambda_1^{(c)}$. If the coherence index $\left[V^{(c)}\right]$ is within the required threshold, the vector would be considered valid $I_c^{(c)}$ as representative of the weight or importance of each characteristic for the purposes of the decision. This vector plays the weighting role, for which it is important to normalize it with a sum equal to the unit. The vector $\left[V^{(c)}\right]$ will become a normalized vector $\left[V^{(c)}\right]$, which can be represented like this:

$\left[N^{(c)}\right]$

Once the matrix $N^{(c)} = \begin{array}{c|c} c_1 & p_1 \\ c_2 & p_2 \\ & \cdots \\ c_n & p_n \end{array}$ and the normalized vector $\left[V\right]$ are obtained, it will suffice to multiply $\left[N^{(c)}\right]$ to find the new vector $\left[V\right]*\left[N^{(c)}\right]$ whose values $\left[D\right]$ will allow an ordering of the objects, taking into account the relative importance assigned to each characteristic.
They will be:

$s_i, i = 1,2,\ldots,m$

Finally, to obtain the dominant eigenvalue and the corresponding eigenvector, the following procedure is followed:

It starts from a square and reciprocal matrix $\left[D\right] = \left[V\right]*\left[N^{(c)}\right] = \begin{array}{c|c} P_1 & s_1 \\ P_2 & s_2 \\ & \cdots \\ P_m & s_m \end{array}$:

$\left[M\right]$

The process starts by multiplying the matrix $\left[M\right] = \begin{array}{c|cccc} & P_1 & P_2 & & P_m \\ \hline P_1 & 1 & {}_{12}\mu & \cdots & {}_{m1}\mu \\ P_2 & {}_{21}\mu & 1 & \cdots & {}_{m2}\mu \\ & \cdots & \cdots & \cdots & \cdots \\ P_m & {}_{1m}\mu & {}_{2m}\mu & \cdots & 1 \end{array}$

by the unit vector $\left[M\right]$. Obtaining the vector $\left[1\right]$:

$\left[W_1\right]$

Every value of the vector

$$[M]*[1] = \begin{array}{c|cccc} & P_1 & P_2 & \cdots & P_m \\ \hline P_1 & 1 & \mu_{12} & \cdots & \mu_{1m} \\ P_2 & \mu_{21} & 1 & \cdots & \mu_{2m} \\ & \cdots & \cdots & \cdots & \cdots \\ P_m & \mu_{m1} & \mu_{m2} & \cdots & 1 \\ P_1 & w_1^{(1)} \\ P_2 & w_2^{(1)} \\ & \cdots \\ P_m & w_m^{(1)} \end{array} * \begin{array}{c|c} P_1 & 1 \\ P_2 & 1 \\ & \cdots \\ P_m & 1 \end{array} = \begin{array}{c|c} P_1 & v_1^{(1)} \\ P_2 & v_2^{(1)} \\ & \cdots \\ P_n & v_m^{(1)} \end{array} = [1] = [W_1] \text{ is}$$

divided by the largest of them, meaning by: $\left[W_1\right]^{)}$. Thus, a normalized vector is found in the sense of the fuzzy subsets. The new values are:

$$w_1^{(1)} \vee w_2^{(1)} \vee \ldots \vee w_m^{(1)}$$

Therefore:

$$V_1^{(1)} = \left(\frac{w_1^{(1)}}{w_1^{(1)} \vee w_2^{(1)} \vee \ldots \vee w_m^{(1)}}\right), V_2^{(1)} = \left(\frac{w_2^{(1)}}{w_1^{(1)}} \vee w_2^{(1)} \vee \ldots \vee w_m^{(1)}\right), \ldots$$

Where at least one

$$\left[W_1\right] = \left(w_1^{(1)} \vee w_2^{(1)} \vee \ldots \vee w_m^{(1)}\right) * \begin{array}{c|c} P_1 & s_1 \\ P_2 & s_2 \\ & \cdots \\ P_m & s_m \end{array} = \left(w_1^{(1)} \vee w_2^{(1)} \vee \ldots \vee w_m^{(1)}\right) * \left[V_1\right] \text{is}$$

equal to the unit.

Then, the multiplication is carried out $v_i^{(1)}, i = 1, 2, \ldots, m,$

$$\left[M\right] * \left[V_1\right]:$$

$$\begin{array}{l|l} P_1 & v_1^{(1)} \\ P_2 & v_2^{(1)} \\ & \cdots \\ P_m & v_m^{(1)} \\ P_1 & w_1^{(2)} \\ P_2 & w_2^{(2)} \\ & \cdots \\ P_m & w_m^{(2)} \end{array}$$

It will continue like this until a value is found, such as:

$$\left[W_2\right] = \left(w_1^{(r)} \vee w_2^{(r)} \vee \ldots \vee w_m^{(r)}\right) * \cong \left(w_1^{(s)} \vee w_2^{(s)} \vee \ldots \vee w_m^{(s)}\right) \text{with r= s-1}$$

When this happens, is the dominant eigenvalue $\left(w_1^{(s)} \vee w_2^{(s)} \vee \ldots \vee w_m^{(s)}\right)$. If the coherence coefficient λ_1 is acceptably small, the matrix can be considered to be almost coherent.

FINDINGS

Multidimensional Analysis by State in Mexico

For the multidimensional study by state, secondary data provided by the Government of Mexico through the National Institute of Statistics and Geography (INEGI) published in the repository of the National Information System of Sustainable Development Goals (SIODS, 2021) is considered. Data was collected in November 2021. All the indicators that include the breakdown by state and that are currently fed into the SIODS platform for Sustainable Development Goal 5 are analyzed.

The set of objects is made up of the 32 states of the Mexican Republic ordered alphabetically (see Table 2), and the set of characteristics is made up of 3 indicators (see Table 3).

The SP method assumes the premise that "more is better", therefore, for some indicators, the scale was inverted through the stochastic oscillator statistical metric (Díaz, 2001).

Table 2. Group of objects

Identifier	Object
R1	Aguascalientes
R2	Baja California
R3	Baja California Sur
R4	Campeche
R5	Coahuila de Zaragoza
R6	Colima
R7	Chiapas
R8	Chihuahua
R9	Mexico City
R10	Durango
R11	Guanajuato
R12	Guerrero
R13	Hidalgo
R14	Jalisco
R15	State of Mexico
R16	Michoacán de Ocampo
R17	Morelos
R18	Nayarit
R19	Nuevo León
R20	Oaxaca
R21	Puebla
R22	Querétaro
R23	Quintana Roo
R24	San Luis Potosí
R25	Sinaloa
R26	Sonora
R27	Tabasco
R28	Tamaulipas
R29	Tlaxcala
R30	Veracruz de Ignacio de la Llave
R31	Yucatán
R32	Zacatecas

Table 3. Group of characteristics

Identifier	Characteristic / Indicator	Invert Scale	Type of Indicator	Description
C1	5.2.1	Yes	G, E	Proportion of women and girls aged 15 and over who have suffered physical, sexual, or psychological violence at the hands of their current or former partner in the last 12 months, broken down by the form of violence and age.
C2	5.2.2	Yes	G, E	Proportion of women and girls aged 15 and over who have suffered sexual violence at the hands of people other than their partner in the last 12 months, broken down by age and place of the act.
C3	5n.3.1	Yes	N, E	Proportion of women and girls 15 years of age and older who have experienced physical or sexual violence by an aggressor other than their partner and requested support from an institution or filed a complaint or report with an authority.

G: Indicator of the global framework of the SDGs; N: Specific indicator for Mexico; E: Breakdown by state.

Once the SP method has been applied, Table 4 presents the result of the ranking, where the maximum value represents the state with the lowest incidence of gender violence, and the lowest value represents the state with the highest incidence of gender violence.

As can be seen in Table 4, Chiapas is the state with the lowest incidence, followed by Guerrero, Tamaulipas, Nuevo León, and Tabasco. On the other hand, Mexico City has the highest incidence of gender violence, followed by Aguascalientes, the state of Mexico, Querétaro, and Jalisco.

It is important to identify that between the state with the lowest incidence and the state with the highest incidence, there is a gap of 0.8118, therefore, it is important to consider strategies that allow the gap to be reduced in the short, medium, and long term. Similarly, it is observed that only 3.12% of the states present values between 9,000 and 1,000; 34.37% present values between 7,000 and 8,999; 40.62% present values between 3,000 and 4,999; 15.62% present values between 3,000 and 4.9999, and 6.25% of the states present values between 0.000 and 2.9999.

Additionally, two more indicators are analyzed by state (see Table 5).

As can be seen in Figure 3, in most of the states of the Mexican Republic, women show that they use the mobile phone in a higher proportion than men, with the exception of states such as Baja California, Baja California Sur, Chiapas, Quintana Roo and Yucatán.

With respect to the average real labor income, it is observed in Figure 4 that, in most of the states of the Mexican Republic, men show a higher income than women,

Table 4. Sorting result, where the maximum value represents a lower incidence

Identifier	Object	Resulting Value
R7	Chiapas	**1.0000**
R12	Guerrero	**0.8936**
R28	Tamaulipas	**0.8914**
R19	Nuevo León	**0.8045**
R27	Tabasco	**0.8004**
R4	Campeche	**0.7904**
R18	Nayarit	**0.7741**
R3	Baja California Sur	**0.7660**
R30	Veracruz de Ignacio de la Llave	**0.7144**
R16	Michoacán de Ocampo	**0.7124**
R13	Hidalgo	**0.7095**
R25	Sinaloa	**0.7009**
R11	Guanajuato	**0.6967**
R24	San Luis Potosí	**0.6882**
R2	Baja California	**0.6792**
R32	Zacatecas	**0.6698**
R29	Tlaxcala	**0.6590**
R20	Oaxaca	**0.6577**
R26	Sonora	**0.6333**
R6	Colima	**0.6031**
R17	Morelos	**0.5834**
R21	Puebla	**0.5633**
R23	Quintana Roo	**0.5358**
R10	Durango	**0.5260**
R5	Coahuila de Zaragoza	**0.5050**
R31	Yucatán	**0.4916**
R8	Chihuahua	**0.4826**
R14	Jalisco	**0.3999**
R22	Querétaro	**0.3767**
R15	State of Mexico	**0.3489**
R1	Aguascalientes	**0.2249**
R9	Mexico City	**0.1882**

Table 5. Additional indicators disaggregated by sex

Indicator	Type of Indicator	Description
5.b.1	G, E	Proportion of people who own a mobile phone, broken down by sex
5n.1.4	N, E	Average real labor income of employed people according to sex

G: Indicator of the global framework of the SDGs; N: Specific indicator for Mexico; E: Breakdown by state.

Figure 3. Proportion of people who own a mobile phone
W: Women; M: Men

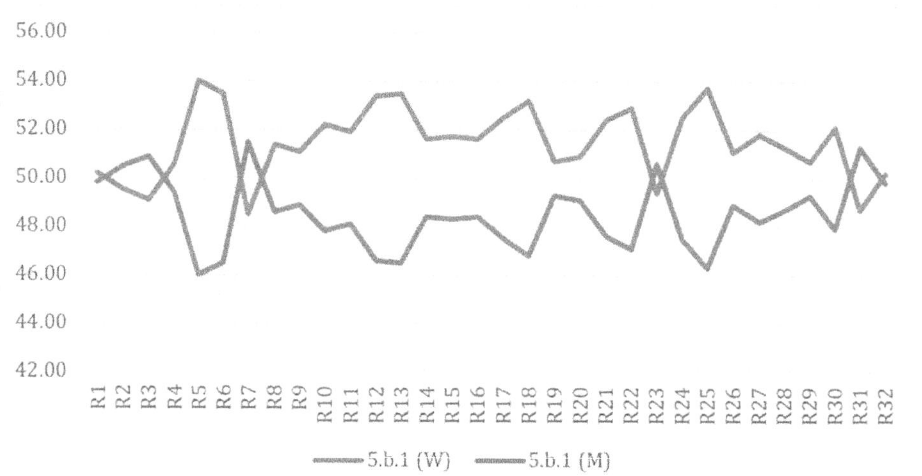

Figure 4. Average real labor income
W: Women, M: Men

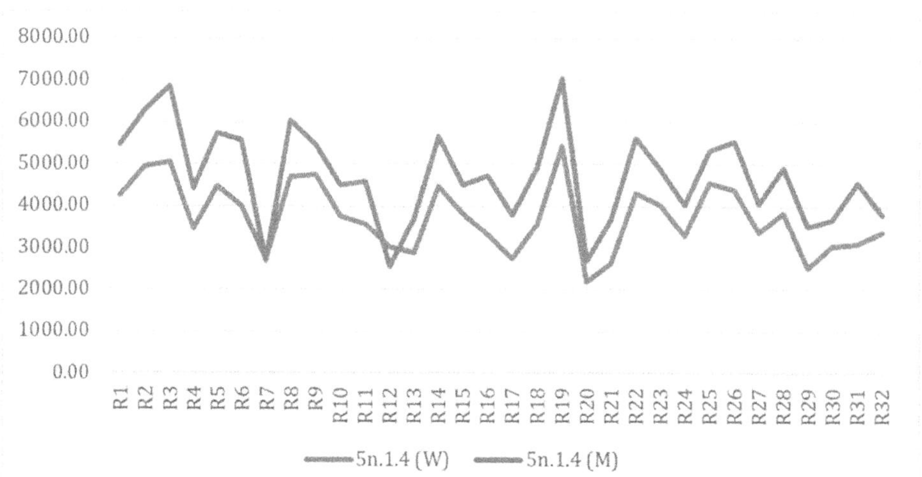

with the exception of states such as Chiapas and Guerrero, where it is observed a higher income in the women.

Global Multidimensional Analysis

For the global multidimensional study, secondary data provided by the United Nations Department of Economics and Social Affairs published in the SDG Global Data Base repository (UN-b, 2021) is considered. The countries of America chosen were those that have information in the database and in all the indicators considered for the study, countries such as Argentina, Chile, and Colombia were not considered because they did not have information available in the system for all the indicators used in the analysis. Data was collected in November 2021.

The set of objects is made up of 12 countries in the American continent ordered alphabetically (see Table 6), and the set of characteristics is made up of 9 indicators (see Table 7).

Once the PS method has been applied, Table 8 presents the result of the ranking, where the maximum value represents the country with the lowest incidence of gender violence, and the lowest value represents the country with the highest incidence of gender violence.

As can be seen in Table 8, Costa Rica is the country with the lowest incidence, followed by Peru, Ecuador, and Mexico. On the other hand, Guatemala is the country with the highest incidence of gender violence, followed by Honduras, Brazil, and

Table 6. Group of objects

Identifier	Object
P1	Bolivia
P2	Brazil
P3	Costa Rica
P4	Ecuador
P5	El Salvador
P6	Guatemala
P7	Honduras
P8	Mexico
P9	Panama
P10	Paraguay
P11	Peru
P12	Uruguay

Table 7. Group of characteristics

Identifier	Characteristic	Invert scale	Description
C1	5.1.1 (1)	No	Legal frameworks that promote, enforce, and monitor gender equality (percentage of achievement, 0 - 100). Area 3: employment and economic benefits.
C2	5.1.1 (2)	No	Legal frameworks that promote, enforce, and monitor gender equality (percentage of achievement, 0 - 100). Area 1: overarching legal frameworks and public life.
C3	5.1.1 (3)	No	Legal frameworks that promote, enforce, and monitor gender equality (percentage of achievement, 0 - 100). Area 4: marriage and family
C4	5.1.1 (4)	No	Legal frameworks that promote, enforce, and monitor gender equality (percentage of achievement, 0 - 100). Area 2: violence against women.
C5	5.2.1	Yes	Proportion of ever-partnered women and girls subjected to physical and/or sexual violence by a current or former intimate partner in the previous 12 months, by age (%).
C6	5.3.1 (1)	Yes	Proportion of women aged 20-24 years who were married or in a union before age 15 (%).
C7	5.3.1 (2)	Yes	Proportion of women aged 20-24 years who were married or in a union before age 18 (%).
C8	5.5.1	No	Proportion of seats held by women in national parliaments (% of the total number of seats).
C9	5.5.2	No	Proportion of women in managerial positions (%).

Table 8. Sorting result, where the maximum value represents a lower incidence

Identifier	Object	Resulting Value
P3	Costa Rica	**1.0000**
P11	Peru	**0.9668**
P4	Ecuador	**0.9633**
P8	Mexico	**0.9436**
P12	Uruguay	**0.9400**
P10	Paraguay	**0.9085**
P5	El Salvador	**0.8700**
P1	Bolivia	**0.8243**
P9	Panama	**0.7729**
P2	Brazil	**0.7399**
P7	Honduras	**0.7097**
P6	Guatemala	**0.6911**

Panama. The gap between the country with the lowest incidence and the country with the highest incidence is 0.3089. 50% of the countries analyzed have values that are between 0.9000 and 1.000; 16.6% is in the range of 0.8000 to 0.8999; 25% is in the range of 0.7000 to 0.7999, and 8.33% is in the range of 0.6000 to 0.6999.

SOLUTIONS AND RECOMMENDATIONS

During the current health emergency derived from the COVID-19 pandemic, the visibility of violence has intensified since confinement conditions have pronounced gender inequalities in the lives of women and girls. In Mexico, according to data from INMUJERES (2021), as of March 2020, emergency calls to 911 related to requests for help due to violence against women increased compared to those registered in the year prior, they went from 197,693 to 260,067 calls, which shows an approximate increase of 31.5%.

Faced with this situation that the world is currently experiencing, it is essential to work together globally and nationally to identify areas of opportunity as well as to design strategies from different areas of government (federal, state, and local) to meet the needs of women and girls when developing public policies focused on reducing gender violence, achieving the Goal 5 proposed in the 2030 Sustainable Development Goals and achieving gender equality, as well as achieving the empowerment of all women and girls.

FUTURE RESEARCH DIRECTIONS

It is of interest for future research to follow up on this analysis, integrating the updated information, as well as increasing the indicators studied depending on how the information is integrated into the different data repositories. The follow-up will allow to analyze how Mexico is progressing in reducing gender violence both nationally and globally.

In the same way, it will be important to contrast the results obtained in this study, increasing the number of countries in America and in other continents to identify the progress of Mexico with regards to gender violence, to the extent that the information is available in the repositories used.

Finally, it will be significant to analyze data from the last two years, the period in which the COVID-19 pandemic was experienced, to identify the impact on gender-based violence compared to the results obtained. The information from the last two years is not yet reflected in the databases used for this study.

CONCLUSION

Violence against women and girls is one of the most prevalent human rights violations, and its impact is immeasurable. The conditions created by the pandemic, including lockdowns, reduced mobility, increased isolation, stress, and economic uncertainty, have led to a significant increase in gender-based violence against women (UN Women 2021a). Poverty and its effects on social cohesion can also lead to increased violence. In this sense, violence against women during the pandemic is linked to different negative outcomes such as affecting emotional and mental health, vulnerability, and even despair, and in some cases, it even correlated with post-traumatic stress disorders.

Mexico has been plagued by violence against women (Hootsen, 2020); it has been a *historic pandemic*, yet COVID-19 made the situation more apparent (CIVICUS, 2020). Domestic violence and violence against women were considered as part of the public health crisis in Mexico, being the home where women experienced the most violence (Mayen-Huerta, 2020). The country has the highest number of femicides in the region after Brazil, and gender-based violence has been an overlooked issue. In fact, before the pandemic, Mexico was considered a country with a permanent risk of violence against women.

At the national level, as can be seen in the results of Table 4, Mexico City, Aguascalientes, Mexico, Querétaro, and Jalisco are the states of the Mexican Republic with the highest prevalence of gender violence; these results are consistent with those presented by INMUJERES (2021). Similarly, the resulting data are consistent with those published by INEGI (2016) since they are mainly urban states, with a minority indigenous population, and with a high level of higher education. On the other hand, the states with the lowest prevalence of gender violence are Chiapas and Guerrero, mainly rural states with a high percentage of indigenous population.

At a global level, very close values are observed, ranging from 1,000 to 0.9085 (see Table 8) among the first six countries, Costa Rica, Peru, Ecuador, Mexico, Uruguay, and Paraguay. Mexico is located in the fourth position with a gap of -0.0564 with respect to Costa Rica, which is located in the first position.

Sadly enough, government officials in Mexico, including President López Obrador (Löhr, 2021), have been underscoring the importance of eliminating discrimination and gender violence against women (UN Meetings Coverage and Press Releases, 2021). A government campaign to delegitimize the victims was in place, and budgets for women shelters and victim aid for women suffering violence were cut (Mayen-Huerta, 2020).

The problem attracted international attention, and Amnesty International has issued a report accusing Mexican authorities of using illegal force and sexual violence to silence women protesting violence against women (Lozano, 2021). Women are being killed in Mexico at unprecedented rates, but the government is calling most emergency calls false (Gallón, 2020). There is a dire lack of public and transparent information that would allow to clearly assess the impact of lockdown and the COVID crisis on violence against women in Mexico (EQUIS, 2020). Authorities have failed victims, and structural violence against women has been normalized (Manríque de Lara & Medina -Arellano, 2020).

This analysis presents objective information to identify areas of opportunity and work on public policies that are focused on reducing the prevalence of gender violence. In the same way, it allows to globally identify those countries that have generated better conditions to reduce gender violence.

REFERENCES

Alvarado, M., & Guerra, N. (2012). Gender-based violence is a public health problem [La violencia de género un problema de salud pública]. *Revista de Trabajo Social, 2*(2), 97–106.

Barber, B. (1995). All Economies Are 'Embedded' The Career of a Concept and Beyond. *Social Research, 62*(2), 387–413.

Beneria, L. (1999). Globalization, Gender And The Davos Man. *Feminist Economics, 5*(3), 61–83. doi:10.1080/135457099337815

Bravo, E. (2004). Gender violence and health. *DiálFil, 20*(59), 261–274.

Carreras, A.I. (2019). *Legal concept of gender violence* [Concepto jurídico de violencia de género]. Dykinson, S.L.

CIDOB. (2022). *The SDG measurement and monitoring system* [El sistema de medición y seguimiento de los ODS]. https://www.cidob.org/es/publicaciones/documentacion/dossiers/dossier_ods_2015_2030/objetivos_de_desarrollo_sostenible_la_agenda_2030_del_compromiso_a_la_practica/el_sistema_de_medicion_y_seguimiento_de_los_ods

CIVICUS. (2020*). MEXICO: 'Violence against women is a historical pandemic'. Interview with Wendy Figueroa.* https://www.civicus.org/index.php/media-resources/news/interviews/4466-mexico-violence-against-women-is-a-historical-pandemic

de México, G. (2021). 2030 Agenda. https://www.gob.mx/agenda2030

Díaz, A. (2001). The %K and %R oscillators of the stock market technical analysis and a proposal to improve the %R [Los osciladores %K y %R del análisis técnico bursátil y una propuesta para mejorar el %R]. *Contaduría y Administración, 203*, 5–26.

Dinh, X. B. (1984). A method for estimating the membership function of a fuzzy set. *Revue Busefal, L.S.I. University Paul Sabatier*, *19*, 68–82.

EQUIS. (2020). *The two pandemics: Violence against women in Mexico amidst COVID-19*. https://equis.org.mx/wp-content/uploads/2020/08/report_thetwopandemicsF.pdf

European Institute for Gender Equality (EIGE). (2017). *Glossary of definitions of rape, femicide and intimate partner violence*. Publication Office of the European Union.

Faludi, J., & Crosby, M. (2021). The Digital Economy of the Sourdough. Housewifisation in the Time of COVID-19. *tripleC: Communication, Capitalism & Critique*, *19*(1), 113–124.

Felbab-Brown, V. (2020). *Opinion | COVID-19 can augment violence to Mexican women*. Mexico Today: Reforma. https://mexicotoday.com/2020/04/10/opinion-covid-19-can-augment-violence-to-mexican-women/

Fernández, B. (2021). *COVID-19: The patriarchal pandemic*. https://www.aljazeera.com/opinions/2021/3/22/covid-19-the-patriarchal-pandemic

Fry, W. (2020). 2019 was the most violent year on record for women in Mexico, report finds. *San Diego Tribune*. https://www.sandiegouniontribune.com/news/border-baja-california/story/2020-08-06/violence-women-mexico

Gallón, N. (2020). *Women are being killed in Mexico ar record rates but the president says most emergency calls are false*. CNN. https://edition.cnn.com/2020/06/05/americas/mexico-femicide-coronavirus-lopez-obrador-intl/index.html

Gil-Aluja, J. (1999). *Elements for a theory of decisions in uncertainty* [Elementos para una teoría de decisiones en la incertidumbre]. Milladoiro. doi:10.1007/978-1-4757-3011-1

Gil-Lafuente, A., Torres, A., Boria, S., & Amiguet, L. (2019). *Gender equity index of the autonomous communities of Spain, a multidimensional analysis* [Índice de equidad de género de las comunidades autónomas de España, un análisis multidimensional]. Real Academia de Ciencias Económicas y Financieras.

Gil-Lafuente, A. M., & Alexánder-López, G. A. (2015). *Algorithms for the evaluation and selection of adaptation strategies to climate change in Computational Data Analysis Techniques in Economics and Finance*. Nova Science Publishers, Inc.

Granovetter, M. (1985). Economic action and social structure: The problem of embeddedness. *American Journal of Sociology*, *91*(3), 481–510. doi:10.1086/228311

Guerra-Lund, R., Manica, S., & Mânica, G. (2020). Collateral issues in times of covid-19: child abuse, domestic violence and femicide. *Revista Brasileira de Odontologia Legal, 7*(2).

Hootsen, J. A. (2020). *Domestic violence epidemic hits Mexico during coronavirus lockdown.* https://www.americamagazine.org/politics-society/2020/08/06/domestic-violence-epidemic-hits-mexico-during-coronavirus-lockdown

Instituto Nacional de Estadística y Geografía INEGI. (2016). *National Survey on the Dynamics of Relationships in Households* [Encuesta Nacional sobre la Dinámica de las Relaciones en los Hogares]. https://www.inegi.org.mx/programas/endireh/2016/

Instituto Nacional de Estadística y Geografía INEGI. (2020a). *National Survey of Urban Public Security ENSU* [Encuesta Nacional de Seguridad Pública Urbana ENSU]. https://www.inegi.org.mx/programas/ensu/

Instituto Nacional de Estadística y Geografía INEGI. (2020b). *Statistics. On the Occasion of the International Day for the Elimination of Violence against Women* [Estadísticas. A propósito del día internacional de la eliminación de la violencia contra la mujer]. Author.

Instituto Nacional de Estadística y Geografía INEGI. (2021). *Statistics on the International Day for the Elimination of Violence against Women* [Estadísticas a propósito del día internacional de la eliminación de la violencia contra la mujer]. https://www.inegi.org.mx/contenidos/saladeprensa/aproposito/2020/Violencia2020_Nal.pdf

Instituto Nacional de Estadística y Geografía INEGI. (2021). *System of Indicators of the Sustainable Development Goals* [Sistema de Indicadores de los Objetivos de Desarrollo Sostenible]. https://agenda2030.mx/#/home

Instituto Nacional de las Mujeres INMUJERES. (2007). *Gender glossary* [Glosario de género]. http://cedoc.inmujeres.gob.mx/documentos_download/100904.pdf

Instituto Nacional de las Mujeres INMUJERES. (2021). *Women and violence in times of pandemic* [Las mujeres y la violencia en los tiempos de pandemia]. http://cedoc.inmujeres.gob.mx/documentos_download/BA7N03%20Para%20Publicar%20con%20vo%20bo.pdf

Kaufmann, A., & Gil Aluja, J. (1986). *Introduction to fuzzy subsets theory in business management*. Ed. Milladoiro.

Löhr, N. (2021). The Shadow Pandemic: Policy Efforts on Gender-Based Violence during COVID-19 in the Global South. *GIGA Focus Global, 6*. https://www.unidas.world/es/node/267

Lozano, A. V. (2021). *Despite some gains, violence against women remains a global 'pandemic'*. NBC News. https://www.nbcnews.com/news/world/despite-some-gains-violence-against-women-remains-global-pandemic-n1261361

Marnrique de Lara, A., & Mediina-Arellano, M. D. J. (2020). The Covid-19 pandemic and ethics in Mexico through a gender lens. *Journal of Bioethical Inquiry*, *17*(4), 613–617.

Márquez-Guajardo, A. (2020). Mexico's other pandemic: Murdered women. *The Wire*. https://thewire.in/world/mexico-murdered-women-domestic-violence-coronavirus

Mayen-Huerta, C. (2020). *Covid-19 and Mexico's domestic violence crisis. Almost half of all women in Mexico experience domestic abuse and the global COVID-19 pandemic has made the situation even worse*. University of Melbourne. https://pursuit.unimelb.edu.au/articles/covid-19-and-mexico-s-domestic-violence-crisis

Meier, B. (2008). The Great Transformation: The Political and Economic Origins of Our Time (2001) by Karl Polanyi. Book Review. *Social Thought & Research*, *29*, 155–160. https://dx.doi.org/10.17161/STR.1808.5695

Murray, C. (2021). *Emergency calls on violence against women spiked in Mexico in 2020*. Thomson Reuters Foundation. https://news.trust.org/item/20210125201102-i73x7

Peck, J. (2013). Disembedding Polanyi: Exploring Polanyian economic geographies. *Environment & Planning A*, *45*(7), 1536–1544.

Pinto-López, I. N., Montaudon-Tomas, C. M., & Gil-Lafuente, A. M. (2022). Mexico and the Challenges of Achieving the 2030 Sustainable Development Goals in Computational and Decision Methods in Economics and Business. *Lecture Notes in Networks and Systems*, *388*, 29–45.

Polanyi, K. (1944). *The great transformation* (Vol. 2). Beacon Press.

Prusa, A., García-Nice, B., & Soledad, O. (2020). *Pandemic of Violence: Protecting Women during COVID-19- OCHA Services*. https://reliefweb.int/report/mexico/pandemic-violence-protecting-women-during-covid-19

Raygada, G., & Mendoza, M. (2021). *Combating gender-based violence during the pandemic*. Inter-American Development Bank. https://www.iadb.org/en/improvinglives/combatting-gender-based-violence-during-pandemic

Saaty, T. L. (1978). Exploring the interface between hierarchies, multiple objectives and fuzzy sets. *Fuzzy Sets and Systems*, *1*(1), 57–68.

Sánchez, E., & Rodríguez, L. (2020). *Femicide on the Rise in Mexico During the COVID-19 Pandemic*. Global Citizen. https://www.globalcitizen.org/en/content/mexico-cuts-womens-institute-budget-femicide-rises/

SIODS. (2021). *Information System of Sustainable Development Goals, Mexico*. https://agenda2030.mx/index.html?lang=en#/home

STATISTA. (2021). https://www.statista.com/statistics/1113975/gender-violence-growth-coronavirus-latin-america/

Stephen, L. M. (2020). *A pandemic within a pandemic across Latinamerica*. US News. https://www.usnews.com/news/best-countries/articles/2020-08-24/violence-against-latin-american-women-increases-during-pandemic

UN Meetings Coverage and Press Releases. (2021). *As Violence against Women Grows in Shadow of Pandemic, Third Committee Experts Cite Need for Data Collection, Strong Policy Responses*. https://www.un.org/press/en/2021/gashc4318.doc.htm

United Nations UN. (2018). *Department of Economic and Social Affairs*. SDG Indicators Database. https://unstats.un.org/sdgs/dataportal

United Nations UN. (2019). *Fourteenth meeting of the HLG-PCCB*. https://unstats.un.org/sdgs/meetings/hlg-meeting-14

United Nations UN. (2020). *Cape Town Global Action Plan for Sustainable Development Data*. https://unstats.un.org/sdgs/hlg/Cape-Town-Global-Action-Plan/

United Nations UN. (2021a). *Una de cada tres mujeres en el mundo sufre violencia física o sexual desde que es muy joven*. https://news.un.org/es/story/2021/03/1489292

United Nations UN. (2021b). *SDG Global Data Base*. https://unstats.un.org/sdgs/unsdg

United Nations UN. (2021c). *Gender equalit*. [Igualdad de género.] https://www.un.org/es/global-issues/gender-equality

Usher, K., Bradbury Jones, C., Bhullar, N., Durkin, D. J., Gyamfi, N., Fatema, S. R., & Jackson, D. (2021). COVID-19 and family violence: Is this a perfect storm? *International Journal of Mental Health Nursing*, *30*, 1022–1032.

Valencia-Londoño, P. A., Martínez-González, E. N., Bruno-Solera, C., & Sorm-Paz, P. (2021). The exacerbation of violence against women as a form of discrimination in the period of the COVID-19 pandemic. *Heliyon*, *7*(3), e06491.

Weil, S. (2020). Two global pandemics: femicide and Covid-19. *Trauma and Memory*, *8*(2), 110-112.

Women, U. N. (2020). *SDG 5: Achieve gender equality and empower all women and girls*. https://www.unwomen.org/en/news/in-focus/women-and-the-sdgs/sdg-5-gender-equality

Women, U. N. (2021a). *Frequently asked questions: types of violence against women and girls*. United Nations. https://www.unwomen.org/en/what-we-do/ending-violence-against-women/faqs/types-of-violence

Women, U. N. (2021b). *Measuring the shadow pandemic. Violence against women during COVID-19*. https://data.unwomen.org/sites/default/files/documents/Publications/Measuring-shadow-pandemic.pdf

Women, U. N. (2021c). *Women and the Sustainable Development Goals* [Las mujeres y los Objetivos de Desarrollo Sostenible]. https://www.unwomen.org/es/news/in-focus/women-and-the-sdgs

World Health Organization. (2002). *Informe mundial sobre la violencia y la salud*. https://www.who.int/violence_injury_prevention/violence/world_report/en/abstract_es.pdf

World Health Organization. (2021). *La violencia contra la mujer es omnipresente y devastadora: la sufren una de cada tres mujeres*. https://www.who.int/es/news/item/09-03-2021-devastatingly-pervasive-1-in-3-women-globally-experience-violence

Yourke, M. (2021). Violence Against Women in Mexico Rises. *Fair Observer*. https://www.fairobserver.com/region/latin_america/mat-youkee-violence-against-mexican-women-mexico-femicide-coronavirus-lockdown-world-news-60178/

ADDITIONAL READING

Caprioli, M., & Boyer, M. A. (2001). Gender, violence, and international crisis. *The Journal of Conflict Resolution*, *45*(4), 503–518. doi:10.1177/0022002701045004005

Chapleau, K. M., Oswald, D. L., & Russell, B. L. (2008). Male rape myths: The role of gender, violence, and sexism. *Journal of Interpersonal Violence*, *23*(5), 600–615. doi:10.1177/0886260507313529 PMID:18259049

Lombardi, E. L., & Malouf, D. (2001). Gender violence: Transgender experiences with violence and discrimination. *Journal of Homosexuality*, *42*(1), 89–101. doi:10.1300/J082v42n01_05 PMID:11991568

Merry, S. E. (2001). Spatial governmentality and the new urban social order: Controlling gender violence through law. *American Anthropologist*, *103*(1), 16–29. doi:10.1525/aa.2001.103.1.16

Morales-Rodríguez, F. M. (2021). Effectiveness of a program to improve attention towards affective-sexual, bodily and gender diversity in university students. *European Journal of Investigation in Health, Psychology and Education*, *11*(4), 1205–1220. doi:10.3390/ejihpe11040088 PMID:34698121

Pronyk, P. M., Kim, J. C., Abramsky, T., Phetla, G., Hargreaves, J. R., Morison, L. A., Watss, C., Busza, J., & Porter, J. D. (2008). A combined microfinance and training intervention con reduce HIV risk behaviour in young female participants. *AIDS (London, England)*, *22*(13), 1659–1665. doi:10.1097/QAD.0b013e328307a040 PMID:18670227

Ringrose, J., & Renold, E. (2010). Normative cruelties and gender deviants: The performative effects of bully discourses for girls and boys in school. *British Educational Research Journal*, *36*(4), 573–596. doi:10.1080/01411920903018117

Rojas-Fernández, V., Altamirano-Benítez, V., & Moreira-Aguirre, D. G. (2022). Treatment of Gender Violence in Digital Newspapers of the Andean Region. *Smart Innovation Systems and Technologies*, *29*, 534–543. doi:10.1007/978-981-16-5792-4_53

Steffensmeier, D., Schwartz, J., Zhong, H., & Ackerman, J. (2005). An assessment of recent trends in girls' violence using diverse longitudinal sources: Is the gender gap closing? *Criminology*, *43*(2), 355–406. doi:10.1111/j.0011-1348.2005.00011.x

Chapter 9
(Un)Learned Resilience:
Impact of the COVID-19 Pandemic on Post-Yugoslav and Post-Soviet Female Immigrants in Austria and Hungary

Sanja (Szonja) Tepavcevic (Tepavcsevics)
https://orcid.org/0000-0001-5752-4698
Institute of Advanced Studies, Koszeg, Hungary

ABSTRACT

Since the times that Karl Polanyi named "the great transformation" and up to the pre-COVID-19 era, the market has played the central role in organization of the society. Such a system has affected women more profoundly: to be officially paid, they had to compromise professional and family life. The COVID-19 pandemic lockdowns added even more burden to them, returning education and childcare to the household realm. This chapter draws on the rich empirical data featuring post-Yugoslav and post-Soviet female immigrants' experiences of the COVID-19 pandemic in Austria and Hungary. The analysis reveals the ways in which experiences with previous global crises that represented radical changes influenced their resilience throughout the COVID-19 pandemic.

INTRODUCTION

Global crises such as the world system change in 1989-1991, the Great Recession of the 2007-2009, and the COVID-19 pandemic, do not equally affect everyone. For example, the collapse of the Socialist bloc of the early 1990s more heavily affected the population of the former socialist countries, than the rest of the world's population.

DOI: 10.4018/978-1-6684-2364-6.ch009

Two former socialist multinational federations collapsed in 1991: Yugoslavia through a series of violent conflicts, and the Soviet Union (SU) first by local and soon after 'frozen' conflicts, and then with long-term emerging and lasting ones (such as the current war in Ukraine). Collapses of both Yugoslavia and the SU had generated significant migration flows, as demonstrated in Tables 1 and 2.

Table 1. Emigration from former Yugoslavia in selected years Source: UNHCR 2006 Annual Statistics

Year	1996	2000	2005
Number of emigrants	1,473,834	1,051,829	78,571

Table 2. Emigration from the former Soviet republics in selected years Sources: IOM Migration Reports 2015/2018/2020

Sending Country/ Number of Emigrants (in Millions/Year)	2000	2015	2019
Russian Federation	12.1	11	10
Ukraine	5.9	6	6
Kazakhstan	3.5	3	2,5

Contrary to most previous global crises, due to almost simultaneous lockdowns in nearly all parts of the globe, the COVID-19 pandemic has so far heavily limited "the number of people crossing borders, especially on permanent or a long-term basis" (Gamlen, 2020, p. 10). Migrants have been seen simultaneously as key spreaders and as the most vulnerable population for a lack of access to appropriate accommodation and healthcare (Tagliacozzo et al., 2020). Moreover, the COVID-19 pandemic has also negatively affected the daily life of women, enforcing the reconsideration of some established socio-economic norms and structures. In the context of the pandemic lockdowns, women across the globe have experienced

[t]he new forms of exploitation and housewifisation in digital capitalism (...) The outsourcing of schooling and social services along with the home office has created a new trend of housewifisation. (...) Modern families have found themselves locked

in their homes in a family structure that turned out to be efficient and dysfunctional at the same time in so many ways (Faludi & Crosby, 2020, pp. 113-117).

While the emerging literature on the COVID-19 pandemic tackles problems that migrants and women encounter across the globe, the literature so far overlooked the conditions of the particular intersection of these two groups traditionally considered as vulnerable – female immigrants. As Castles et al. (2018, p. 61) point out,

Today, migrant women still tend to be overrepresented in the least desirable occupations, such as repetitive factory work, and lower-skilled positions in the personal care and other services sectors, although there has also been increased mobility into white-collar jobs. Complex patterns of division of labor and ethnic and gender lines have developed. (…) Today, in many countries, women who enter as dependents or marriage migrants do not have an entitlement to residence in their own right and may face deportation if they get divorced.

The insights into the experiences and coping strategies of the female immigrants during the COVID-19 pandemic are particularly important because they are able to reflect on the resilience mechanisms of the population that is more likely to have previous personal life-changing experiences through other global crises. To examine such experiences, through this chapter the author explores the following questions: whether and to what extent have the experiences from previous global crises affected the reactions and adaptation strategies of female immigrants during the COVID-19 pandemic? How do these experiences differ, if any, across 'older' and 'newer' European Union (EU) member states?

Whilst the present chapter aims to contribute to the discussion on the impact of COVID-19 on female immigrants in the three following ways. First, the study gives female immigrants direct voices. Second, it compares these voices across two immigrant groups – former Yugoslav and former Soviet female immigrants in older and newer EU member states. Third, the chapter reflects on their experiences from two previous global crises – the collapse of the socialist system and the global financial crisis. The analysis starts with the review of existing studies about female migrants, and post-Yugoslav and post-Soviet immigrant communities, and then continues with a description of major concepts. Section 2 describes in detail the major methods of inquiry, and the data collected. Section 3 first provides the analysis of experiences and coping strategies of the two female immigrant groups – post-Yugoslav and post-Soviet (former citizens of the two multinational federations) – in Hungary and Austria during the COVID-19 pandemic. Then it reflects on how experiences from previous global crises assisted, or impeded thereof, these immigrant women to overcome challenges posed by the COVID-19 pandemic. The last section situates the findings into the existing literature and provides some conclusions.

LITERATURE REVIEW: FEMALE MIGRANTS – INHERENTLY VULNERABLE, OR ENFORCED BY MIGRATION?

As Degani and De Stefani (2020, p. 113) rightly notice, "women's voices and experiences of subordination and oppression are often overlooked. Too often, the different overlapping of discriminatory grounds are taken into account separately, without capturing the complexity of experiences they face". Migration literature generally portrays female immigrants as inherently vulnerable. On the one hand, as Phizacklea (1983) notes, ascribing inferiority to female migrant workers was facilitated by their primary roles in patriarchal societies that were defined as wife and mother, dependent on the male breadwinner. As a result, they were paid lower wages and were controlled more easily than men. On the other hand, Phizacklea (1998) and later Dannecker and Cakir (2016) also suggest that female migration:

...can reinforce the exploitation of women, but can also help women from patriarchal societies to gain more control over their lives. (...) This frequently makes women reluctant to return to their countries of origin to avoid losing their new-won rights and freedoms (cited in Castles et al. 2018, p. 62).

Therefore, the inherited vulnerability of female immigrants (Phizacklea, 1983; Degani & DeStefani, 2020) serves as the first underlying theoretical assumption. Female emigration as reinforcement of rights and freedoms (Phizacklea, 1998; Dannecker & Cakir, 2016) serves as the major competing theoretical assumption for the analysis in this chapter. The following review of the literature on post-Yugoslav and post-Soviet migrants, including female immigrants, reveals major complementing propositions about the female immigrant resilience in the times of radical changes to these competing general assumptions about female migrants.

Female Migrants and Mechanisms of Resilience

Scholarly literature on post-Yugoslav and post-Soviet migrants belongs to different disciplines and fields within social sciences, and it roughly composes two thematic blocs. The first focuses on the psychological and cultural aspects of migration and integration, tackling questions of nationalism, national and cultural identities through the relationship between the place of origin and the place of destination. The analyses belonging to this thematic bloc are concerned with migrants' political and cultural vulnerabilities and resilience. For instance, Kovacevic-Bielicki (2017) describes that the war and migration experiences have shaped the identities of former children/former refugees/from former Yugoslavia in Norway with a profound and long-lasting effect expressed in the Bosnian-Croatian-Serbian proverb "neither on the earth nor in the sky". Her work, thus, points towards post-Yugoslav migrants' psychological, social and cultural vulnerabilities posed by the forced migration, and translates the basic assumption about female immigrants' vulnerability to a larger migrant population. This serves as the third - complementing – assumption to the underlying female immigrants' vulnerability thesis. In contrast to Kovacevic-Bielicki (2017), exploring the Bosnian diaspora around the world, a group of scholars found that Bosnians' mobility (Valenta & Ramet, 2011) and adaption of old identities to new spaces (Halilovich, 2011) served them major integration and resilience strategies. These findings also translate the second basic assumption about female migration as an enforcement mechanism for a larger migrant population. Simultaneously, this later proposition complements the second general assumption that migration enforces (female) migrants' rights and freedoms.

The second thematic bloc focuses on socio-economic aspects of migration and integration, such as channels of integration to labor markets that constitute the central topic of the immigrant entrepreneurship field of studies. Consequently, the analyses within this thematic bloc reflect on migrants' socio-economic vulnerabilities and resilience. For instance, Castles, de Haas, and Miller (2018) point out, that community ties play a crucial role in migration decisions and geographical directions of migration flows. Furthermore, due to having usually less privileged positions in host countries and in their labor markets, in particular, immigrants represent a vulnerable social group, that usually addresses this socio-economic vulnerability by conducting entrepreneurship that serves their compatriot immigrant group or community (Portes, 1997; Mesch & Czamanski, 1997).

Immigrants typically turn to friends, acquaintances, and relatives in the immigrant community (…) Through these ties, new arrivals learn about job opportunities, find affordable housing, and master the informal and formal rules of the game as they adapt to the host society (Kim, 2014, p. 352).

Confirming such tendency, Tepavcevic (2021) points out that the social and economic integration of immigrants from the post-Soviet countries in Austria and Hungary usually happens through the common-culture-based post-Soviet, Russian-speaking immigrant community.

Similarly, focusing on Russian-speaking female immigrants in Hungary, Zueva (2005) demonstrated that some of them founded companies and became entrepreneurs mostly in order to obtain residency permits. Thus, entrepreneurship turned out to be their multiple - legal and socio-economic - resilience mechanism. Similarly, Munkejord (2017) focuses on local and transnational networks of Russian female entrepreneurs in the Finnmark area of Norway and points out that, being a part of the mainstream economy and support of family ties were the most striking features of their immigrant entrepreneurship. On the other side of the spectrum, examining Russian-speaking former Soviet female immigrants in Italy, Cvajner (2012) points out that they usually arrive in Italy illegally and serve as social care providers to the Italian elderly. Considering it as downgrading in contrast to their previous positions and level of education, these women conduct entrepreneurship to regain their social status and human dignity that had suffered through illegal migration and social care provision. This argument suggests that entrepreneurship represents not only socio-economic but also psychological resilience mechanisms for female immigrants.

As becomes evident from this brief review, the act of migration is fairly considered a radical change or transformation of one's life. This radical change generates vulnerability on one hand and resilience on the other. Thus, the vulnerability of being an immigrant in general and female immigrant in particular usually produces two broad types of resilience mechanisms. The first comprises 'soft' psychological, cultural, and sociopolitical elements, and usually manifests itself in psychological adaptation and reconsideration of national/cultural/geographical and even professional identities. The second type of resilience mechanism comprises 'hard' meaning legal and socio-economic aspects, and it usually materializes through entrepreneurship. The next subsection describes the ways in which the two central concepts of this chapter – resilience and transformation – are adapted and applied in methodological and empirical sections of this chapter.

Major Concepts and Operationalization

The COVID-19 pandemic can be interpreted and conceptualized as kind of transformation. Similar to Karl Polanyi's "transformation as a certain political-economic moment of radical rupture, a type of political revolution and short-term change, which might accelerate ongoing profound transformations" (Novy, 2021, p. 60). Nevertheless, as Novy (2021) keenly points out, the short-term cannot be understood without contextualizing it within the long-term transformation, Therefore, this chapter puts the COVID-19 pandemic – as a radical change – into the long-term context of post-Yugoslav and post-Soviet female migrants' experiences with previous global crises and forms of resilience acquired through them.

As noted earlier, 'soft' resilience constitutes psychological and cultural aspects of adaptation to radical change. In this 'soft' form, it represents mostly coping with the crisis, and psychological recovery from the crisis. Discussing it in the context of mental illness, Foulkes (2021) defines resilience as "psychological immunization':

"the idea of stress inoculation is that (mildly) stressful challenges teach us ways to cope. When future stressors arise, we are then more likely to believe they are manageable" (Foulkes, 2021, p. 203). Foulkes (2021) also suggests that in contrast to mild stress that generates psychological immunity, high stress results in psychological vulnerability. Based on this definition, the chapter explores the ways that the post-Yugoslav and post-Soviet female immigrants' experiences from previous global crises provide "psychological immunization'. Foulkes points out that during the pandemic people between the ages of 18 and 41 suffered most severely because of the isolation and lockdowns. The chapter checks this statement by dividing the post-Yugoslav and post-Soviet female immigrants – respondents and interlocutors - into the three age groups: the youngest between 18 and 35 years old, a middle group between 36 and 50, and the most mature respondents between 51 and 65.

Regarding 'hard' resilience, the migration literature suggests migrant community networks and entrepreneurship as major responses to socio-economic and legal vulnerabilities of female migrants. The present chapter examines whether, and if so, to what extent female immigrants applied these mechanisms during the COVID-19 pandemic lockdowns.

METHODS OF INQUIRY AND DATA

Post-Yugoslavs represent the second largest immigrant group in Austria, where citizens of Serbia, Bosnia, and Croatia together count for about a million of the current Austrian population. Since 2013, when Croatia joined the EU, Croatian citizens who migrated to Austria have been included in Austrian migration statistics as EU citizens. In contrast to citizens of former Yugoslavia, the overall number of post-Soviet immigrants in Austria is about 33,000, and the majority of them are women. In Hungary, counting only about 6,000, more than half of these post-Yugoslav immigrants in Hungary are female. They have resided for more than a decade in Hungary and have fully integrated into the Hungarian society. Post-Soviets are the second largest immigrant group in Hungary. The current number of immigrants from the former Soviet Union in Hungary is approximately 15000, with also more than half being women.

Autoethnography served a major theory-building strategy in collecting data about their experiences of the COVID-19 pandemic. With that in mind, Adams et al. (2017, pp. 1-4) define it as a research approach,

Autoethnography uses personal experience ("auto") to describe and interpret ("graphy") cultural texts, experiences, beliefs, and practices ("ethno"). (...) Given the focus on personal experience, autoethnographers also describe moments of

everyday experience that cannot be captured through more traditional research methods. Doing autoethnographic fieldwork allows what we see, hear, think, and feel to become part of the "field".

In this chapter, autoethnography was applied in two ways. First, the research was conducted through the author's personal experience of the COVID-19 pandemic as a post-Yugoslav female immigrant, native Bosnian-Croatian-Serbian speaker, and a close-to-native Russian speaker, who studied and worked in Russia for almost two decades. Many of her acquaintances and friends are also (female) immigrants from the former Soviet Union and former Yugoslavia, and she is embedded in these communities. Such a position provided her with genuine insights into her fellow post-Yugoslav and post-Soviet female immigrants in Hungary and Austria. Personal notes and reflections from face-to-face and online conversations with fellow female immigrants during and after the COVID-19 pandemic lockdowns serve as the first form of data used in this chapter. Such communication resulted in 10 conversations with post-Yugoslav female immigrants – four in Austria, six in Hungary, and 12 post-Soviet female immigrants, five in Austria, and seven in Hungary. Only the most illustrative of these narratives were directly quoted in the empirical section. In the text, they were referred to as personal communication with demographic characteristics of the interlocutor: country of origin, country of current residence, and age at the time of conversation taking place. These conversations were frequent and continuous in the period between February 2020 and February 2022.

Second, with regard to such positionality, the author is also a member of numerous post-Yugoslav and post-Soviet Facebook public groups initiated and administrated by and for immigrants from former Yugoslavia and the former Soviet Union in the EU, for example, "Ours in Austria", "Russians in Austria", "Russian-speaking Women in Hungary", and "Serbs in Hungary" to name few. As a member of these groups, the author observed the content of discussions, and actively participated in them. In addition, led by the propositions derived from the scholarly literature about female immigrants' double vulnerability, the author created anonymous online questionnaires and posted them into these groups. Driven by the propositions from the literature, these questionnaires included the following questions: how did the pandemic influence your life, a) in terms of work and income, b) in terms of your personal well-being, c) in terms of your family life, if any? The questionnaire also included the inquiry into how the experiences of previous global crises influenced their coping and resilience mechanisms during the COVID-19 pandemic. The respondents were also asked about their gender, age group (choosing among three options – 18-35,36-50, and 51-65), time of arrival to the host country, and the country of origin. These online questionnaires were conducted during the March-April 2021 lockdowns.

An online survey of former Yugoslav immigrants in Austria resulted in 60 respondents, of whom 48 were female. The online survey placed on the Russian-speaking immigrant groups in Austria resulted in significantly fewer, 20 responses, out of which 14 were women. Such a result was expected, given the much smaller size of the post-Soviet Russian-speaking community in Austria in comparison to the post-Yugoslav one. The results of online surveys in Hungary were reversed: 25 responses to the online questionnaire posed in post-Soviet Russian-speaking groups, with 18 of them from female respondents, and only 10 responses in post-Yugoslav groups, out of which only four were from female respondents. These results are also expectable considering the numbers of both immigrant communities in two host countries. In sum, the inquiries resulted in rich qualitative data about the experiences of both analyzed female immigrant groups that are presented in the following section.

IMPACT OF COVID-19 PANDEMIC ON POST-YUGOSLAV AND POST-SOVIET FEMALE IMMIGRANTS IN AUSTRIA AND HUNGARY

When in the early spring of 2020 one after another the governments introduced lockdowns to prevent the spread of COVID-19, most communication and social activities moved to the online regime. While digitalization of all contacts increased rapidly, for migrants this way of communication boomed as the only available channel of communication with their families and friends. Simultaneously, the significance of social media groups created and used by immigrants rapidly increased as accessible platforms for communication, exchange of experiences, and advice in coping with the pandemic in the contexts of host countries and localities. This practice confirmed the proposition about migrant community ties as a 'hard' resilience mechanism, and it continued throughout the stages and waves of the COVID-19 pandemic. Taking alone the results of online surveys in post-Yugoslav groups, about 60% answered that the pandemic did not influence their employment and financial statuses, as illustrated in the following response.

The pandemic did not change my financial situation. I find it relatively easy to accept the situation with the pandemic having experienced the war (a female immigrant from Bosnia, aged between 35 and 50).

The respondents providing this type of answer usually reported being middle-level managers of Austrian firms or multinational corporations based in Austria or working in the educational sector. Only two of the post-Yugoslav female immigrants in Austria reported that they lost their jobs due to the pandemic and that in searching for new employment, they turned to Austria's official labor market bureau. Simultaneously, they received minimal financial support from the state. Those employed as blue-collar workers in factories that had to stop working due to pandemic reported that they also received the state's financial support. Prior to the pandemic, seven of these respondents worked in trade, five worked in medical services, and five in the education sector. Before the pandemic, only three respondents of the survey from this immigrant group in Austria worked in tourism. Furthermore, all pointed out that the pandemic has made their lives even more complex due to not being able to travel back to their home countries to visit their families. Here is the comment that illustrates the frustration of one of the female Bosnian immigrants in Austria:

These lockdowns are catastrophic, as now I have to take a three-week vacation to spend one week with my parents (aged between 35 and 50).

Another general response received from the majority of the post-Yugoslav female immigrants in Austria regarding the impact of the pandemic on their lives was that they reduced their expenditures to non-essentials; others pointed out that they reduce their spending on everything. In contrast, other post-Yugoslav female immigrants' responses received through online surveys and personal communication, revealed positive aspects of the pandemic.

It might not sound nice to say, but my work flourished during the pandemic: it is much easier to organize an event online. We got more customers and increased activities and profits (personal communication, female immigrant from Croatia in Austria aged 38).

Most discussions among female immigrants evolved around restrictions on movement and travel, the remote work with the lack of the technical equipment, and for parenting, female immigrants topics related to simultaneous childcare and remote work in the same space. Personal communication provided deep insights into these situations and the emotions related to them.

To me working remotely is a huge relief because I can spend more time with my children, and I feel that I fulfill my parental duties better than before the pandemic. At the same time, all burden of parenting is on me. My husband works as technical support in a factory, and he is at work the whole day. Therefore, apart from my work, I take care of the kids, cook for them, and ensure that they are ready and on time for online classes. (…) Now even thinking of returning to the office seems like a nightmare… Of course, for the kids, online schooling had its tradeoffs, because before the pandemic they never used to study at home. Now they are accustomed to it (personal communication, a female immigrant from Bosnia in Austria aged 46).

This insight suggests that female immigrants in Austria, who have families and hold white-collar positions, have perceived the pandemic relatively calmly because it paved the way back to their personal integrity of being professionals and parents simultaneously. As many of them admitted, such calmness relates to the fact that simultaneously they have received the pre-pandemic level of income. In parallel, during the pandemic, the family had come to the focus of their daily activities. In turn, the time spent on childcare balanced the absence of commuting to work. Thus, regardless of their age and the time of arrival to Austria, former Yugoslav female immigrants in Austria seem to perceive the changes brought by the pandemic as a new routine or temporary obstacle, thus, for them, the pandemic is only another stage of the gradual transformation.

Furthermore, analysis of the content of the social media groups revealed that female immigrants – whether coming from former Yugoslavia or from the former SU, who live with partners but have no kids and hold white-collar positions, have had the calmest and most positive reaction to remote work and the pandemic lockdowns. For example, they have continuously posted photographs of their desks, sunny working rooms, and balconies with flowers onFacebook, commenting that possibility to spend the day working in such an environment is the positive aspect of remote work and the pandemic lockdowns.

At the same time, the research revealed that there have been more entrepreneurs among post-Soviet female immigrants than among their post-Yugoslav counterparts. Post-Soviet women immigrants usually hold positions in information technologies (IT), in education, and in marketing. This suggests that most of the respondents have kept their jobs and the level of salaries during the pandemic. Those who worked as entrepreneurs and were not able to continue their work remotely received state support during the lockdowns. For example, the director of the languages and art school located in Vienna shared the challenges faced in her work during the pandemic:

Our school currently works 40% of the pre-pandemic capacity (…) it is hard to teach children arts or music remotely. (…) Parents are afraid of the virus. Without the Austrian state'ssupport, we would not be able to survive the pandemic (personal communication, female immigrant from Russia in Austria, aged 53).

Another respondent framed the pandemic as an opportunity to find a job in a different sector of the economy.

I moved to work for another company and to a better position: before the pandemic, I worked in tourism as a medium-level professional, and now I work in marketing as a top manager (online survey, immigrant from Russia in Austria, aged between 18 and 35).

Similar to their counterparts from former Yugoslavia, most post-Soviets in Austria reported that during the pandemic the biggest challenge for them was "the ban on air (and other) travel to visit the family" (online survey, immigrant from Russia in Austria, aged between 35 and 50). Others found the travel ban difficult for much simpler reasons: it did not allow for "a change in the environment and scenery" (online survey, immigrant from Russia in Austria, aged between 18 and 35). With a couple of important exceptions, the overall impression from the surveys and interviews conducted in Austria among both former Yugoslav and post-Soviet immigrants (in this case, including both genders and age groups) is that during the pandemic their incomes and their socio-economic situations have not significantly changed. Still, this factor seems insufficient in completely neutralizing the negative psychological influence of the pandemic.

In Hungary, the pandemic had a greater socio-economic impact on female immigrants than in Austria. First, a much higher percentage of respondents from post-Yugoslav and post-Soviet female immigrant groups reported that they either lost their jobs during the pandemic (30% of respondents in Hungary from former Yugoslavia, and 12% among the female respondents from the former SU), or that they changed the sphere of work or profession (12%). As reported through personal communication and surveys, in the pre-pandemic period most female immigrants worked in the tourism sector (25% of immigrants from former Yugoslavia and even 36% of their post-Soviet counterparts). The following quotation provides a personal insight.

I had worked as a tourist guide ever since I came to Hungary in the early 1990s. My business partners and customers have always been from the Balkans – from the former Yugoslavia. The pandemic stopped travel, and both my business partners and I have temporarily lost our incomes. My savings help me to survive financially. … Nevertheless, I have kept myself busy supporting my kids: I became a grandma during the pandemic, and I help in bringing up my grandchild (personal communication, immigrant from Croatia in Hungary aged 65).

Another, post-Yugoslav interlocutor aged 31 lost her job in the textile industry during the first lockdown in the spring of 2020. She used all her personal and professional networks to find a new job, and two months later, she got a managerial position in the IT industry. At the same time, only one of the female respondents in

Hungary reported that she received financial support from the state. Furthermore, some of the immigrants explained that the pandemic negatively affected them through their households due to the loss of jobs of their family members.

My Hungarian husband lost his job in the movie industry temporarily, though the taxes remained the same and there were no compensations or state support, so it was heavily challenging to survive having only my salary (online survey, female immigrant from Russia in Hungary, aged between 18 and 35).

Similarly, another female immigrant from Russia aged 37, who before the pandemic held a top-manager position in the tourism sector, noted that she would not survive during the pandemic without finding an additional job. As a result, she reported that she became a private entrepreneur and a cosmetologist. This example also confirms the proposition from the immigrant entrepreneurship field of literature portraying entrepreneurship and self-employment of female immigrants as socio-economic resilience mechanisms. Simultaneously, the post-Soviet immigrants in Hungary, including both women and men, working in the financial (20%), IT (20%), and marketing (4%) sectors as employees of international corporations seem to have been the least affected by the pandemic in socio-economic terms.

A similar argument can be made for female immigrants from former Yugoslavia in Hungary, who have been working in the IT and education sectors. Neither had they reported losing their jobs, nor a change in their income and socio-economic status. At the same time, some detailed responses reflected that the pandemic has also had a positive impact on the personal lives of some immigrants.

Prior to the lockdown, I met a man that I liked. During the lockdown, we moved in together and a couple of months later we got married (online survey, female immigrant from Russia in Hungary, aged between 18 and 35).

Similar to responses from Austria, responses in Hungary showed that the lockdowns have had a major impact on immigrant households. In Hungary, several female immigrants complained about the difficulties that their kids experienced with remote learning. The following quote from personal communication sheds light on the scale and depth of such a problem.

Despite the teachers' promises that there will be remote classes during the lockdowns, my kids' school did not provide them properly. The teachers sent homework in emails, and they had some online meetings for 20 minutes once a week. As a result, I spent all of the lockdown teaching my kids. I never studied in Hungarian and I have limited knowledge of this language. That was a nightmare (personal communication, female immigrant from Russia in Hungary, aged between 35 and 50).

This quotation from the personal communication reveals triple vulnerability: being female, a mother, and a migrant during the COVID-19 pandemic, confirming the argument about the concept of 'superwomanization' during the pandemic lockdowns put by Faludi and Crosby (2020). Therefore, this concept is also applicable to immigrant women. Simultaneously, it confirms the female migrant vulnerability thesis raised by the scholarly literature on migration. Whilst, during the pandemic lockdowns, in certain cases, both state and market structures failed to provide elementary education to migrants' kids, turning the migrant mothers into educators. Other female immigrant parents, whose working schedules did not allow for homeschooling along with the remote work, solved this problem in a different way.

When the lockdown was announced, we used the social media Russian-language groups in Hungary to find a bilingual tutor for our two kids. We found her quite quickly, and in a couple of days, she started to work with the kids. It was relatively costly, but the only efficient way for us to solve this problem (personal communication, immigrant from Russia in Hungary, aged between 35 and 50).

At the same time, there was a significant number of post-Soviet female immigrants, who came to Hungary as labor migrants and during the lockdowns felt isolated and alone. The situation explained in the citation below reveals the lack of social protection in Hungary during the lockdowns in economic, social, and psychological aspects.

We have been working remotely for almost two years now. In Hungary, I live alone, I have only neighbors and friends, and working from home and being isolated is so depressing. At the beginning of the pandemic, we used our own technical equipment, which was barely sufficient for the tasks at work, but we were required to continue to work online. (…) We were not allowed to travel to our home countries and work remotely from there. Therefore, we organized a small trade union within the company to compensate us for electricity and equipment. (…) Our CEO was constantly sending letters asking us to be mindful of our colleagues who have small kids. Being single, I felt invisible and forgotten (…) In response to one of such letters from the CEO, my colleague wrote that those who suffer from lockdowns are not only those colleagues who have small kids, but also those who live alone that face psychological challenges because of isolation. When I saw this letter, I finally felt that my pain was recognized, and I started to cry (personal communication, female immigrant from Russia in Hungary, aged between 35 and 50).

The situation described in this quotation demonstrates that both 'soft' elements – communication with co-workers, colleagues, and broader professional community, and 'hard' elements of resilience – the creation of a trade union to compensate for the costs of the remote work - had an important positive influence on the respondent. It is also significant that these aspects of resilience appeared in response to the lack of the states and company-led social protection throughout the pandemic.

Overall, the most striking difference in terms of the socio-economic impact of the pandemic on the post-Yugoslav and post-Soviet female immigrants, considering their responses in Hungary and Austria, is the frequency and the quality of the state's support during the pandemic in Austria, and the lack of it in Hungary. Another striking difference between the situations considering female immigrants in these two countries is in the sector of their employment: while there are only a few former Yugoslav and post-Soviet immigrants in Austria, who before the pandemic worked in the tourism sector, these numbers are significant in Hungary, especially among the post-Soviet female immigrants. Finally, the ban on travel and lockdowns seemed to have negative psychological impacts on both groups of female immigrants in Austria and Hungary reflected in the following two responses from the online surveys.

Life has changed tremendously because before the pandemic we traveled a lot: on business trips, vacations, and back to home countries (online survey, female immigrant from Ukraine in Hungary aged between 18 and 35).

The obstacles to traveling home during the year and visits of my family have had a strong negative impact on my psychological condition (online survey, female immigrant from Russia in Austria, aged between 18 and 35).

Lessons From Previous Global Crises Applied During the COVID-19 Pandemic

The differences in regulations of social protection and other socio-economic settings in Austria and Hungary as well as in sizes and times of formations of the former Yugoslav and post-Soviet migrant communities, and responses from the post-Yugoslav and post-Soviet female immigrants serve the striking examples of the emergence and levels of 'psychological immunization' (Foulkes, 2021). Considering the following comment, it seems that the relatively harsh experiences of the former Yugoslav female immigrants from previous global crises resulted in their relatively strong 'soft' resilience.

Growing up in a destroyed and devastated country during and after the war formed my worldview on the pandemic. With regard to the pandemic, my financial situation has not changed; it is much easier to accept the current situation having such experiences from the past (online survey, female immigrant from Bosnia in Austria, aged between 18 and 35).

Simultaneously, this testimony reflects the effect of previously experienced crises in shaping personal identity. At the same time, it confirms that stable income contributes to a higher level of 'soft' resilience.

Nothing is in scarcity, I have enough of everything (food, flat, WiFi), and all that we did not have during the war (online survey, female immigrant from Bosnia in Austria, aged between 35 and 50).

Like their counterparts in Austria, immigrants from former Yugoslavia who reside in Hungary have reported mild levels of stress because of the pandemic, again in comparison to the war experiences. One of the key reasons for being calm seems to be the possibility to communicate and work remotely.

In contrast to the war, during the pandemic lockdowns, we constantly have had water and electricity; we have had constant channels of communication via Internet platforms, so I kept in contact with my family and friends… I spent much more time with my kid, and I became much more productive at work, as there was no need to commute to the office and back (personal communication, female immigrant from Croatia in Hungary, aged 42).

Contrary to all other respondents from former Yugoslavia, one female immigrant, who was among the most senior respondents of the online survey (aged between 50 and 65) and who came to Austria as a refugee responded that she has never experienced any situation like the pandemic. She noted that, apart from decreased mobility, the pandemic did not change her life much. Her response also suggests that various types of global crises generate different experiences, but also that perception depends equally on one's personality.

In contrast to most former Yugoslavs, the post-Soviet immigrants in both Austria and Hungary stated that the pandemic is a unique situation for them that they cannot compare to any previous experiences. Only two of total 32 survey female respondents, residing either in Austria or in Hungary, related their experience from the pandemic with previously experienced global crises.

I survived all the crises, starting from 1985. I hope that I will survive this crisis too. Our knowledge and skills are our only treasure (online survey, female immigrant from Russia in Hungary, aged between 50 and 65).

In my life, there were many worse situations than this pandemic (online survey, female Russian immigrant in Austria, aged between 35 and 50).

These responses reflect on relatively high level of both 'soft' and 'hard' aspects of resilience developed through the previous global crises. Table 3 and 4 summarize these findings.

Table 3. Impact of COVID-19 on post-Yugoslav and post-Soviet female migrants in Austria

Vulnerabilities and Forms of Resilience During COVID-19 Pandemic Among Female Immigrants in Austria	**18-35 Age Group**	**35-50 Age Group**	**50-65 Age Group**
Post-Yugoslav female immigrants	a) inability to travel to home country/ the loss of job; b) the use of online communication platforms to keep in touch with family/ friends/ search of jobs through official bureau	a) the loss of job; b) the state's financial support	a) inability to travel; b) online communication
Post-Soviet female immigrants	a) inability to travel to home country/ job loss/; b) online communication/ change of profession and/or industry	a) inability to travel to home country and depression; b) online communication with family and friends	a) radically decreased income; b) state's financial support

Table 4. Impact of COVID-19 pandemic on post-Yugoslav and post-Soviet female immigrants in Hungary, Retained Vulnerabilities and Lessons from the COVID-19 Pandemic

Vulnerabilities and Forms of Resilience During COVID-19 Pandemic Among Female Immigrants in Hungary	18-35 Age Group	35-50 Age Group	50-65 Age Group
Post-Yugoslav female immigrants	a) the loss of job; b) using professional networks to get a new job and change of industry;	a) lack of appropriate remote schooling/ lack of technical equipment and compensations for remote work; b) home schooling/ renting technical equipment from a school	a) the loss of income; b) family support in childcare and use of savings in bridging the income gap
Post-Soviet female immigrants	a) inability to travel to home country/ the loss of job; b) online communication and increasing sport activities/ cutting spending	a) lack of appropriate remote schooling/ the loss of job; lack of technical equipment and compensations for remote work; b) home schooling and hiring a tutor/ entrepreneurship and self-employment/ organizing trade union to compensate for costs of remote work	a) inability to travel to home country; b) online communication

Though rare, some responses to online surveys from post-Yugoslav female immigrants in Austria reflected negative effect of the COVID-19 pandemic on their lives. Many of them referred to the phenomenon of ‘infodemic’: they noted that uncertainty, lack of information and even – as one of them noted – wearing the mask – were difficulties that COVID-19 pandemic brought to their lives. Some even expressed widespread tendency to believe that the pandemic is a conspiracy:

If there really were a pandemic, it would not have such a strong impact on my brain. This seems like butchering sheep before killing them (online survey, immigrant from Bosnia in Austria aged between 18 and 35).

The most elderly of online surveys’ former Yugoslav female respondents was 60 years old and she worked as the head of a supermarket. She has resided in Austria since 1992, and she noted that the “pandemic brought more stress because it disabled me to do my job in the usual way” and highlighted that “insecurity, the lack of knowledge, restrictions to travel home, and the misinformation" have made her increasingly anxious (immigrant from Bosnia in Austria, aged 60). These examples second Foulkes' (2021) argument that high stress results in psychological vulnerability.

Several post-Soviet female survey respondents from mostly from aged between 35 and 50 mentioned that the lockdowns prompted them to think about changing the lifestyle and the place of living again.

During the lockdowns, I was working all the time, even more than before the pandemic ... After this pandemic, I think of moving away from the city, somewhere closer to the nature. Even statistics demonstrate that people who own large houses somewhere closer to the nature overcame the lockdown much easier than those, who live in the flats (personal communication, immigrant from Ukraine, aged between 35 and 50).

Talking about mechanisms of resilience, many respondents referred to skills obtained, and habits developed during the pandemic.

The pandemic ... is merely the possibility to revise my views and habits (online survey, immigrant from Russia in Hungary, aged between 35 and 50);

I try to keep myself maximally active: I do sports and take courses, I bought a dog (online survey, immigrant from Ukraine in Hungary, aged between 18 and 35);

Looking at the positive side of each situation, taking responsibility for your own mood, health, and finances (online survey, immigrant from Russia in Hungary aged between 18 and 35).

Though most of the female immigrants cited above noted that they have not experienced anything like COVID-19 pandemic before, they seem to build psychological immunization or 'soft' resilience throughout the current crisis. On one hand, one can interpret this resilience mechanism as a combination of personal and generational characteristics. On the other hand, the pandemic turned out to be a learning experience generating 'soft' resilience. In sum, through communication with fellow female immigrants, the author reinforced the view that each person is unique and their behavior in the crisis depends on peculiarities of the situations in which they faced the crisis. Nevertheless, their testimonies shown that the time of immigration, age, and family status play most important roles in the ways in which the pandemic has influenced their lives. Furthermore, their experiences from the previous global crises influenced their perceptions of the pandemic to be seen as a temporary inconvenience, rather than the real problem.

CONCLUSION

The COVID-19 pandemic has played a role of catalyzer for almost all aspects and levels of female immigrants' lives: health, finances, society, and family. The findings of the present chapter lead to several important conclusions and theoretical implications. In general, the chapter demonstrated that female immigrants' vulnerability and enforcement in the face of global crises depends on several key factors.

The first is their employment and income status. In Austria, where the state provided stable social protection during the lockdowns practically all examined female immigrants from both groups experienced minimal negative impact of the crisis. In Hungary such protection turned to be either minimal, or absent. As a result, both post-Yugoslav and post-Soviet female immigrants in Hungary experienced significant negative impact of the pandemic in the form of job and income losses. Consequentially, psychological or 'soft' resilience expressed through the perception of it as temporary inconvenience was much more frequently present among female immigrants in Austria, than in Hungary. This finding demonstrates that both vulnerability of female immigrants and their mobility as an enforcement is heavily dependent on formal institutions of a host country, especially its' social protection regulations, meaning that the more social protection there is, the stress is lesser, and higher is the 'soft' resilience. This finding confirms Foulkes' (2021) argument that the mild level of stress results in 'psychological immunization'.

The second related influential factor regarding female immigrants' vulnerability and enforcement is the industry of employment and the type of employer. As the analysis in this chapter demonstrated, the employment in financial and IT industries and in large multinational corporations, as well as in some educational organizations proved to provide a better social security during the pandemic, than other sectors and types of employment. Examined post-Yugoslav and post-Soviet female immigrants in both Austria and Hungary experienced little if any change in their jobs and incomes. Quite the contrary, most of the explored female immigrants who prior to the pandemic were employed or self-employed in tourism industry, experienced either radical decrease or the loss of income during the lockdowns. Such experiences were mostly present in Hungary and change of profession and additional self-employment were major female immigrants' 'hard' resilience mechanisms. This finding correlates with the proposition derived from the immigrant entrepreneurship field of scholarly literature, stating that immigrant entrepreneurship is 'hard' resilience response to radical change (Zueva, 2005; Munkejord, 2017).

Third important factor influencing female immigrants' vulnerability, and/or enforcement thereof, is their marital/family status. In this dimension, the analysis provided in this chapter demonstrated that both 'soft' and 'hard' resilience mechanisms of examined post-Yugoslav and post-Soviet female immigrants heavily depended on whether they were single, living with a partner, or mothers of underage children. These three situations combined with their employment statuses, in turn, fell into four categories: first, those, who have long-term or permanent contracts; second, those, who have their businesses/ are entrepreneurs; third, those, who have project-based short-term jobs or are individual entrepreneurs, and the last – unemployed 'housewives'. Pandemic has changed these statuses for at least one third of respondents in both Austria and Hungary. The exploration conducted in Austria revealed that some immigrant mothers of underage kids, during the lockdowns experienced vulnerability of 'housewifeization'. In Hungary, this phenomenon was accompanied either with job and income losses or with the lack of technical equipment for work from home. An acute problem for some immigrant mothers in Hungary was poorly organized online schooling. The 'countermovement' – enforcement or 'hard' resilience in such cases took two forms: either immigrant mothers took the role of (usually insufficiently qualified) home teachers, or they turned for support to their immigrant communities by hiring fellow immigrant instructors. The implication of such trend is that the process of commodification of the female employment, that started long before the pandemic, has continued during the pandemic, while unpaid home schooling and social services were added responsibilities. This finding, thus, confirms Foulkes (2021) argument, that, in contrast to mild stress that generates psychological immunity, high stress results in psychological vulnerability: this seems applicable to female immigrants who worked as blue-collar workers, and who lost their jobs due to the pandemic. Confirming Foulkes' finding, others less severely exposed to the pandemic in socio-economic terms, demonstrated a relatively high level of resilience.

These findings lead to the last major conclusion about the female immigrants' resilience mechanisms during the COVID-19 pandemic. As the analysis revealed, both post-Yugoslav and post-Soviet female immigrants in Austria and in Hungary actively participated in formation of online communities in social media and in their discussions. Through these channels of communication, they received moral support from their families, friends, and especially from their fellow female immigrants. This finding contributes to the assumption from the migration literature, stating that in challenging situation the support comes from the immigrant community (Kim, 2014; Tepavcevic, 2021). The findings of the present analysis also have significant extension to this proposition. Namely, along with immigrant communities, professional communities in host countries and in the places of employment and cooperation with them in times of crises serve equally important element of 'hard' resilience. During COVID-19 pandemic, this support has transformed to the support of digital immigrant and professional communities that continue to play important role in the early post-pandemic era.

Finally, these findings are limited to the comparisons of post-Yugoslav and post-Soviet female immigrants living in Austria and Hungary. Further research in various municipal and national contexts and exploration of other immigrant groups would provide valuable contribution to the research presented in this chapter.

ACKNOWLEDGMENT

This research was financially supported by the Individual Research Fellowship of the Polanyi Centre, Institute of Advanced Studies Kőszeg, Hungary. The author also wants to thank her female family members, fellow female migrant friends and colleagues in Austria and Hungary, administrators of social media groups, anonymous respondents of online questionnaires, and anonymous reviewers for their comments and suggestions.

REFERENCES

Adams, T., Ellis, C., & Holman, J. S. (2017). Autoethnography. In C. S. Davis & R. F. Potter (Eds.), *The International Encyclopedia of Communication Research Methods* (pp. 1–11). John Wiley & Sons.

Castles, S., de Haas, H., & Miller, M. (2018). *The Age of Migration. International Population Movements in the Modern World*. Palgrave MacMillan.

Cvajner, M. (2012). The Presentation of Self in Emigration: Eastern European Women in Italy. *The Annals of the American Academy of Political and Social Science, 624*(1), 186–198.

Dannecker, P., & Cakir, A. (2016). Female Migrant Entrepreneurs in Vienna. Mobility and its Embeddedness. *Osterreichische Zeitschrift fur Soziologie, 41*(1), 97–113. doi:10.100711614-016-0193-y

Degani, P., & De Stefani, P. (2020). Addressing Migrant Women's Intersecting Vulnerabilities. Refugee Protection, Anti-trafficking and Anti-violence Referral Patterns in Italy. *Peace Human Rights Governance, 4*(1), 113–152.

Faludi, J., & Crosby, M. (2020). The Digital Economy of the Sourdough: Housewifisation in the Time of COVID-19. *TripleC, 19*(1), 113–124.

Foulkes, L. (2021). *Losing Our Minds. What Mental Illness Really Is, and What it isn't*. Penguin Books.

Gamlen, A. (2020). Migration and mobility after the 2020 pandemic: The end of an age? In *Covid-19 and Transformation, Migration and Mobility Globally*. International Organization of Migration.

Halilovich, H. (2011). (Per)Forming "Trans-Local" Homes: Bosnian Diaspora in Australia. In M. Valenta & S. Ramet (Eds.), *The Bosnian Diaspora: Integration in Transnational Communities* (pp. 63–81). Ashgate Publishing Limited.

International Organization of Migration (IOM). (2005). *World Migration Report 2005*. Retrieved from: https://publications.iom.int/system/files/pdf/wmr_2005_3.pdf?language=en

International Organization of Migration (IOM). (2018). *World Migration Report 2018*. Retrieved from: https://publications.iom.int/system/files/pdf/wmr_2018_en.pdf

International Organization of Migration (IOM). (2020). *World Migration Report 2020*. Retrieved from: https://publications.iom.int/system/files/pdf/wmr_2020.pdf

Kim, H. H. (2014). Immigrant Network Structure and Perceived Social Capital: A Study of the Korean Ethnic Enclave in Uzbekistan. *Development and Society*, *43*(2), 351–379.

Kovacevic-Bielicki, D. (2017). *Born in Yugoslavia- Raised in Norway: Former Child Refugees and Belonging*. Novus Press.

Mesch, G., & Czamanski, D. (1997). Occupational closure and immigrant entrepreneurship: Russian Jews in Israel. *Journal of Socio-Economics*, *26*(6), 597–610.

Munkejord, M. C. (2017). Local and transnational networking among female immigrant entrepreneurs in peripheral rural contexts: Russian female entrepreneurs in Norway. *European Urban and Regional Studies*, *24*(1), 7–20.

Novy, A. (2021). The political trilemma of contemporary social-ecological transformation – lessons from Karl Polanyi's 'The Great Transformation'. *Globalizations*, 1–23. doi:10.1080/14747731.2020.1850073

Phizacklea, A. (1983). *One Way Ticket? Migration and Female Labour*. Routledge.

Phizacklea, A. (1998). Migration and Globalization: A Feminist Perspective. In K. Koser & H. Lutz (Eds.), *The New Migration in Europe*. Palgrave Macmillan., doi:10.1007/978-1-349-26258-8_2

Polanyi, K. (1944). *The Great Transformation. The Political and Economic Origins of Our Time*. Beacon Press.

Portes, A. (1997). Immigration Theory for a New Century: Some Problems and Opportunities. *The International Migration Review*, *31*(4), 799–825.

Reliefweb. (2019). *Women and migration: vulnerability in the face of abuse and discrimination*. Retrieved from: https://reliefweb.int/report/world/women-and-migration-vulnerability-face-abuse-and-discrimination

Tagliacozzo, S., Pisacane, L., & Kilkey, M. (2020). The interplay between structural and systemic vulnerability during the COVID-19 pandemic: Migrant agricultural workers in informal settlements in Southern Italy. *Journal of Ethnic and Migration Studies*, *47*(9), 1903–1921.

Tepavcevic, S. (2021). Changing Geography, Retaining the Mentality: Social and Economic Integration of Post-Soviet Immigrants in Austria and Hungary. *Review of Economic Theory and Policy*, *3*, 137–154.

United Nations Higher Committee for Refugees (UNHCR). (2006). *Annual Statistics 2006*. Retrieved from: https://www.unhcr.org/statistics/%20STATISTICS/4486ceb12.pdf

Valenta, M., & Ramet, S. (Eds.). (2011). *The Bosnian Diaspora. Integration in Transnational Communities*. Routledge.

Zueva, A. (2005). *Gendered experiences in migration from Russia to Hungary*. Retrieved from: https://migrationonline.cz/en/genderedexperiences-in-migration-from-russia-to-hungary-in-the-gender

Compilation of References

Acemoglu, D., Robinson, J. A., & Santos, R. J. (2013). The monopoly of violence: Evidence from Colombia. *Journal of the European Economic Association*, *11*(suppl_1), 5–44. doi:10.1111/j.1542-4774.2012.01099.x

Adams, T., Ellis, C., & Holman, J. S. (2017). Autoethnography. In C. S. Davis & R. F. Potter (Eds.), *The International Encyclopedia of Communication Research Methods* (pp. 1–11). John Wiley & Sons.

Adeniyi-Ogunyankin, G. (2012). “When will I get my rest?” Neo-liberalism, women, class and ageing in Ibadan, Nigeria. *Agenda: Empowering Women for Gender Equity*, *26*(4), 29–36. doi: 10.1080/10130950.2012.758426

Ağar, C. C., & Böhm, S. (2018). Towards a pluralist labor geography: Constrained grassroots agency and the socio-spatial fix in Dêrsim, Turkey. *Environment and Planning A. Economy and Space*, *50*(6), 1228–1249.

Ahrendt, D., Cabrita, J., Clerici, E., Hurley, J., Leončikas, T., Mascherini, M., Riso, S., & Sándor, E. (2020). *Living, working and COVID-19* (report COVID-19 series). Publications Office of the European Union. https://www.eurofound.europa.eu/publications/report/2020/living-working-and-covid-19

Ajzen, I., & Fishbein, M. (1974). Factors influencing intentions and the intentionbehavior relation. *Human Relations*, *27*(1), 1–15. doi:10.1177/001872677402700101

Akerlof, G. A. (1982). Labor contracts as partial gift exchange. *The Quarterly Journal of Economics*, *97*(4), 543–569. doi:10.2307/1885099

Akerlof, G. A., & Kranton, R. A. (2000). Economics and identity. *The Quarterly Journal of Economics*, *115*(3), 715–753. doi:10.1162/003355300554881

Alon, T., Doepke, M., Olmstead-Rumsey, J., & Tertilt, M. (2020). *The Impact of COVID-19 on Gender Equality*. National Bureau of Economic Research. doi:10.3386/w26947

Alvarado, M., & Guerra, N. (2012). Gender-based violence is a public health problem [La violencia de género un problema de salud pública]. *Revista de Trabajo Social*, *2*(2), 97–106.

Andrade, C., & Lobo Fernandes, J. (2021). Role boundary management during COVID-19 pandemic: A qualitative analysis of focus group data with working-student mothers. *Psicologia*, *35*(1), 175–162. doi:10.17575/psicologia.v35i1.1694

Antunes, R. (2013). *The Meanings of Work* (Vol. 43). Academic Press.

Armiero, M. (2008). Seeing like a protester: Nature, power, and environmental struggles. *Left History*, *13*(1). Advance online publication. doi:10.25071/1913-9632.24610

Armiero, M., & D'Alisa, G. (2012). Rights of resistance: The garbage struggles for environmental justice in Campania, Italy. *Capitalism, Nature, Socialism*, *23*(4), 52–68. doi:10.1080/10455752.2012.724200

Armiero, M., & D'Alisa, G. (2013). Voices, clues, numbers: Roaming among waste in Campania. *Capitalism, Nature, Socialism*, *24*(4), 7–16. doi:10.1080/10455752.2013.851262

Bacchiega, A., & Borzaga, C. (2001). Social enterprises as incentive structures. An economic analysis. In C. Borzaga & J. Defourny (Eds.), *The emergence of social enterprises (pp* (pp. 273–295). Routledge.

Banks, M., Lovatt, A., O'Connor, J., & Raffo, C. (2000). Risk and trust in the cultural industries. *Geoforum*, *31*(4), 453–464. doi:10.1016/S0016-7185(00)00008-7

Barber, B. (1995). All Economies Are 'Embedded' The Career of a Concept and Beyond. *Social Research*, *62*(2), 387–413.

Bar-Haim, A. (2002). *Participation programs in work organizations: past, present, and scenarios for the future*. Praeger.

Baruch, Y. (2000). Teleworking: Benefits and pitfalls as perceived by professionals and managers. *New Technology, Work and Employment*, *15*(1), 34–49. doi:10.1111/1468-005X.00063

Bathelt, H., Malmberg, A., & Maskell, P. (2004). Clusters and knowledge: Local buzz, global pipelines and the process of knowledge creation. *Progress in Human Geography*, *28*(1), 31–56. doi:10.1191/0309132504ph469oa

Bell, E., & Taylor, S. (2004). 'From outward bound to inward bound': The prophetic voices and discursive practices of spiritual management development. *Human Relations*, *57*(4), 439–466. doi:10.1177/0018726704043895

Beneria, L. (1999). Globalization, Gender And The Davos Man. *Feminist Economics*, *5*(3), 61–83. doi:10.1080/135457099337815

Ben-Ner, A., & Jones, D. C. (1995). Employee participation, ownership and productivity: A theoretical framework. *Industrial Relations*, *34*(4), 532–554. doi:10.1111/j.1468-232X.1995.tb00387.x

Benson, J., & Brown, M. (2007). Knowledge workers: What keeps them committed; what turns them away. *Work, Employment and Society*, *21*(1), 121–141. doi:10.1177/0950017007073623

Benston, M. (1989). The political economy of women's liberation. *Monthly Review (New York, N.Y.)*, *41*(7), 31–44. doi:10.14452/MR-041-07-1989-11_5

Berruti, G., & Palestino, M. F. (2020). Contested land and blurred rights in the Land of Fires (Italy). *International Planning Studies*, *25*(3), 277–288. doi:10.1080/13563475.2019.1584551

Berrutti, G., & Palestino, M. (2019). Contested land and blurred rights in the Land of Fires (Italy). In International Planning Studies. Routledge.

Bhansing, P. V., Hitters, E., & Wijngaarden, Y. (2018). Passion inspires: Motivations of creative entrepreneurs in creative business centres in the Netherlands. *The Journal of Entrepreneurship*, *27*(1), 1–24. doi:10.1177/0971355717738589

Blagoev, B., Costas, J., & Kärreman, D. (2019). 'We are all herd animals': Community and organizationality in coworking spaces. *Organization*, *26*(6), 894–916. doi:10.1177/1350508418821008

Blau, G. (1999). Testing the longitudinal impact of work variables and performance appraisal satisfaction on subsequent overall job satisfaction. *Human Relations*, *52*(8), 1099–1113. doi:10.1177/001872679905200806

Block, F. (2003). Karl Polanyi and the writing of the Great Transformation. *Theory and Society*, *32*(3), 275–306. doi:10.1023/A:1024420102334

Block, F., & Somers, M. (2014). *The Power of Market Fundamentalism: Karl Polanyi's Critique*. Harvard University Press. doi:10.4159/harvard.9780674416345

Bobby Banerjee, S. (2008). Necrocapitalism. *Organization Studies*, *29*(12), 1541–1563. doi:10.1177/0170840607096386

Borg, V., Kristensen, T. S., & Burr, H. (2000). Work environment and changes in self-rated health: A five-year follow-up study. *Stress Medicine*, *16*(1), 37–47. doi:10.1002/(SICI)1099-1700(200001)16:1<37::AID-SMI830>3.0.CO;2-O

Bradley, H. (1989). *Men's work, women's work: A sociological history of the sexual division of labour in employment*. University of Minnesota Press.

Bravo, E. (2004). Gender violence and health. *DiálFil*, *20*(59), 261–274.

Browne, J. H. (2000). Benchmarking HRM practices in healthy work organisations. *American Business Review*, *18*(2), 54–61.

Byrnes, K. G., Kiely, P. A., Dunne, C. P., McDermott, K. W., & Coffey, J. C. (2021). Communication, collaboration and contagion: "Virtualisation" of anatomy during COVID-19. *Clinical Anatomy (New York, N.Y.)*, *34*(1), 82–89. doi:10.1002/ca.23649 PMID:32648289

Böhm, S., & Pascucci, S. (2020). It's Not Just About the Mafia! Conceptualizing Business–Society Relations of Organized Violence. *The Academy of Management Perspectives*, *34*(4), 546–565. doi:10.5465/amp.2019.0029

Cangiani, M. (2011). Karl Polanyi's institutional theory: Market society and its "disembedded" economy. *Journal of Economic Issues*, *45*(1), 177–198. doi:10.2753/JEI0021-3624450110

Carreras, A.I. (2019). *Legal concept of gender violence* [Concepto jurídico de violencia de género]. Dykinson, S.L.

Castles, S., de Haas, H., & Miller, M. (2018). *The Age of Migration. International Population Movements in the Modern World*. Palgrave MacMillan.

Cavotta, V., Palazzo, G., & Vaccaro, A. (2021). Mobilizing After Corporate Environmental Irresponsibility in a Community of Place: A Framing Microprocess Perspective. *Journal of Business Ethics*, 1–15. doi:10.100710551-021-04983-1

Cerrato, J., & Cifre, E. (2018). Gender inequality in household chores and work-family conflict. *Frontiers in Psychology*, *9*(1330), 1–11. doi:10.3389/fpsyg.2018.01330 PMID:30123153

Chadeau, A. (1992). *What is a Households' Non-market Production Worth*. Organisation for Economic Co-operation and Development.

CIDOB. (2022). *The SDG measurement and monitoring system* [El sistema de medición y seguimiento de los ODS]. https://www.cidob.org/es/publicaciones/documentacion/dossiers/dossier_ods_2015_2030/objetivos_de_desarrollo_sostenible_la_agenda_2030_del_compromiso_a_la_practica/el_sistema_de_medicion_y_seguimiento_de_los_ods

Ciolfi, L., Gray, B., & Pinatti de Carvalho, A. F. (2020). Making home work places. *Proceedings of 18th European Conference on Computer-Supported Cooperative Work*. 10.18420/ecscw2020_ep10

CIVICUS. (2020). *MEXICO: 'Violence against women is a historical pandemic'. Interview with Wendy Figueroa*. https://www.civicus.org/index.php/media-resources/news/interviews/4466-mexico-violence-against-women-is-a-historical-pandemic

Clark, S. C. (2000). Work/family border theory: A new theory of work/family balance. *Human Relations*, *53*(6), 747–770.

Clark, S. C. (2000). Work/Family Border Theory: A New Theory of Work/Family Balance. *Human Relations*, *53*(6), 747–770. doi:10.1177/0018726700536001

Clegg, C., & Wall, T. D. (1981). A note on some new scales for measuring aspects of psychological wellbeing at work. *Journal of Occupational Psychology*, *54*(3), 221–225. doi:10.1111/j.2044-8325.1981.tb00062.x

Coleman, J. S. (1990). *Foundations of Social Theory*. Harvard University Press.

Collins, C., Landivar, L. C., Ruppanner, L., & Scarborough, W. J. (2021). COVID-19 and the Gender Gap in Work Hours. *Gender, Work and Organization*, *28*(1), 549–560. doi:10.1111/gwao.12506 PMID:32837019

Collins, R. (2020). Social distancing as a critical test of the micro-sociology of solidarity. *American Journal of Cultural Sociology*, *8*(3), 477–497. doi:10.105741290-020-00120-z PMID:33101676

Commons, J. R. (1931). Institutional economics. *The American Economic Review*, *21*(4), 648–657.

Costas, J., & Grey, C. (2019). Violence and organization studies. *Organization Studies*, *40*(10), 1573–1586. doi:10.1177/0170840618782282

Cvajner, M. (2012). The Presentation of Self in Emigration: Eastern European Women in Italy. *The Annals of the American Academy of Political and Social Science*, *624*(1), 186–198.

D'Alisa, G., Burgalassi, D., Healy, H., & Walter, M. (2010). Conflict in Campania: Waste emergency or crisis of democracy. *Ecological Economics*, *70*(2), 239–249. doi:10.1016/j.ecolecon.2010.06.021

D'Alisa, G., Germani, A. R., Falcone, P. M., & Morone, P. (2017). Political ecology of health in the Land of Fires: A hotspot of environmental crimes in the south of Italy. *Journal of Political Ecology*, *24*(1), 59–86.

D'Amato, A., Mazzanti, M., & Nicolli, F. (2015). Waste and organized crime in regional environments. *Resource and Energy Economics*, *41*, 185–201. doi:10.1016/j.reseneeco.2015.04.003

D'Amato, A., & Zoli, M. (2012). Illegal waste disposal in the time of the mafia: A tale of enforcement and social wellbeing. *Journal of Environmental Planning and Management*, *55*(5), 637–655. doi:10.1080/09640568.2011.620324

Dacin, M. T., Ventresca, M. J., & Beal, B. D. (1999). The embeddedness of organizations: Dialogue & directions. *Journal of Management*, *25*(3), 317–356. doi:10.1177/014920639902500304

Dannecker, P., & Cakir, A. (2016). Female Migrant Entrepreneurs in Vienna. Mobility and its Embeddedness. *Osterreichische Zeitschrift fur Soziologie*, *41*(1), 97–113. doi:10.100711614-016-0193-y

Davis, J. H., Schoorman, F. D., & Donaldson, L. (1997). Toward a stewardship theory of management. *Academy of Management Review*, *22*(1), 20–47. doi:10.2307/259223

de México, G. (2021). 2030 Agenda. https://www.gob.mx/agenda2030

Deci, E. L., & Ryan, R. M. (2000). Self-determination theory and the facilitation of intrinsic motivation, social development and well-being. *The American Psychologist*, *55*(1), 68–78. doi:10.1037/0003-066X.55.1.68 PMID:11392867

Deci, E. L., & Ryan, R. M. (2008a). Facilitating optimal motivation and psychological well-being across life's domains. *Canadian Psychology*, *49*(1), 14–23. doi:10.1037/0708-5591.49.1.14

Deci, E. L., & Ryan, R. M. (2008b). Self-determination theory: A macrotheory of human motivation, development, and health. *Canadian Psychology*, *49*(3), 182–185. doi:10.1037/a0012801

Degani, P., & De Stefani, P. (2020). Addressing Migrant Women's Intersecting Vulnerabilities. Refugee Protection, Anti-trafficking and Anti-violence Referral Patterns in Italy. *Peace Human Rights Governance*, *4*(1), 113–152.

Dejours, C. (2012). *From the psychopathology to the psychodynamics of work*. Academic Press.

Dejours, C., & Deranty, J. (2010). The Centrality of Work. *Critical Horizons*, *11*(2), 167–180. doi:10.1558/crit.v11i2.167

Demaegdt, C., & Rolo, D. (2013). Psychopathology and psychodynamics of work [Psychopathologie et psychodynamique du travail]. *Pathologie Professionnelle et de l'environnement, 3*(8), 1–11.

Dén-Nagy, I. (2014). A Double-Edged Sword? A Critical Evaluation of the Mobile Phone in Creating Work–Life Balance. *New Technology, Work and Employment*, *29*(2), 193–211. doi:10.1111/ntwe.12031

Dewey, J. (1930). *The quest for certainty. A study of the relations of knowledge and action.* Allen and Unwin.

Díaz, A. (2001). The %K and %R oscillators of the stock market technical analysis and a proposal to improve the %R [Los osciladores %K y %R del análisis técnico bursátil y una propuesta para mejorar el %R]. *Contaduría y Administración*, *203*, 5–26.

Dinh, X. B. (1984). A method for estimating the membership function of a fuzzy set. *Revue Busefal, L.S.I. University Paul Sabatier*, *19*, 68–82.

Drake, G. (2003). 'This place gives me space': Place and creativity in the creative industries. *Geoforum*, *34*(4), 511–524. doi:10.1016/S0016-7185(03)00029-0

Duxbury, L., Higgins, C., Smart, R., & Stevenson, M. (2014). Mobile Technology and Boundary Permeability. *British Journal of Management*, *25*(3), 570–588. doi:10.1111/1467-8551.12027

Duzgun, E. (2020). Ecology, democracy, and COVID-19. In J. M. Ryan (Ed.), *COVID-19: Global Pandemic, Societal Responses, Ideological Solutions* (pp. 54–67). Routledge. doi:10.4324/9781003142089-7

Earl, J. (2003). Tanks, Tear Gas, and Taxes: Toward a Theory of Movement Repression. *Sociological Theory*, *21*(1), 44–68. doi:10.1111/1467-9558.00175

Eddleston, K. A., & Mulki, J. (2017). Toward understanding remote workers' management of work–family boundaries: The complexity of workplace embeddedness. *Group & Organization Management*, *42*(3), 346–387. doi:10.1177/1059601115619548

Eilam, G. (2003). The Philosophical Foundations of Aleksandr R. Luria's Neuropsychology. *Science in Context, 16*(4), 551–577. doi:10.1017/S0269889703000966

Eisenhardt, K. M., & Graebner, M. E. (2007). Theory building form cases: Opportunities and challenges. *Academy of Management Journal*, *50*(1), 25–32. doi:10.5465/amj.2007.24160888

Ekers, M., & Prudham, S. (2017). The metabolism of socioecological fixes: Capital switching, spatial fixes, and the production of nature. *Annals of the Association of American Geographers*, *107*(6), 1370–1388. doi:10.1080/24694452.2017.1309962

Elmer, T., Mepham, K., & Stadtfeld, C. (2020). Students under lockdown: Comparisons of students' social networks and mental health before and during the COVID-19 crisis in Switzerland. *PLoS One*, *15*(7), e0236337. doi:10.1371/journal.pone.0236337 PMID:32702065

Engels, F. (1934). *Dialectics of Nature*. Progress Publishers.

EQUIS. (2020). *The two pandemics: Violence against women in Mexico amidst COVID-19*. https://equis.org.mx/wp-content/uploads/2020/08/report_thetwopandemicsF.pdf

Erdal, E. (2011). *Beyond the corporation: Humanity working*. The Bodley Head.

Esping-Andersen, G., & Kolberg, J. E. (1991). Decommodification and work absence in the welfare state. *International Journal of Sociology*, *21*(3), 77–111. doi:10.1080/15579336.1991.11770014

Ettlinger, N. (2003). Cultural economic geography and a relational and microspace approach to trusts, rationalities, networks, and change in collaborative workplaces. *Journal of Economic Geography*, *3*(2), 145–171. doi:10.1093/jeg/3.2.145

Eurofound. (2020). *Living, working and COVID-19*. Retrieved March 7, 2022, from https://www.eurofound.europa.eu/publications/report/2020/living-working-and-covid-19

European Commission. (n.d.). *SURE A szükséghelyzeti munkanélküliségi kockázatokat mérséklő ideiglenes támogatást nyújtó európai eszköz (SURE)*. Retrieved May 26, 2022, from https://ec.europa.eu/info/business-economy-euro/economic-and-fiscal-policy-coordination/financial-assistance-eu/funding-mechanisms-and-facilities/sure_hu

European Institute for Gender Equality (EIGE). (2017). *Glossary of definitions of rape, femicide and intimate partner violence*. Publication Office of the European Union.

Evans, P., & Bartolomé, F. (1984). The changing pictures of the relationship between career and family. *Journal of Occupational Behaviour*, *5*(1), 9–21. doi:10.1002/job.4030050103

Falcone, P. M., D'Alisa, G., Germani, A. R., & Morone, P. (2020). When all seemed lost. A social network analysis of the waste-related environmental movement in Campania, Italy. *Political Geography*, *77*, 102114. doi:10.1016/j.polgeo.2019.102114

Faludi, J., & Crosby, M. (2020). The Digital Economy of the Sourdough: Housewifisation in the Time of COVID-19. *TripleC*, *19*(1), 113–124.

Faludi, J., & Crosby, M. (2021). The Digital Economy of the Sourdough. Housewifisation in the Time of COVID-19. *TripleC*, *19*(1), 113–124. doi:10.31269/triplec.v19i1.1222

Faludi, J., & Crosby, M. (2021). The Digital Economy of the Sourdough. Housewifisation in the Time of COVID-19. *tripleC: Communication, Capitalism & Critique*, *19*(1), 113–124.

Felbab-Brown, V. (2020). *Opinion | COVID-19 can augment violence to Mexican women*. Mexico Today: Reforma. https://mexicotoday.com/2020/04/10/opinion-covid-19-can-augment-violence-to-mexican-women/

Fernández, B. (2021). *COVID-19: The patriarchal pandemic.* https://www.aljazeera.com/opinions/2021/3/22/covid-19-the-patriarchal-pandemic

Fodor, É., Gregor, A., Koltai, J., & Kováts, E. (2021). The impact of COVID-19 on the gender division of childcare work in Hungary. *European Societies, 23*(1), 95–110. doi:10.1080/14616696.2020.1817522

Folbre, N. (1982). Exploitation comes home: A critique of the Marxian theory of family labour. *Cambridge Journal of Economics, 6*(4), 317–329.

Foss, N. J., & Weber, L. (2016). Moving opportunism to the back seat: Bounded rationality, costly conflict, and hierarchical forms. *Academy of Management Review, 41*(1), 61–69. doi:10.5465/amr.2014.0105

Foster, J. (2017). The Meaning of Work in a Sustainable Society. *Monthly Review (New York, N.Y.), 69*(4), 1. doi:10.14452/MR-069-04-2017-08_1

Foulkes, L. (2021). *Losing Our Minds. What Mental Illness Really Is, and What it isn't.* Penguin Books.

Freudenberger, H. J. (1980). *Burnout: The High Cost of High Achievement.* Anchor Press.

Frey, B. S. (1997). *Not just for the money. An economic theory of personal motivation.* Edward Elgar.

Frey, B. S., & Osterloh, M. (1999). Yes, managers should be paid like bureaucrats. *Journal of Management Inquiry, 14*(1), 96–111. doi:10.1177/1056492604273757

Fry, W. (2020). 2019 was the most violent year on record for women in Mexico, report finds. *San Diego Tribune.* https://www.sandiegouniontribune.com/news/border-baja-california/story/2020-08-06/violence-women-mexico

Gabris, G. T., & Ihrke, D. M. (2001). Does performance appraisal contribute to heightened levels of employee burnout? The results of one study. *Public Personnel Management, 30*(2), 157–172. doi:10.1177/009102600103000203

Galanti, T., Guidetti, G., Mazzei, E., Zappalà, S., & Toscano, F. (2021). Work From Home During the COVID-19 Outbreak: The Impact on Employees' Remote Work Productivity, Engagement, and Stress. *Journal of Occupational and Environmental Medicine, 63*(7), e426–e432. doi:10.1097/JOM.0000000000002236 PMID:33883531

Galeano, E. (1973). *Open Veins of Latin America. Five Centuries of the Pillage of a Continent* (C. Belfrage, Trans.). Monthly Review Press.

Gallón, N. (2020). *Women are being killed in Mexico ar record rates but the president says most emergency calls are false.* CNN. https://edition.cnn.com/2020/06/05/americas/mexico-femicide-coronavirus-lopez-obrador-intl/index.html

Gamlen, A. (2020). Migration and mobility after the 2020 pandemic: The end of an age? In *Covid-19 and Transformation, Migration and Mobility Globally*. International Organization of Migration.

Ganem, V. (2011). Relato de uma experiência de terreno de intervenção em Psicodinâmica do Trabalho [Field experience report on Psychodynamics of Work]. *Laboreal (Porto)*, *7*(1). Advance online publication. doi:10.4000/laboreal.8304

Gehman, J., Glaser, V. L., Eisenhardt, K. M., Gioia, D., Langley, A., & Corley, K. G. (2018). Finding theory–method fit: A comparison of three qualitative approaches to theory building. *Journal of Management Inquiry*, *27*(3), 284–300. doi:10.1177/1056492617706029

Gertler, M. S. (2001). Best practice? Geography, learning, and the institutional limits to stro convergence. *Journal of Economic Geography*, *1*(1), 5–26. doi:10.1093/jeg/1.1.5

Gertler, M. S. (2008). Buzz Without Being There? Communities of Practice in Context 1. In *Community, Economic Creativity, and Organization*. Oxford University Press. doi:10.1093/acprof:oso/9780199545490.003.0009

Geszler, N. (2012). *A munka és család konfliktusának forrásai az európai férfiak életében* [Unpublished MA Thesis]. Corvinus University of Budapest, Budapest, Hungary.

Geurts, S. A., & Demerouti, E. (2003). Work/non-work interface: A review of theories and findings. In M. J. Schabraco, A. M. Winnubst, & C. L. Cooper (Eds.), *The handbook of work and health psychology* (pp. 279–312). John Wiley & Sons.

Gil-Aluja, J. (1999). *Elements for a theory of decisions in uncertainty* [Elementos para una teoría de decisiones en la incertidumbre]. Milladoiro. doi:10.1007/978-1-4757-3011-1

Gil-Lafuente, A. M., & Alexánder-López, G. A. (2015). *Algorithms for the evaluation and selection of adaptation strategies to climate change in Computational Data Analysis Techniques in Economics and Finance*. Nova Science Publishers, Inc.

Gil-Lafuente, A., Torres, A., Boria, S., & Amiguet, L. (2019). *Gender equity index of the autonomous communities of Spain, a multidimensional analysis* [Índice de equidad de género de las comunidades autónomas de España, un análisis multidimensional]. Real Academia de Ciencias Económicas y Financieras.

Glazer-Malbin, N. (1976). Housework. *Signs (Chicago, Ill.)*, *1*(4), 905–922. doi:10.1086/493308

Glazer, N. Y. (1984). Servants to Capital: Unpaid Domestic Labor and Paid Work. *The Review of Radical Political Economics*, *16*(1), 60–87. doi:10.1177/048661348401600106

Glazer, N. Y. (1990). The Home as Workshop: Women as Amateur Nurses and Medical Care Providers. *Gender & Society*, *4*(4), 479–499. doi:10.1177/089124390004004004

Goodin, R. E., Rice, J. M., Parpo, A., & Eriksson, L. (2008). *Discretionary Time: A New Measure of Freedom*. Cambridge University Press. doi:10.1017/CBO9780511611452

Goodwin, G. (2018). Rethinking the double movement: Expanding the frontiers of Polanyian analysis in the Global South. *Development and Change*, *49*(5), 1268–1290. doi:10.1111/dech.12419

Goodwin, G. (2022). Double movements and disembedded economies: A response to Richard Sandbrook. *Development and Change*, *53*(3), 676–702. doi:10.1111/dech.12698

Gopinah, R. (2020). Prominence of Self-Actualization in Organization. *International Journal of Advanced Science and Technology*, *29*(3), 11591–11602.

Gorski, P. S. (2013). Beyond the fact/value distinction: *Ethical naturalism and the social sciences. Society*, *50*(6), 543–553. doi:10.100712115-013-9709-2

Gould, S. J. (2011). *I Have Landed: The End of a Beginning in Natural History*. Belknap Press: An Imprint of Harvard University Press.

Gouveia, V. V., & Ros, M. (2000). Hofstede and Schwartz's models for classifying individualism at the cultural level: Their relation to macro-social and macro-economic variables. *Psicothema*, *12*(Suppl), 25–33.

Grabher, G., & König, J. (2020). Disruption, Embedded. A Polanyian Framing of the Platform Economy. *Sociologica*, *14*(1), 95–118. doi:10.6092/issn.1971-8853/10443

Granovetter, M. (1973). The strength of weak ties. *American Journal of Sociology*, *78*(6), 1360–1380. doi:10.1086/225469

Granovetter, M. (1985). Economic action and social structure: The problem of embeddedness. *American Journal of Sociology*, *91*(3), 481–510. doi:10.1086/228311

Grant, A. M., & Berg, J. M. (2012). Prosocial motivation. In K. S. Cameron & G. M. Spreitzer (Eds.), *The Oxford handbook of positive organizational scholarship* (pp. 28–44). Oxford University Press.

Gregory-Smith, I., & Main, B. (2015). Heads I win, tails you lose? A career analysis of executive pay and corporate performance. *Cambridge Journal of Economics*, *39*(5), 1373–1398. doi:10.1093/cje/beu049

Grespan, J. (2021). *Marx: An Introduction* [Marx: Uma introdução]. Boitempo.

Guerra-Lund, R., Manica, S., & Mânica, G. (2020). Collateral issues in times of covid-19: child abuse, domestic violence and femicide. *Revista Brasileira de Odontologia Legal*, *7*(2).

Guest, D. (2002). Human resource management, corporate performance and employee wellbeing: Building the worker into HRM. *The Journal of Industrial Relations*, *4*(3), 335–358. doi:10.1111/1472-9296.00053

Habermas, J. (1971). *Toward a rational society: Student protest, science, and politics*. Beacon Press.

Habermas, J. (2016). *Time of transitions*. John Wiley & Sons.

Hackman, J. R., & Oldham, G. R. (1980). *Work redesign*. Addition-Wesley.

Halilovich, H. (2011). (Per)Forming "Trans-Local" Homes: Bosnian Diaspora in Australia. In M. Valenta & S. Ramet (Eds.), *The Bosnian Diaspora: Integration in Transnational Communities* (pp. 63–81). Ashgate Publishing Limited.

Hansmann, H. (1988). Ownership of the firm. *Journal of Law Economics and Organization*, *4*(2), 267–304.

Hansmann, H. (1996). *The Ownership of Enterprise*. Belknap Press Harvard University.

Han, W.-J., & Hart, J. (2021). Job precarity and economic prospects during the COVID-19 public health crisis. *Social Science Quarterly*, *102*(5), 1–18. Advance online publication. doi:10.1111squ.13031 PMID:34908614

Harvey, D. (2002). *Spaces of capital: Towards a critical geography*. Routledge. doi:10.4324/9780203821695

Herzberg, F. (1968). One more time. How do you motivate employees. *Harvard Business Review*, *81*(1), 87–96. PMID:12545925

Hjálmsdóttir, A., & Bjarnadóttir, V. S. (2021). "I have turned into a foreman here at home": Families and work–life balance in times of COVID-19 in a gender equality paradise. *Gender, Work and Organization*, *28*(1), 268–283. doi:10.1111/gwao.12552 PMID:33041540

Hobson, B., Fahlén, S., & Takács, J. (2011). Agency and Capabilities to Achieve a Work-Life Balance: A Comparison of Sweden and Hungary. *Social Politics*, *18*(2), 168–198. doi:10.1093p/jxr007 PMID:21966697

Hodgson, G. M. (2004). Opportunism is not the only reason why firms exist: Why an explanatory emphasis on opportunism may mislead management strategy. *Industrial and Corporate Change*, *13*(2), 401–418. doi:10.1093/icc/dth016

Hofstede, G. (1980). Motivation, leadership, and organization: Do American theories apply abroad? *Organizational Dynamics*, *9*(1), 42–63. doi:10.1016/0090-2616(80)90013-3

Hofstede, G. (1991). *Cultures and organizations: software of the mind*. McGraw-Hill.

Hofstede, G. (1998). Think locally, act globally: Cultural constraints in personnel management. *MIR*, *38*(2), 7–26. doi:10.1007/978-3-322-90989-3_2

Hofstede, G., & Bond, M. H. (1988). The Confucian connection: From cultural roots to economic growth. *Organizational Dynamics*, *16*(4), 5–21. doi:10.1016/0090-2616(88)90009-5

Hofstede, G., Neuijen, B., Daval Ohayv, D., & Sanders, G. (1990). Measuring organizational cultures: A qualitative and quantitative study across twenty cases. *Administrative Science Quarterly*, *35*(2), 286–316. doi:10.2307/2393392

Hootsen, J. A. (2020). *Domestic violence epidemic hits Mexico during coronavirus lockdown*. https://www.americamagazine.org/politics-society/2020/08/06/domestic-violence-epidemic-hits-mexico-during-coronavirus-lockdown

Hu, Y., & Qian, Y. (2021). COVID-19, Inter-household Contact and Mental Well-Being Among Older Adults in the US and the UK. *Frontiers in Sociology*, *6*, 143. doi:10.3389/fsoc.2021.714626 PMID:34381838

Iengo, I., & Armiero, M. (2017). The politicization of ill bodies in Campania, Italy. *Journal of Political Ecology*, *24*(1), 44–58. doi:10.2458/v24i1.20781

Instituto Nacional de Estadística y Geografía INEGI. (2016). *National Survey on the Dynamics of Relationships in Households* [Encuesta Nacional sobre la Dinámica de las Relaciones en los Hogares]. https://www.inegi.org.mx/programas/endireh/2016/

Instituto Nacional de Estadística y Geografía INEGI. (2020a). *National Survey of Urban Public Security ENSU* [Encuesta Nacional de Seguridad Pública Urbana ENSU]. https://www.inegi.org.mx/programas/ensu/

Instituto Nacional de Estadística y Geografía INEGI. (2020b). *Statistics. On the Occasion of the International Day for the Elimination of Violence against Women* [Estadísticas. A propósito del día internacional de la eliminación de la violencia contra la mujer]. Author.

Instituto Nacional de Estadística y Geografía INEGI. (2021). *Statistics on the International Day for the Elimination of Violence against Women* [Estadísticas a propósito del día internacional de la eliminación de la violencia contra la mujer]. https://www.inegi.org.mx/contenidos/saladeprensa/aproposito/2020/Violencia2020_Nal.pdf

Instituto Nacional de Estadística y Geografía INEGI. (2021). *System of Indicators of the Sustainable Development Goals* [Sistema de Indicadores de los Objetivos de Desarrollo Sostenible]. https://agenda2030.mx/#/home

Instituto Nacional de las Mujeres INMUJERES. (2007). *Gender glossary* [Glosario de género]. http://cedoc.inmujeres.gob.mx/documentos_download/100904.pdf

Instituto Nacional de las Mujeres INMUJERES. (2021). *Women and violence in times of pandemic* [Las mujeres y la violencia en los tiempos de pandemia]. http://cedoc.inmujeres.gob.mx/documentos_download/BA7N03%20Para%20Publicar%20con%20vo%20bo.pdf

International Labour Organization. (1944). *Declaration of Philadelphia*. ILO.

International Organization of Migration (IOM). (2005). *World Migration Report 2005*. Retrieved from: https://publications.iom.int/system/files/pdf/wmr_2005_3.pdf?language=en

International Organization of Migration (IOM). (2018). *World Migration Report 2018*. Retrieved from: https://publications.iom.int/system/files/pdf/wmr_2018_en.pdf

International Organization of Migration (IOM). (2020). *World Migration Report 2020*. Retrieved from: https://publications.iom.int/system/files/pdf/wmr_2020.pdf

Ipsen, C., van Veldhoven, M., Kirchner, K., & Hansen, J. P. (2021). Six Key Advantages and Disadvantages of Working from Home in Europe during COVID-19. *International Journal of Environmental Research and Public Health, 18*(4), 1826. doi:10.3390/ijerph18041826 PMID:33668505

Ivtzan, I., Gardner, H. E., Bernard, I., Sekhon, M., & Hart, R. (2013). Wellbeing through self-fulfilment: Examining developmental aspects of self-actualization. *The Humanistic Psychologist, 41*(2), 119–132. doi:10.1080/08873267.2012.712076

Jahn, K., Klesel, M., Lemmer, K., Weigel, A., & Niehaves, B. (2016). Individual Boundary Management: An Empirical Investigation on Technology-related Tactics. *PACIS 2016 Proceedings*, 268–271.

Jefferson, T., & King, J. E. (2001). "Never intended to be a theory of everything": Domestic labor in neoclassical and Marxian economics. *Feminist Economics, 7*(3), 71–101. doi:10.1080/13545700110103504

Jensen, M., & Meckling, W. (1976). Theory of the firm: Managerial behavior, agency costs and ownership structure. *Journal of Financial Economics, 3*(4), 305–360. doi:10.1016/0304-405X(76)90026-X

Jevons, W. S. (1871). *The Match Tax: A Problem in Finance*. E. Stanford.

Kangal, K. (2020). Engels's Emergentist Dialectics. *Monthly Review: An Independent Socialist Magazine, 72*(6), 18–27. https://stanford.idm.oclc.org/login?url=https://search.ebscohost.com/login.aspx?direct=true&site=eds-live&db=aph&AN=146780847

Kaufmann, A., & Gil Aluja, J. (1986). *Introduction to fuzzy subsets theory in business management*. Ed. Milladoiro.

Kerman, K., Korunka, C., & Tement, S. (2021). Work and home boundary violations during the COVID-19 pandemic: The role of segmentation preferences and unfinished tasks. *Applied Psychology*, 1–23. Advance online publication. doi:10.1111/apps.12335 PMID:34548734

Khan, D. B. (2020). Economic Impact of Covid-19 and Change in Value System. *LC International Journal of STEM, 1*(2), 23–31.

Kilby, J. (2013). Introduction to special issue: Theorizing violence. *European Journal of Social Theory, 16*(3), 261–272. doi:10.1177/1368431013476579

Kim, H. H. (2014). Immigrant Network Structure and Perceived Social Capital: A Study of the Korean Ethnic Enclave in Uzbekistan. *Development and Society, 43*(2), 351–379.

Koós, B., Kovács, Zs. S., Páger, B., & Uzzoli, A. (2020). Az új koronavírus-járvány társadalmi-gazdasági hatásai és ezek területi következményei. In M. Czirfusz (Ed.), Területi kihívások és területi politikák Magyarországon, 2010-2020 (pp. 123-131). Közgazdaság- és Regionális Tudományi Kutatóközpont Regionális Kutatások Intézete

Kovacevic-Bielicki, D. (2017). *Born in Yugoslavia- Raised in Norway: Former Child Refugees and Belonging*. Novus Press.

Krippner, G. R. (2001). The elusive market: Embeddedness and the paradigm of economic sociology. *Theory and Society*, *30*(6), 775–810. doi:10.1023/A:1013330324198

Lacher, H. (1999). The politics of the market: Re-reading Karl Polanyi. *Global Society*, *13*(3), 313–326. doi:10.1080/13600829908443193

Langley, A. (1999). Strategies for theorizing from process data. *Academy of Management Review*, *24*(4), 691–710. doi:10.5465/amr.1999.2553248

Langley, A. N. N., Smallman, C., Tsoukas, H., & Van de Ven, A. H. (2013). Process studies of change in organization and management: Unveiling temporality, activity, and flow. *Academy of Management Journal*, *56*(1), 1–13. doi:10.5465/amj.2013.4001

Leibenstein, H. (1966). Allocative VS "X-efficiency. *The American Economic Review*, *56*(3), 392–415.

Leibenstein, H. (1978). *General X-efficiency theory and economic development*. Oxford University Press.

Lengyel, G. (2016). Embeddedness, redistribution and double dependence: Polanyi-reception reconsidered. *Intersections. East European Journal of Society and Politics*, *2*(2), 13–37. doi:10.17356/ieejsp.v2i2.184

Liegl, M. (2014). Nomadicity and the Care of Place—On the Aesthetic and Affective Organization of Space in Freelance Creative Work. *Computer Supported Cooperative Work*, *23*(2), 163–183. doi:10.100710606-014-9198-x

Loasby, B. (2006). Industrial organization. In T. Raffaelli, G. Becattini, & M. Dardi (Eds.), *The Elgar Companion to Alfred Marshall* (pp. 371–378). Edward Elgar.

Löhr, N. (2021). The Shadow Pandemic: Policy Efforts on Gender-Based Violence during COVID-19 in the Global South. *GIGA Focus Global, 6*. https://www.unidas.world/es/node/267

Lozano, A. V. (2021). *Despite some gains, violence against women remains a global 'pandemic'*. NBC News. https://www.nbcnews.com/news/world/despite-some-gains-violence-against-women-remains-global-pandemic-n1261361

Lucchini, F., & Membretti, A. (2016). The land of fires. Evaluating a state law to restore the narrative power of local communities. *Partecipazione e conflitto, 9*(2), 640-665.

Luhmann, N. (1995). *Social systems*. Stanford University Press.

Mann, S., & Holdsworth, L. (2003). The psychological impact of teleworking: Stress, emotions and health. *New Technology, Work and Employment*, *18*(3), 196–211. doi:10.1111/1468-005X.00121

Marlow, S. L., Lacerenza, C. N., & Salas, E. (2017). Communication in virtual teams: A conceptual framework and research agenda. *Human Resource Management Review*, *27*(4), 575–589. doi:10.1016/j.hrmr.2016.12.005

Marnrique de Lara, A., & Mediina-Arellano, M. D. J. (2020). The Covid-19 pandemic and ethics in Mexico through a gender lens. *Journal of Bioethical Inquiry*, *17*(4), 613–617.

Márquez-Guajardo, A. (2020). Mexico's other pandemic: Murdered women. *The Wire*. https://thewire.in/world/mexico-murdered-women-domestic-violence-coronavirus

Martinengo, G. (2007), *Gender differences and similarities in the work-family interface: The importance of considering family life stages* [PhD dissertation, Brigham Young University]. Theses and Dissertations.

Marx, K. (n.d.). *Economic Philosophic Manuscripts*. Academic Press.

Marx, K. (1973). *Karl Marx on society and social change: With selections by Friedrich Engels*. University of Chicago Press. doi:10.7208/chicago/9780226173788.001.0001

Maslow, A. H. (1998). Maslow on management. New York, NY: Wiley.

Maslow, A. H. (1943). A Theory of human motivation. *Psychological Review*, *50*(4), 370–396. doi:10.1037/h0054346

Maslow, A. H. (1962). *Towards a psychology of being*. D. Van Nostrand. doi:10.1037/10793-000

Matulevicius, S. A., Kho, K. A., Reisch, J., & Yin, H. (2021). Academic medicine faculty perceptions of work-life balance before and since the COVID-19 pandemic. *JAMA Network Open*, *4*(6), 1–10. doi:10.1001/jamanetworkopen.2021.13539 PMID:34129021

Mayen-Huerta, C. (2020). *Covid-19 and Mexico's domestic violence crisis. Almost half of all women in Mexico experience domestic abuse and the global COVID-19 pandemic has made the situation even worse*. University of Melbourne. https://pursuit.unimelb.edu.au/articles/covid-19-and-mexico-s-domestic-violence-crisis

Mayo, E. (1933). *The human problems of an industrial civilization*. Macmillan.

McDonough, P. (2000). Job insecurity and health. *International Journal of Health Services*, *30*(3), 453–476. doi:10.2190/BPFG-X3ME-LHTA-6RPV PMID:11109176

McGregor, D. M. (1960). *The human side of enterprise*. McGraw-Hill.

Meier, B. (2008). The Great Transformation: The Political and Economic Origins of Our Time (2001) by Karl Polanyi. Book Review. *Social Thought & Research*, *29*, 155–160. https://dx.doi.org/10.17161/STR.1808.5695

Merton, R. K. (1968). *Social Theory and Social Structure*. Free Press.

Mesch, G., & Czamanski, D. (1997). Occupational closure and immigrant entrepreneurship: Russian Jews in Israel. *Journal of Socio-Economics*, *26*(6), 597–610.

Mills, C. W. (1959). *The sociological imagination*. Oxford University Press.

Minkov, M. (2009). Predictors of differences in subjective well-being across 97 nations. *Cross-Cultural Research, 43*(2), 152–179. doi:10.1177/1069397109332239

Minkov, M., & Hofstede, G. (2011). The evolution of Hofstede's doctrine. *Cross Cultural Management, 18*(1), 10–20. doi:10.1108/13527601111104269

Misangyi, V. F., Weaver, G. R., & Elms, H. (2008). Ending corruption: The interplay among institutional logics, resources, and institutional entrepreneurs. *Academy of Management Review, 33*(3), 750–770. doi:10.5465/amr.2008.32465769

Molinier, P. (2013). The Work of Care [Le travail du care]. Paris: La Dispute.

Mols, A., & Pridmore, J. (2021). Always available via WhatsApp: Mapping everyday boundary work practices and privacy negotiations. *Mobile Media & Communication, 9*(3), 1–19. doi:10.1177/2050157920970582

Montuori, A., & Purser, R. (2014). Humanistic psychology in the workplace. In K. J. Schneider, J. F. Pierson, & J. F. T. Bugental (Eds.), *The handbook of humanistic psychology: Theory, research, and practice* (pp. 723–734). Russel Sage.

Morrison-Smith, S., & Ruiz, J. (2020). Challenges and barriers in virtual teams: A literature review. *SN Applied Sciences, 2*(6), 1096. doi:10.100742452-020-2801-5

Mullarkey, S., Jackson, P. R., Wall, T. D., Wilson, J. R., & Grey-Taylor, S. M. (1997). The impact of technology characteristics and job control on worker mental health. *Journal of Organizational Behavior, 18*(5), 471–489. doi:10.1002/(SICI)1099-1379(199709)18:5<471::AID-JOB810>3.0.CO;2-V

Munkejord, M. C. (2017). Local and transnational networking among female immigrant entrepreneurs in peripheral rural contexts: Russian female entrepreneurs in Norway. *European Urban and Regional Studies, 24*(1), 7–20.

Murray, C. (2021). *Emergency calls on violence against women spiked in Mexico in 2020*. Thomson Reuters Foundation. https://news.trust.org/item/20210125201102-i73x7

Neher, A. (1991). Maslow's theory of motivations. *Journal of Humanistic Psychology, 31*(3), 89–112. doi:10.1177/0022167891313010

Nippert-Eng, C. E. (1996). *Home and Work: Negotiating Boundaries Through Everyday Life*. University of Chicago Press. doi:10.7208/chicago/9780226581477.001.0001

Nonaka, I. (2007). The Knowledge-Creating Company. *Harvard Business Review*. https://hbr.org/2007/07/the-knowledge-creating-company

Nooteboom, B. (2000). Learning by Interaction: Absorptive Capacity, Cognitive Distance and Governance. *The Journal of Management and Governance, 4*(1), 69–92. doi:10.1023/A:1009941416749

Novy, A. (2021). The political trilemma of contemporary social-ecological transformation – lessons from Karl Polanyi's 'The Great Transformation'. *Globalizations*, 1–23. doi:10.1080/14747731.2020.1850073

O'Hara, P. A. (1995). Household Labor, the Family, and Macroeconomic Instability in the United States: 1940s—1990s. *Review of Social Economy*, *53*(1), 89–120. doi:10.1080/00346769500000004

OECD. (2021). *Caregiving in Crisis: Gender inequality in paid and unpaid work during COVID-19*. Retrieved March 7, 2022, from https://www.oecd.org/coronavirus/policy-responses/caregiving-in-crisis-gender-inequality-in-paid-and-unpaid-work-during-covid-19-3555d164/

Ostrom, E. (1990). *Governing the commons. The evolution of institutions for collective action*. Cambridge University Press. doi:10.1017/CBO9780511807763

Ostrom, E. (2002). Crowding out citizenship. *Scandinavian Political Studies*, *23*(1), 3–16. doi:10.1111/1467-9477.00028

Ostrom, E., & Basurto, X. (2011). Crafting analytical tools to study institutional change. *Journal of Institutional Economics*, *7*(3), 317–343. doi:10.1017/S1744137410000305

Otonkorpi-Lehtoranta, K., Salin, M., Hakovirta, M., & Kaittila, A. (2021). Gendering boundary work: Experiences of work–family practices among Finnish working parents during COVID-19 lockdown. *Gender, Work and Organization*, gwao.12773. Advance online publication. doi:10.1111/gwao.12773 PMID:34898870

Pagh, J. (2020). Managing Context Collapses: The Internet as a Conditioning Technology in the Organization of Practices. *International Journal of Communication*, *12*, 2810–2827. https://ijoc.org/index.php/ijoc/article/view/11872

Paksi, V., Sebők, Cs., & Szalma, I. (2008). A párkapcsolatban élők háztartási munkamegosztásának főbb meghatározói. *Társadalmi Regiszter*, *2*, 79–106.

Patomäki, H. (2014). On the dialectics of global governance in the twenty-first century: A Polanyian double movement? *Globalizations*, *11*(5), 733–750. doi:10.1080/14747731.2014.981079

Peck, J. (2013). Disembedding Polanyi: Exploring Polanyian economic geographies. *Environment & Planning A*, *45*(7), 1536–1544.

Phizacklea, A. (1983). *One Way Ticket? Migration and Female Labour*. Routledge.

Phizacklea, A. (1998). Migration and Globalization: A Feminist Perspective. In K. Koser & H. Lutz (Eds.), *The New Migration in Europe*. Palgrave Macmillan., doi:10.1007/978-1-349-26258-8_2

Pinto-López, I. N., Montaudon-Tomas, C. M., & Gil-Lafuente, A. M. (2022). Mexico and the Challenges of Achieving the 2030 Sustainable Development Goals in Computational and Decision Methods in Economics and Business. *Lecture Notes in Networks and Systems*, *388*, 29–45.

Polanyi, M. (2009). *The Tacit Dimension*. The University of Chicago Press. https://press.uchicago.edu/ucp/books/book/chicago/T/bo6035368.html

Polanyi, K. (1944). *The great transformation* (Vol. 2). Beacon Press.

Polanyi, K. (1944). *The Great Transformation*. Beacon.

Polanyi, K. (1944). *The Great Transformation. The Political and Economic Origins of Our Time*. Beacon Press.

Polanyi, K. (1944). *The great transformation: the political and economic origins of our time*. Farrar & Rinehart.

Portes, A. (1997). Immigration Theory for a New Century: Some Problems and Opportunities. *The International Migration Review*, *31*(4), 799–825.

Prendergast, C. (1999). The provision of incentives in firms. *Journal of Economic Literature*, *37*(1), 7–63. doi:10.1257/jel.37.1.7

Prusa, A., García-Nice, B., & Soledad, O. (2020). *Pandemic of Violence: Protecting Women during COVID-19- OCHA Services*. https://reliefweb.int/report/mexico/pandemic-violence-protecting-women-during-covid-19

Qian, Y., & Hu, Y. (2021). Couples' changing work patterns in the United Kingdom and the United States during the COVID-19 pandemic. *Gender, Work and Organization*, *28*(S2), 535–553. doi:10.1111/gwao.12661 PMID:34230781

Raab, J., & Milward, H. B. (2003). Dark networks as problems. *Journal of Public Administration: Research and Theory*, *13*(4), 413–439. doi:10.1093/jopart/mug029

Rantanen, J. (2008). *Work-Family Interface and Psychological Well-Being: A Personality and Longitudinal Perspective*. University of Jyväskylä.

Raygada, G., & Mendoza, M. (2021). *Combating gender-based violence during the pandemic*. Inter-American Development Bank. https://www.iadb.org/en/improvinglives/combatting-gender-based-violence-during-pandemic

Reliefweb. (2019). *Women and migration: vulnerability in the face of abuse and discrimination*. Retrieved from: https://reliefweb.int/report/world/women-and-migration-vulnerability-face-abuse-and-discrimination

Rhoades, L., Eisenberger, R., & Armeli, S. (2001). Affective commitment to the organization: The contribution of perceived organizational support. *The Journal of Applied Psychology*, *86*(5), 825–836. doi:10.1037/0021-9010.86.5.825 PMID:11596800

Ricardo, D. (1821). *On the principles of political economy*. J. Murray.

Rodríguez-Ruiz, Ó. (2014). The history of human resource management in Spain: An autocratic legacy beyond the waves of rational and normative control. *Management & Organizational History*, *9*(3), 256–271. doi:10.1080/17449359.2013.878251

Rudnicka, L., Gupta, M., Kassir, M., Jafferany, M., Lotti, T., Sadoughifar, R., & Goldust, M. (2020). Priorities for global health community in COVID-19 pandemic. *Dermatologic Therapy*, *33*(4), 1–4. doi:10.1111/dth.13361 PMID:32239578

Saaty, T. L. (1978). Exploring the interface between hierarchies, multiple objectives and fuzzy sets. *Fuzzy Sets and Systems*, *1*(1), 57–68.

Sacchetti, S. (2015). Inclusive and exclusive social preferences: A Deweyan framework to explain governance heterogeneity. *Journal of Business Ethics*, *126*(3), 473–485. doi:10.100710551-013-1971-0

Sacchetti, S., & Borzaga, C. (2021). The Foundations of the "Public Organisation": Governance failure and the problem of external effects. *The Journal of Management and Governance*, *25*(3), 731–758. doi:10.100710997-020-09525-x

Sacchetti, S., & Sugden, R. (2009). The organization of production and its publics: Mental proximity, markets and hierarchies. *Review of Social Economy*, *67*(3), 289–311. doi:10.1080/00346760802621906

Sánchez, E., & Rodríguez, L. (2020). *Femicide on the Rise in Mexico During the COVID-19 Pandemic*. Global Citizen. https://www.globalcitizen.org/en/content/mexico-cuts-womens-institute-budget-femicide-rises/

Scaff, L. A. (1992). *Fleeing the Iron Cage: Culture, Politics, and Modernity in the Thought of Max Weber*. University of California Press.

Scafuto, F., & La Barbera, F. (2016). Protest against waste contamination in the 'Land of Fires': Psychological antecedents for activists and non-activists. *Journal of Community & Applied Social Psychology*, *26*(6), 481–495. doi:10.1002/casp.2275

Schieman, S., Badawy, P. J. A., Milkie, M., & Bierman, A. (2021). Work-Life Conflict During the Covid-19 Pandemic. *Socius: Sociological Research for a Dynamic World*, *7*, 1–19. doi:10.1177/2378023120982856

Schwartz, S. H. (1990). Individualism-collectivism: Critique and proposed refinements. *Journal of Cross-Cultural Psychology*, *21*(2), 139–157. doi:10.1177/0022022190212001

Seccombe, W. (1980). The Expanded Reproduction Cycle of Labour Power in Twentieth Century Capitalism. In B. Fox (Ed.), *Hidden in the Household: Women's Domestic Labour Under Capitalism* (pp. 217–266). The Women's Press.

SIODS. (2021). *Information System of Sustainable Development Goals, Mexico*. https://agenda2030.mx/index.html?lang=en#/home

Smith, A. (1937). *The wealth of nations: An inquiry into the nature and causes*. Modern Library.

Spector, P. E. (1986). Perceived control by employees: A meta-analysis of studies concerning autonomy and participation at work. *Human Relations*, *39*(11), 1005–1016. doi:10.1177/001872678603901104

Spector, P. E. (1987). Interactive effects of perceived control and job stressors on affective reactions and health outcomes for clerical workers. *Work and Stress*, *1*(2), 155–162. doi:10.1080/02678378708258497

Srnicek, N. (2017). *Platform Capitalism*. John Wiley & Sons.

Staines, G. L. (1980). Spillover versus compensation: A review of the literature on the relationship between work and non-work. *Human Relations*, *33*(2), 111–129. doi:10.1177/001872678003300203

Stanfield, J. R. (1986). *The Economic Thought of Karl Polanyi: Lives and Livelihood*. St. Martin's Press. doi:10.1007/978-1-349-18434-7

STATISTA. (2021). https://www.statista.com/statistics/1113975/gender-violence-growth-coronavirus-latin-america/

StatLine—Arbeidsdeelname; kerncijfers. (2021, November 16). *CBS*. https://opendata.cbs.nl/statline/#/CBS/nl/dataset/82309NED/table?dl=56E36

Stephen, L. M. (2020). *A pandemic within a pandemic across Latinamerica*. US News. https://www.usnews.com/news/best-countries/articles/2020-08-24/violence-against-latin-american-women-increases-during-pandemic

Straume, L. V., & Vittersø, J. (2012). Happiness, inspiration and the fully functioning person: Separating hedonic and eudaimonic well-being in the workplace. *The Journal of Positive Psychology*, *7*(5), 387–398. doi:10.1080/17439760.2012.711348

Supiot, A. (2019). *Work is not a commodity. Content and meaning of work in the 21st century* [Le travail n'est pas une marchandise.Contenu et sens du travail au xxie siècle]. Collège de France.

Szántó, Z. (1994). A gazdaság társadalmi beágyazottsága. *Szociologiai Szemle*, *3*, 141–145.

Tagliacozzo, S., Pisacane, L., & Kilkey, M. (2020). The interplay between structural and systemic vulnerability during the COVID-19 pandemic: Migrant agricultural workers in informal settlements in Southern Italy. *Journal of Ethnic and Migration Studies*, *47*(9), 1903–1921.

Takács, J. (2008). Ha a mosogatógép nem lenne, már elváltunk volna…" Férfiak és nők otthoni munkamegosztása, európai összehasonlításban. *Esély*, *6*, 51–73.

Taylor, J. C. (1977). Experiments in work system design: Economic and human results. Part II. *Personnel Review*, *6*(4), 21–34. doi:10.1108/eb055345

Taylor, S. E., & Lobel, M. (1989). Social comparison activity under threat: Downward evaluation and upward contacts. *Psychological Review*, *96*(4), 569–575. doi:10.1037/0033-295X.96.4.569 PMID:2678204

Tepavcevic, S. (2021). Changing Geography, Retaining the Mentality: Social and Economic Integration of Post-Soviet Immigrants in Austria and Hungary. *Review of Economic Theory and Policy*, *3*, 137–154.

Terpe, S. (2020). Working with Max Weber's 'spheres of life': An actor-centred approach. *Journal of Classical Sociology*, *20*(1), 22–42. doi:10.1177/1468795X18789328

Thelwall, M., & Thelwall, S. (2020). *Covid-19 Tweeting in English: Gender Differences.* ArXiv: 2003. 11090v1

Thrash, T. M., Maruskin, L. A., Cassidy, S. E., Fryer, J. W., & Ryan, R. M. (2010). Mediating between the muse and the masses: Inspiration and the actualization of creative ideas. *Journal of Personality and Social Psychology*, *98*(3), 469–487. doi:10.1037/a0017907 PMID:20175625

Tietze, I. N., & Shakeshaft, C. (1982). *Toward a reconstruction of organizational theory: Androcentric bias in A. H. Maslow's* Theory of Human Motivation and Self-Actualization. Paper presented at the Annual Meeting of the American Educational Research Association, New York, NY. https://files.eric.ed.gov/fulltext/ED216440.pdf

TNO. (2021). Bijna een kwart van de thuiswerkers wil ook na corona grotendeels thuis blijven werken [Almost a quarter of the homeworkers wants to work mostly from home even after corona]. *TNO.* Retrieved 22 September 2021, from https://www.tno.nl/nl/over-tno/nieuws/2021/2/kwart-thuiswerkers-na-corona-deels-thuis-blijven-werken/

Tortia, E. C., & Valentinov, V. (2018). Internal organization and governance. In B. A. Seaman & D. Young (Eds.), Handbook of Research on Nonprofit Economics and Management (2nd ed., pp. 285–299). Edward Elgar. doi:10.4337/9781785363528.00022

Tortia, E. C. (2008). Worker well-being and perceived fairness: Survey-based findings from Italy. *Journal of Socio-Economics*, *37*(5), 2080–2094. doi:10.1016/j.socec.2007.10.005

Tortia, E. C. (2022). Employment protection regimes and dismissal of members in worker cooperatives. *Scandinavian Journal of Management*, *38*(3), 101213. doi:10.1016/j.scaman.2022.101213

Tsouri, M., & Pegoretti, G. (2021). Structure and resilience of local knowledge networks: The case of the ICT network in Trentino. *Industry and Innovation*, *28*(7), 860–879. doi:10.1080/13662716.2020.1775070

UN Meetings Coverage and Press Releases. (2021). *As Violence against Women Grows in Shadow of Pandemic, Third Committee Experts Cite Need for Data Collection, Strong Policy Responses.* https://www.un.org/press/en/2021/gashc4318.doc.htm

United Nations Higher Committee for Refugees (UNHCR). (2006). *Annual Statistics 2006.* Retrieved from: https://www.unhcr.org/statistics/%20STATISTICS/4486ceb12.pdf

United Nations UN. (2018). *Department of Economic and Social Affairs.* SDG Indicators Database. https://unstats.un.org/sdgs/dataportal

United Nations UN. (2019). *Fourteenth meeting of the HLG-PCCB.* https://unstats.un.org/sdgs/meetings/hlg-meeting-14

United Nations UN. (2020). *Cape Town Global Action Plan for Sustainable Development Data.* https://unstats.un.org/sdgs/hlg/Cape-Town-Global-Action-Plan/

United Nations UN. (2021a). *Una de cada tres mujeres en el mundo sufre violencia física o sexual desde que es muy joven.* https://news.un.org/es/story/2021/03/1489292

United Nations UN. (2021b). *SDG Global Data Base.* https://unstats.un.org/sdgs/unsdg

United Nations UN. (2021c). *Gender equalit.* [Igualdad de género.] https://www.un.org/es/global-issues/gender-equality

Usher, K., Bradbury Jones, C., Bhullar, N., Durkin, D. J., Gyamfi, N., Fatema, S. R., & Jackson, D. (2021). COVID-19 and family violence: Is this a perfect storm? *International Journal of Mental Health Nursing, 30*, 1022–1032.

Vaccaro, A., & Palazzo, G. (2015). Values against violence: Institutional change in societies dominated by organized crime. *Academy of Management Journal, 58*(4), 1075–1101. doi:10.5465/amj.2012.0865

Vaggi, G., & Groenewegen, P. (2003). Léon Walras, 1834–1910: The Notion of General Equilibrium. In G. Vaggi & P. Groenewegen (Eds.), *A Concise History of Economic Thought: From Mercantilism to Monetarism* (pp. 217–226). Palgrave Macmillan. doi:10.1057/9780230505803_21

Valencia-Londoño, P. A., Martínez-González, E. N., Bruno-Solera, C., & Sorm-Paz, P. (2021). The exacerbation of violence against women as a form of discrimination in the period of the COVID-19 pandemic. *Heliyon, 7*(3), e06491.

Valenta, M., & Ramet, S. (Eds.). (2011). *The Bosnian Diaspora. Integration in Transnational Communities.* Routledge.

Valentinov, V. (2013). Veblen and instrumental value: A systems theory perspective. *Journal of Economic Issues, 47*(3), 673–688. doi:10.2753/JEI0021-3624470304

Van Dijck, J., Poell, T., & De Waal, T. (2018). *The Platform Society: Public Values in a Connective World.* Oxford University Press. doi:10.1093/oso/9780190889760.001.0001

Vančura, M. (2011). *Polanyi's Great Transformation and the concept of the embedded economy.* IES Occasional Paper, No. 2/2011. Charles University in Prague, Institute of Economic Studies (IES).

Vanhala, S., & Tuomi, K. (2003). Individual, organisational and work-related determinants of employee well-being. *EBS Review*, (Autumn), 70–81.

Varela, R., & Pereira, L. (2016). Social Security, work and the State in Portugal [Segurança Social, trabalho e Estado em Portugal]. *Temporalis, 15*, 21. doi:10.22422/2238-1856.2015v15n30p21-52

Veblen, T. (1899). *[1994]. The Theory of the Leisure Class.* Dover Thrift.

Venkatapuram, S. (2020). Human Capabilities and Pandemics. *Journal of Human Development and Capabilities, 21*(3), 280–286. doi:10.1080/19452829.2020.1786028

Vygotsky, L. S. (1978). *Mind in Society*. Harvard University Press. doi:10.2307/j.ctvjf9vz4

Vygotsky, L. S. (2000). *Thought and Language*. MIT Press.

Wahba, M. A., & Bridwell, L. G. (1976). Maslow Reconsidered: A review of research on the need hierarchy theory. *Organizational Behavior and Human Performance*, *15*(2), 212–240. doi:10.1016/0030-5073(76)90038-6

Waizenegger, L., McKenna, B., Cai, W., & Bendz, T. (2020). An affordance perspective of team collaboration and enforced working from home during COVID-19. *European Journal of Information Systems*, *29*(4), 429–442. doi:10.1080/0960085X.2020.1800417

Walsh, F. (1996). The Concept of Family Resilience: Crisis and Challenge. *Family Process*, *35*(3), 261–281. doi:10.1111/j.1545-5300.1996.00261.x PMID:9111709

Weber, M. (1978). *Economy and society: An outline of interpretive sociology* (Vol. 2). University of California Press.

Weber, M. (1978). *Gesammelte Aufsätze zur Religionssoziologie* (Vol. 1). Mohr.

Weil, S. (2020). Two global pandemics: femicide and Covid-19. *Trauma and Memory*, *8*(2), 110-112.

Wheatley, D. (2012). Good to be home? Time-use and satisfaction levels among home-based teleworkers. *New Technology, Work and Employment*, *27*(3), 224–241. doi:10.1111/j.1468-005X.2012.00289.x

Whitley, R. (1999). *Divergent capitalisms: the social structuring and change of business systems*. Oxford University Press.

WHO. (2022). *WHO Coronavirus (COVID-19) Dashboard.* Retrieved May 12, 2022, from https://covid19.who.int

Wicksteed, P. H. (1967). *The Common Sense of Political Economy*. Routledge.

Wijngaarden, Y., Bhansing, P. V., & Hitters, E. (2021). Character trait, context or… create! Innovative practices among creative entrepreneurs. *Industry and Innovation*, *28*(8), 1077–1097. doi:10.1080/13662716.2021.1949964

Wijngaarden, Y., Hitters, E., & Bhansing, P. V. (2020). Cultivating fertile learning grounds: Collegiality, tacit knowledge and innovation in creative co-working spaces. *Geoforum*, *109*, 86–94. doi:10.1016/j.geoforum.2020.01.005

Williamson, O. E. (1975). *Markets and hierarchies: Analysis and Anti-trust implications: A study in the economics of internal organization*. Free Press.

Williamson, O. E. (2000). The new institutional economics: Taking stock, looking ahead. *Journal of Economic Literature*, *38*(3), 595–613. doi:10.1257/jel.38.3.595

Women, U. N. (2020). *SDG 5: Achieve gender equality and empower all women and girls.* https://www.unwomen.org/en/news/in-focus/women-and-the-sdgs/sdg-5-gender-equality

Women, U. N. (2021a). *Frequently asked questions: types of violence against women and girls.* United Nations. https://www.unwomen.org/en/what-we-do/ending-violence-against-women/faqs/types-of-violence

Women, U. N. (2021b). *Measuring the shadow pandemic. Violence against women during COVID-19.* https://data.unwomen.org/sites/default/files/documents/Publications/Measuring-shadow-pandemic.pdf

Women, U. N. (2021c). *Women and the Sustainable Development Goals* [Las mujeres y los Objetivos de Desarrollo Sostenible]. https://www.unwomen.org/es/news/in-focus/women-and-the-sdgs

Wood, A. J., Graham, M., Lehdonvirta, V., & Hjorth, I. (2019). Networked but commodified: The (dis) embeddedness of digital labour in the gig economy. *Sociology, 53*(5), 931–950. doi:10.1177/0038038519828906

World Health Organization. (2002). *Informe mundial sobre la violencia y la salud.* https://www.who.int/violence_injury_prevention/violence/world_report/en/abstract_es.pdf

World Health Organization. (2021). *La violencia contra la mujer es omnipresente y devastadora: la sufren una de cada tres mujeres.* https://www.who.int/es/news/item/09-03-2021-devastatingly-pervasive-1-in-3-women-globally-experience-violence

Yerkes, M. A., André, S. C., Besamusca, J. W., Kruyen, P. M., Remery, C. L., van der Zwan, R., Beckers, D. G. J., & Geurts, S. A. (2020). 'Intelligent' lockdown, intelligent effects? Results from a survey on gender (in) equality in paid work, the division of childcare and household work, and quality of life among parents in the Netherlands during the Covid-19 lockdown. *PLoS One, 15*(11), e0242249. doi:10.1371/journal.pone.0242249 PMID:33253238

Yourke, M. (2021). Violence Against Women in Mexico Rises. *Fair Observer.* https://www.fairobserver.com/region/latin_america/mat-youkee-violence-against-mexican-women-mexico-femicide-coronavirus-lockdown-world-news-60178/

Zedeck, S., & Mosier, K. (1990). Work in the family and employing organization. *The American Psychologist, 45*(2), 240–251. doi:10.1037/0003-066X.45.2.240 PMID:2178504

Zuboff, S. (2019). *The Age of Surveillance Capitalism: The Fight for a Human Future at the New Frontier of Power.* Public Affairs.

Zueva, A. (2005). *Gendered experiences in migration from Russia to Hungary.* Retrieved from: https://migrationonline.cz/en/genderedexperiences-in-migration-from-russia-to-hungary-in-the-gender

Zukin, S., & DiMaggio, P. (Eds.). (1990). *Structures of Capital. The Social Organization of the Economy.* Cambridge University Press.

About the Contributors

Michelle Crosby is an active Social Scientist with background in Research Methods and Evaluation working in the international affairs industry. She is interested in Teaching, Critical Theory and Analysis, Quantitative Research, Qualitative Research and Research Design.

Julianna Faludi, PhD, is Associate Professor and Sociologist at Corvinus University of Budapest. She obtained her PhD in Local Development and Global Dynamics at the University of Trento, and a PhD in Sociology at Corvinus University of Budapest. Julianna Faludi is an active Professor at the Doctoral School of Business and Management, where she is responsible for the expansion of the International Network of scholars. Julianna is a Founding member of the Karl Polanyi Research Center at CUB. She is involved in teaching various courses at international business programmes from MBA, MA, BA. Her publishing activity encompasses fields related to the digital economy, innovation, technology and society. She is an active consultant in the field of social startups, social impact and sustainability. Julianna is a member of several editorial boards.

* * *

Teresa del Giudice is professor in agricultural economics and policy at the University of Naples Federico II (Italy), Department of Agricultural Sciences. Her research interests are related to food and agricultural sectors, with a specific focus on innovation, sustainability, ecosystem services economic evaluation, and rural development with a specific focus on understanding specific drivers of rural environmental and social change.

Ildikó Dén-Nagy is an Economist and economic sociologist with a unique intersection of skill sets from both business management and academia. A published scholar and skilled researcher, familiar with both quantitative and qualitative methods, and an experienced teacher with a focus on Media Communication and Science

& Technology Studies. A demonstrated business leader in Public Relations with significant experience in multicultural work environments.

Imke Greven is an analyst with a passion for entrepreneurship. Prior to this, she completed her Master of Arts in Media and Business from Erasmus University Rotterdam. She is driven by how startups can catalyze innovation, focusing her research on leveraging open innovation and people-centric technologies.

Paula Guerra is Professor of Sociology at the University of Porto and Researcher at the Institute of Sociology of the same University. Paula is Adjunct Associate Professor of the Griffith Centre for Social and Cultural Research in Australia. She is founder/coordinator of the Network All the Arts: Luso-Afro-Brazilian Network of the Sociology of Culture and the Arts. Paula is the founder/coordinator of the KISMIF (kismifconference.com and kismifcommunity.com). Paula is member of the Board of the Research Network of Sociology of Art of ESA. She coordinates several research projects subordinated to the youth cultures, sociology of the arts and culture, co-creation, methodology and research techniques, DIY cultures, among other subjects. She has likewise advised and supervised several Masters, PhD and Post-Doc projects in the aforementioned areas. She is a member of the editorial council of several national and international journals, as well as editor and reviewer of several articles and books on a national and international level (https://www.kismif.conference.com; https://www.kismifcommunity.com).

Elise Lobbedez is a PhD candidate at emlyon business school and at Paris, Sciences et Lettres Research University, Paris-Dauphine University. She is affiliated with the research centers Organizations, Critical and Ethnographic Perspectives (OCE) and Dauphine Recherches en Management-MOST (DRM-MOST). Her dissertation builds on an ethnography of the French yellow vest movement to analyze how actors collectively resist the multiple expressions of organized violence. More broadly, her research interests include social movement organizing and collective action in violent settings, hidden organizing and secrecy and the craft of qualitative research.

Anouk Mols is a postdoctoral researcher in the Media & Communication Department of the Erasmus School of History, Culture, and Communication. She conducts research about privacy and surveillance practices in the context of AI, local communities, workplaces, messaging apps, families, and smart technologies.

Cynthia Montaudon-Tomas is a full-time professor and a business consultant at the Business School at UPAEP. Since September 2018, she became head of the Observatory on Competitiveness and New Ways of Working, which deals with numerous issues related to social problems and creates awareness about current and future social needs. She has obtained a Post Doctorate Certificate In Organizational Leadership from Regent University in Virginia, USA; a Ph.D. in Strategic Planning and Technology Management from UPAEP, in Puebla, Mexico; a Ph.D. in Business from the University of Lincoln in Lincolnshire, UK, and three masters degrees: one in Quality Engineering from the Universidad Iberoamericana in Puebla, Mexico, another in Communication and media from the Jean Moulin, Lyon II University in Lyon, France, and the last one in Business Administration from the Tec de Monterrey in Mexico.

Teresa Panico is an applied economist who developed an interest for value chain analysis and sustainability. Her research focuses on ethical or sustainable consumption and production, especially regarding organic, fair trade and sustainable forestry products. Moreover, currently, she is particularly concerned about how to analyse the behavior of agricultural entrepreneurs in areas characterized by organized violence. She is an associate professor of the University of Naples Federico II, Department of Agricultural Sciences, Agricultural Economics &Policy Group. From 2005-2020 she has been Assistant Professor in Agricultural Economics at the same Department. Regarding the Academic Background: 1990 Ph.D., Agricultural Economics and Policy, University of Naples Federico II, Italy. 1987 Master in Agricultural Economics, Centro di Specializzazione e Ricerche Economico-Agrarie per il Mezzogiorno "Manlio Rossi-Doria", Portici, Italy. 1985 Advanced Degree (Laurea) in Agricultural Science, score 110/110 cum laude, University of Naples, Italy. She has published, among others, in the Agricultural Economics Review, British Food Journal, Forest Policy and Economics.

Stefano Pascucci is professor in Sustainability and Circular Economy – University of Exeter Business School (UK) and visiting professor in Sustainable Business at the University of Auckland Business School (NZ). he also holds a position as Visiting Researcher at the Business Management and Organization Group, Wageningen University (NL). He is a social scientist interested in sustainability and circular economy as a context to develop evidence-based theories and impacts for societal change. He is particularly focused on understanding the role of businesses, communities and other forms of organizing in ensuring transitions and transformations into a more fair and sustainable society. His research explores business and society relations, sustainable innovation and entrepreneurship, as well as value chain configurations. He is still particularly interested in food, agribusiness, sustainability and circular economy. He has published in various academic journals, among others, in the Organization Studies, Academy of Management Perspectives, Journal of Business Venturing, Journal of Business Ethics, and Journal of Cleaner Production.

Ingrid Pinto López is a university professor, researcher and consultor at Business School of UPAEP University, recognized by the National System of Researchers (SNI Conacyt). Ph.D. in Strategic Planning and Technology Management. Currently coordinator of the competitiveness observatory and new forms of work, coordinator of the international arbitration of the Latin American Association of Accounting and Administration Schools ALAFEC, member of Barcelona Economics Network and the Illustrious Latin American Academy of doctors.

Silvia Sacchetti's research at the University of Trento is concerned with the development of inclusive economies and localities with the aim of increasing people well-being. To this end she addresses the governance of enterprises and their networks, the underpinning values and consequences of decision making in private organisations as well as in local development policy. Her aim is to build a body of literature that contributes to explain the impact that taking a cooperative and inclusive approach to business and policy choices can have in terms of development model. Recently she focused on three areas: the third sector (including cooperative firms and social enterprises) social capital and local economic development. One of her current projects studies the involvement of users in the governance of social enterprises that provide health and other welfare services, its outcomes and impacts. Another one focuses on how social enterprises contribute to the regeneration of physical spaces where communities can cooperate and develop new opportunities.

Sanja Tepavcevic (Tepavcsevics Szonja) received her PhD in Political Science, Political Economy Track from the Central European University (CEU), Budapest, in 2014. From 2014 to 2019, she led the Central European University's Rector Series of academic conferences, lectures and seminars, and as Adjunct Lecturer taught MA course in Public Policy at Central European University, Political Science at Budapest Business University, and International Relations at Eotvos Lorand University in Hungary. Since 2020, she works as Research Fellow at Institute of Advanced Studies Koszeg, and Adjunct Lecturer at International Studies MA Programme of the University of Pannonia. She writes and presents widely about the issues of migrations, international relations, global crises, and foreign direct investments from emerging markets.

Ermanno Tortia's researches are focused on the economics of cooperation, organization studies and human resource management, as applied to third sector research (social enterprises, nonprofit organizations, and cooperative enterprises) and local economic development (development of local and welfare systems). He teaches Microeconomics and Economics of Institutions at Trento University. He also teaches Stakeholder Theory and Corporate Social responsibility in the Ph:D. program

Sustainability: Economics, Environment, Management and Society (SusTEEM) at the Doctoral School in Social Sciences at Trento University. He is associated to Euricse (European Research Institute on Cooperative and Social Enterprises, Trento) and is member of the Ph.D. program in Development Economics and Local Systems (DeLOS) at the University of Florence, where he teaches Economics of Institutions. He is also member of the Italian Association for Development Economics (SItES), the Italian Economics Association (SIE), the International Association for Social Economics (ASE) and Ius Cooperativum.

Marloes van Wijnen received a MA-degree in Media and the Creative Industries from Erasmus University Rotterdam in 2020. She wrote her thesis during the Covid pandemic, researching how elements of the workplace encourage self-perceived creativity amongst freelancers in the creative industries – the worldwide crisis, forcing people all over the world to work from their homes on a larger scale than ever in history, once more confirming the relevance of her research topic. After graduating, Marloes has been continuing her freelance work for the digital departments of clients such as LINDA., Vogue Netherlands and NRC.

Raquel Varela is a professor with Habilitation in FCSH/Universidade Nova de Lisboa. Varela is a social historian and a researcher in global labour history. In February 2021, she has done her Habilitation in History in the field of History, with a specialty in Contemporary History, at FCSH / Universidade Nova de Lisboa (unanimously approved). In 2020 wone the Prize of the Ibero-American Communication Association / University of Oviedo, Spain, for her contribution to global labour history and social movements. In 2020, she was the first distinguished with the Simone Veil-Project Europe research grant, University of Munich. In 2021, she was visiting researcher at the Institute of European Global Studies at the University of Basel, Switzerland. She is a researcher at the Foundation for Science and Technology / New University of Lisbon, with a scholarship from the International Institute of Social History (Amsterdam) and since 2011 Group Leader FCSH-UNL. Varela coordinates the Observatory for Living and Working Conditions at FCSH / Nova4Globe. In 2021, she created the Social Data - Digital Platform for Social Sciences at FCSH / Nova4Globe, which she coordinatesShe is author and coordinator of 37 books on global labour history, the welfare state, history of Portugal, history of Europe in the XX Century, history of social movements. Several of her books are translated into German, English and French.

Yosha Wijngaarden is Assistant Professor of Media and Creative Industries at the Erasmus School of History, Culture and Communication, Erasmus University Rotterdam. In 2019, finished her PhD dissertation "Spaces of co-working: Situating

Innovation in the Creative Industries", also at Erasmus University Rotterdam. Her main research interests are work practices, earnings, and inequalities in the creative industries. Yosha also published on innovation in the creative industries, social interactions within and outside of the workplace, and clustering and placemaking.

Index

W

www.ingramcontent.com/pod-product-compliance
Ingram Content Group UK Ltd.
Pitfield, Milton Keynes, MK11 3LW, UK
UKHW051452290926
15471UKWH00008B/1152

9 781668 423653